# IMAGING AND THE AGING BRAIN

ANNALS OF THE NEW YORK ACADEMY OF SCIENCES
*Volume 1097*

# IMAGING AND THE AGING BRAIN

*Edited by Mony J. de Leon, Donald A. Snider, and Howard Federoff*

*Published by Blackwell Publishing on behalf of the New York Academy of Sciences*
*Boston, Massachusetts*
*2007*

Library of Congress Cataloging-in-Publication Data

Imaging and the aging brain / edited by Mony J. de Leon, Howard J. Federoff, and Donald A. Snider.
    p. ; cm. – (Annals of the New York Academy of Sciences, ISSN 0077-8923 ; v. 1097)
    Includes bibliographical references.
    ISBN 978-1-57331-659-0 (alk. paper)
    1. Brain–Aging–Imaging–Congresses. 2. Alzheimer's diseaese–Imaging–Congresses. I. De Leon, Mony J. II. Federoff, Howard. III. Snider, Donald A. IV. New York Academy of Sciences. V. Series.
    [DNLM: 1. Brain Diseases–diagnosis–Congresses. 2. Aging–pathology–Congresses. 3. Alzheimer Disease–pathology–Congresses. 4. Cognition Disorders–pathology–Congresses. 5. Disease Models, Animal–Congresses. 6. Magnetic Resonance Imaging–Congresses. W1 AN626YL v.1097 2006 / WL 300 I305 2006]

    QP356.25.I43 2006
    616.8'0475–dc22

                                                    2006100876

The *Annals of the New York Academy of Sciences* (ISSN: 0077-8923 [print]; ISSN: 1749-6632 [online]) is published 28 times a year on behalf of the New York Academy of Sciences by Blackwell Publishing with offices at 350 Main St., Malden, MA 02148 USA; 9600 Garsington Road, Oxford, OX4 2ZG UK; and 600 North Bridge Rd, #05-01 Parkview Square, 18878 Singapore.

**Information for subscribers:** For new orders, renewals, sample copy requests, claims, changes of address and all other subscription correspondence please contact the Journals Department at your nearest Blackwell office (address details listed above). UK office phone: +44 (0)1865 778315, fax +44 (0)1865 471775; US office phone: 1-800-835-6770 (toll free US) or 1-781-388-8599; fax: 1-781-388-8232; Asia office phone: +65 6511 8000, fax; +44 (0)1865 471775, Email: customerservices@blackwellpublishing.com

**Subscription rates:**
Institutional Premium        The Americas: $4043        Rest of World: £2246
The Premium institutional price also includes online access to full-text articles from 1997 to present, where available. For other pricing options or more information about online access to Blackwell Publishing journals, including access information and terms and conditions, please visit www.blackwellpublishing. com/nyas
*Customers in Canada should add 6% GST or provide evidence of entitlement to exemption.
**Customer in the UK or EU: add the appropriate rate for VAT EC for non-registered customers in countries where this is applicable. If you are registered for VAT please supply your registration number.

**Mailing:** *The Annals of the New York Academy of Sciences* is mailed Standard Rate. Mailing to rest of world by DHL Smart & Global Mail. Canadian mail is sent by Canadian publications mail agreement number 40573520. **Postmaster:** Send all address changes to Annals of the New York Academy of Sciences, Blackwell Publishing Inc., Journals Subscription Department, 350 Main St., Malden, MA 02148-5020.

**Membership information:** Members may order copies of Annals volumes directly from the Academy by visiting www.nyas.org/annals, emailing membership@nyas.org, faxing 212-298-3650, or calling 800-843-6927 (US only), or 212-298-8640 (International). For more information on becoming a member of the New York Academy of Sciences, please visit www.nyas.org/membership. Claims and inquiries on member orders should be directed to the Academy at email: membership@nyas.org or Tel: 212-298-8640 (International) or 800-843-6927 (US only).

Printed in the USA. Printed on acid-free paper.

*Annals* are available to subscribers online at the New York Academy of Sciences and also at Blackwell Synergy. Visit www.blackwell-synergy.com or www.annalsnyas.org to search the articles and register for table of contents e-mail alerts. Access to full text and PDF downloads of *Annals* articles are available to nonmembers and subscribers on a pay-per-view basis at www.blackwell-synergy.com and www.annalsnyas.org.

The paper used in this publication meets the minimum requirements of the National Standard for Information Sciences Permanence of Paper for Printed Library Materials, ANSI Z39.48_1984.

ISSN: 0077-8923 (print); 1749-6632 (online)
ISBN-10: 1-57331-659-8 (paper); ISBN-13: 978-1-57331-659-0 (paper)

A catalogue record for this title is available from the British Library.

ANNALS OF THE NEW YORK ACADEMY OF SCIENCES
Volume 1097
February 2007

# IMAGING AND THE AGING BRAIN

*Editors*
MONY J. DE LEON, DONALD A. SNIDER, AND
HOWARD FEDEROFF

This volume is the result of a meeting entitled **Imaging and the Aging Brain**, sponsored by the New York Academy of Sciences and held on May 16–17, 2006 in New York City.

## CONTENTS

## Part II. *In Vivo* Imaging of Human Aging and the Transition to Cognitive Impairment

## Part III. Diagnostic Applications of Imaging to Alzheimer's Disease

**Financial assistance was received from:**

*Sponsors*

- American Federation for Aging Research

*Supporters*

- International Brain Research Foundation
- The Alzheimer's Association
- GE Global Research
- Pfizer
- Anonymous
- Johnson & Johnson
- Sanofi-Aventis
- Elan
- Ohio Valley Imaging Solutions
- Institute for the Study of Aging

# Foreword

In May 2006, the American Federation of Aging Research (AFAR), under the stewardship of CEO Stephanie Lederman and Scientific Director George Martin, celebrated its 25th anniversary. This venerable philanthropic organization continues in partnership with the National Institutes of Health and other organizations to offer research and training grants. With the New York Academy of Sciences led by Ellis Rubinstein and Rashid Shaikh, AFAR hosted a conference entitled Imaging and the Aging Brain. Perhaps it should also be mentioned that 2006 also marked the 100th anniversary of Alois Alzheimer's presentation of his first case. In 1910 Emile Kraepelin named this dementia, with its characteristic postmortem findings, Alzheimer's disease. Most relevant to this conference is that evolving imaging technology also played a big part in this original discovery. Alzheimer's recognition of neurofibrillary tangles was made possible by the use of the then recently developed Bielschowsky silver preparation. Previously, the senile plaques were observed without stain contrast or even magnification.

From its inception some 30 years ago, *in vivo* tomographic brain imaging research has progressed at a rapid pace. This arena comprises gross anatomical, "molecular" or receptor imaging, and functional neuroanatomical systems. Technological advances in *in vivo* imaging have already greatly enhanced our understandings of normal anatomy and function and of the consequences of pathology associated with age-related disease. The Imaging and the Aging Brain conference that led to this *Annals* was envisioned and implemented by an organizing committee consisting of Howard Federoff, University of Rochester; Joy Hirsch, Columbia University; George Martin, University of Washington; John Morrison, Mount Sinai School of Medicine; Al Snider, the James N. Jarvie Commonweal Service; and myself from New York University.

With the support of AFAR, the New York Academy of Sciences, the NIH-NIA (Neil Buckholtz and Susan Molchan), the Alzheimer's Association, Elan Pharmaceuticals, the Institute for The Study of Aging, the International Brain Research Foundation, Johnson and Johnson, Ohio Valley Imaging Solutions, Pfizer, Sanofi-Aventis, and a generous anonymous donor, we invited a select group of international experts to attend and lecture. In addition, we invited junior and senior scientists working in these general areas to submit posters and attend the two-day conference. With the additional participation of GE Healthcare, we were able to offer four junior investigator prizes for the best poster presentations. The occasion of the meeting also provided opportunity for AFAR to honor and celebrate the lifetime contributions of Robert Terry (the pathology of Alzheimer's disease) and Joshua Lederberg (genetics) to the study of aging.

Ann. N.Y. Acad. Sci. 1097: xi–xii (2007). © 2007 New York Academy of Sciences.
doi: 10.1196/annals.1379.001

The manuscripts included in this volume nicely summarize this dynamic conference, which began with a keynote address by Nobel laureate Eric Kandel. With the enthusiastic participation of nearly all the lecturers, we have produced a summary that captures the current breadth of *in vivo* imaging technologies as applied to the neurobiology of brain aging and Alzheimer's disease. In addition, Judy Illes (Stanford University) was invited to contribute a chapter on the ethical challenges associated with brain imaging. This *Annals* issue is divided into three sections: basic cellular and animal systems studies; normal human aging and transitions to cognitive impairment; and diagnostic applications of imaging to Alzheimer's disease.

We envision that the knowledge acquired by imaging at cellular and mechanistic levels will translate to further improvements in the use of imaging for the early sensitive and specific clinical diagnoses of age-related cognitive disorders. While we trust that the scholarly contributions herein are continuously being updated, our still unrealized goal is to apply early diagnosis in the service of preventing symptomatic expression of those brain diseases that affect the quality of life of so many older individuals.

We dedicate this issue to the memory of the pioneers and patients who taught us.

—MONY J. DE LEON
*New York University School of Medicine*
*New York, New York 10016*

# Making New Memories

## The Role of the Hippocampus in New Associative Learning

WENDY A. SUZUKI

*Center for Neural Science, New York University, New York, New York*

ABSTRACT: Both aging and Alzheimer's disease target the hippocampal formation and can result in mild to devastating memory impairment depending on the severity of the condition. Understanding the normal mnemonic functions of the hippocampus and related structures of the medial temporal lobe is the first step toward the development of diagnostics and treatments designed to ameliorate these potentially devastating age-related memory deficits. Here I describe findings from behavioral neurophysiological studies in which we have investigated the patterns of dynamic neural activity seen in the macaque monkey hippocampus during the acquisition of new associative memories. We report that hippocampal neurons signal the formation of new associations with dramatic changes in their firing rate. Because these learning-related signals can occur just before behavioral learning is expressed, this suggests that these signals play a role in driving the learning process. Implications of these findings for understanding the memory deficits associated with aging and Alzheimer's disease are discussed.

KEYWORDS: relational memory; medial temporal lobe; changing cells; macaque monkey

## INTRODUCTION

Because both aging and Alzheimer's disease target the medial temporal lobe, the study of age-related memory impairment has benefited enormously from basic research on the memory functions of this region. For example, the groundbreaking description of the amnesic patient HM in the 1950s[1] demonstrated definitively for the first time that the structures of the medial temporal lobe are critical for our ability to learn and retain new long-term memories for facts and events. This critical form of memory is referred to as declarative memory in humans[2] and relational memory in animals.[3] The development of powerful animal models of human amnesia in monkeys[4–7] and in

Address for correspondence: Wendy A. Suzuki, Ph.D., Center for Neural Science, New York University, 4 Washington Place Room 809, New York, NY 10003. Voice: 212-998-3734; fax: 212-995-4011. wendy@cns.nyu.edu

Ann. N.Y. Acad. Sci. 1097: 1–11 (2007). © 2007 New York Academy of Sciences. doi: 10.1196/annals.1379.007

rodents,[8–11] together with detailed neuroanatomical studies [12–15] demonstrated definitively that the key medial temporal lobe structures important for declarative/relational memory include the hippocampus together with the surrounding entorhinal, perirhinal, and parahippocampal cortices. While this convergence of studies in humans and animals has provided detailed information about the pattern of memory impairment following damage to the medial temporal lobe (including aging-related damage), less information is available about how individual cells in the intact medial temporal lobe participate in the acquisition, consolidation, or retrieval of various forms of declarative/relational memory.

A large body of evidence suggests that the medial temporal lobe in general and the hippocampus in particular are critically involved in the ability to form fast new associations in memory. For example, amnesic patients with medial temporal lobe damage are impaired in forming fast new associations between stimuli in multiple sensory modalities.[16–19] The importance of the hippocampus for the ability to form fast new associations is also a key feature of recent theories of hippocampal function.[20] Given these convergent findings, an important question is, how does the hippocampus participate in the formation of new associative memories? To address this question, we have used single-unit electrophysiological recording techniques to record neural activity as animals learn new associations "on-line" with trial and error. We find dramatic changes in the firing rate of hippocampal neurons that are highly correlated with the animal's behavioral learning curve. I will first summarize these neurophysiological findings and then discuss some of the implications of these findings for the study of aging and age-related memory impairments.

## Location-Scene Association Task

To examine the patterns of neural activity during the formation of new associative memories, we recorded the activity of individual hippocampal neurons as monkeys performed a location–scene association task.[21] In this task, animals learned to associate a particular target location with a particular complex visual scene for reward. We chose this task because several previous studies had shown that damage to the medial temporal lobe produced impairment in the ability to learn new location–scene associations.[22–27] In this task, each trial started with the monkeys fixating a central fixation point (FIG. 1). The monkeys were then presented with four identical targets superimposed on a complex visual scene. Following a delay interval where the visual scene disappears but the targets remain on the screen, the fixation spot was extinguished, which was the animal's cue to making an eye movement to one of four possible targets. Only one of the targets was rewarded for each new scene. Each day, the animals were presented with a random mix of two to four new scenes (each associated with a different rewarded target location) together with two to four highly familiar "reference" scenes (each also associated with a different rewarded target location). The new location–scene associations were learned in an average of $12 \pm 1$

## Location-scene association task

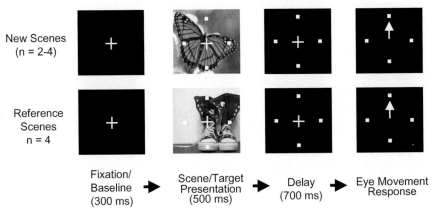

**FIGURE 1.** Location–Scene Association Task. In this task, following fixation, animals were shown a set of four identical visual targets superimposed on a complex visual image (all images used in task were color). Following a delay interval during which time the targets remained on the screen, but the scene disappeared, the animal was cued to make an eye movement response (illustrated schematically by the white arrow) to one of the targets. Only one of the targets was rewarded for each particular scene. Animals learned by trial and error to associate each new scene with a particular eye movement response. Animals were also shown highly familiar "reference" scenes that they had seen many times before and which they performed at ceiling levels.

trials and animals always performed the reference scenes at or near ceiling levels.

### *Learning-Related Neural Activity in the Monkey Hippocampus*

Many isolated hippocampal neurons were engaged in the performance of this task with 61% (89) of the 145 isolated cells responding in a scene-selective fashion during either the scene period, the delay period, or both periods of the task. We hypothesized that the hippocampal cells that signaled learning would change their activity when closely correlated with the animal's behavioral learning curve for particular learned new location–scene associations, but not for the reference scenes with the corresponding rewarded target location. To test this hypothesis, we compared the animal's behavioral performance to the hippocampal cell's firing rate during either the scene or delay period of the task. Behaviorally, the animal's performance typically went from chance levels (i.e., 25% correct) at the beginning of the session to at or near ceiling for all the scenes learned. FIGURE 2A illustrates a trial-by-trial estimate of the animal's probability correct performance (dashed line) together with a trial-by-trial estimate of neural activity (solid line) during the delay interval of the task for the 55 trials that the animal completed for this particular new

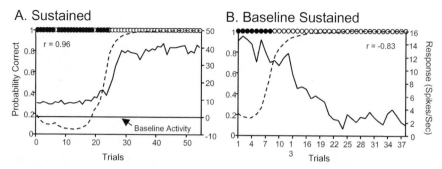

**FIGURE 2.** Illustration of the trial-by-trial probability correct performance (dotted line read from the left axis) as a function of the trial-by-trial activity of cells during either the scene or delay period of the task (solid line read from right axis) for a sustained (**A**) and baseline sustained (**B**) cell. Note the strong positive or negative correlation between neural activity and learning.

location–scene association. The dashed line (associated with the left $y$-axis) shows that the animal exhibited a dramatic increase in behavioral performance at trial 25. The solid line in the same graph (associated with the right $y$-axis) shows that this dramatic shift in behavior was accompanied by an equally dramatic shift in the cell's firing rate during the delay interval of the task. This change in firing rate was highly correlated with learning ($r = 0.96$). We found 18% of the total population of sampled hippocampal cells (or 28% of the cells that responded selectively during at least one phase of the task) signaled new learning with similar dramatic shifts in firing rate that were highly correlated with the animal's behavioral learning curve. We call these cells changing cells. Approximately half the changing cells increased their activity during either the scene or delay periods of the task correlated with learning and this change in neural activity was sustained for as long as we were able to hold the cell (sustained changing cells; FIG. 2A). Some of the sustained changing cells started out with very weak or no response during the early trials of the session and only developed a strong response as the animal learned a particular association. These cells provide some of the most striking examples of dynamic changes in neural activity associated with new learning. The remaining half of the changing cells responded robustly and selectively to a particular scene early in the session before any association was learned. These cells signaled learning by decreasing their firing rate to baseline levels and this decreasing activity was anti-correlated with learning (baseline sustained changing cells FIG. 2B). The responses of both sustained and baseline sustained changing cells were highly selective in that the changes in neural activity only occurred for a particular learned scene.

While we interpreted these changes in neural activity with respect to learn-ing, another possible interpretation is that these changes are related to changes in the animal's motor response. For example, in the changing cell illustrated in FIGURE 2A, the animal almost never makes the correct response (to the north target in this case) before trial 25 and always makes a north response after trial 25. Perhaps the change in neural activity simply reflects a preferred direction of movement. To test this hypothesis, we compared the response of the changing cell during new learning to the response of the same cell to the reference scenes with the same rewarded target location (i.e., the same motor response for both new and reference scenes). In no case did the changing cells respond similarly to the reference scenes suggesting that the changing signal was not simply signaling the direction of movement. To determine if the changing cells signal new learning specific for a particular rewarded target location, we recorded the activity of a changing cell during learning of two different new scenes with the same rewarded target location. Typically, the cell would change in parallel to learning for the first new scene. However, similar changes in activity were never seen for the second new scene with the same rewarded target location. Thus, hippocampal changing cells do not appear to signal new learning in a motor-based or direction-based frame of reference. Instead, these findings suggest that hippocampal cells signal fast associative learning between sensory stimuli and motor responses or target locations. This interpretation is consistent with theories suggesting that the hippocampus plays a fundamental role in forming the random associations or relationships between unrelated items.[3] These kinds of simple associations may be critical to building up the more complex associations between the "what," "where," and "when" information that forms the basis of episodic memory.

### What Does the Change in Neural Activity Represent?

Previous studies have shown that neurons in both the perirhinal cortex and visual area TE (Temporal area "E" of von Bonin and Bailey) signal long-term associations between visual stimuli by responding similarly to the two items that had been paired in memory.[28,29] These findings suggested that the learning of the paired associates may have "tuned" or "shaped" the sensory responses of these cells toward a similar response to the two stimuli paired in memory. Consistent with this idea, several other groups demonstrated that perirhinal neurons show a shift in response selectivity during the associative learning process.[30–32] These findings suggested that the striking changes in neural activity observed during the location–scene association task may represent a change in the cell's stimulus selective response properties with learning. To address this possibility, we examined the average response of a single changing cell to all new scenes and reference scenes over the course of learning. The changing cell illustrated in FIGURE 3A did not differentiate between any of the scenes during the scene period of the task early in the learning

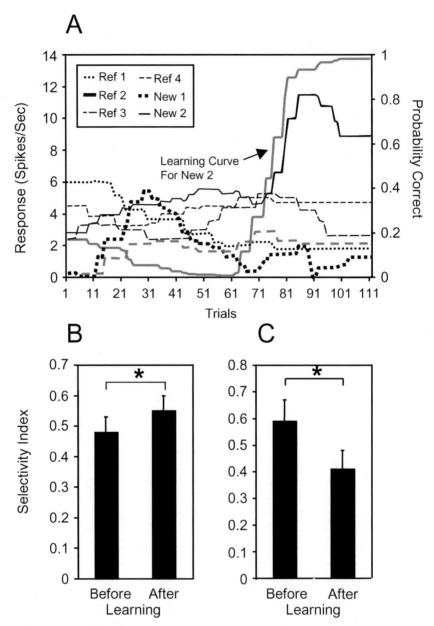

**FIGURE 3. (A)** Average response to four reference scenes and two new scenes over the course of the recording session for a sustained changing cell. The learning curve for New Scene 2 is illustrated as the thick gray line. **(B)** Graph showing the significant increase in the selectivity index for sustained changing cells after learning compared to before learning. **(C)** In contrast, baseline sustained changing cells decreased their selectivity after learning compared to before learning.

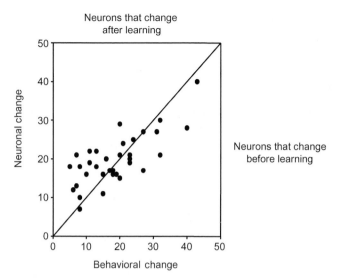

**FIGURE 4.** Scatter plot illustrating the temporal relationship between trial number of behavioral changing (i.e., learning) and trial number of neuronal change. Note that about half the cells change before or at the same time as learning while the remaining half of the cells change before learning.

session. However, this cell appeared to develop a highly selective response to new scene 2 (black line), which occurred in parallel with learning (thick gray line). To quantify this observation across the changing cells, we measured selectivity using a selectivity index[33] to the responses to all new and reference scenes before versus after learning. We analyzed the sustained and baseline sustained changing cells separately. We found that while the sustained cells exhibited a significant increase in selectivity (FIG. 4B) with learning, the baseline sustained cells exhibited a significant decrease in selectivity (FIG. 4C). These findings suggest that hippocampal cells signal new associations with a significant change in their stimulus-selective response properties.

### Timing of the Changing Cells Relative to Learning

While the analyses illustrated in FIGURE 2 show a strong correlation between changing cell activity and learning, a critical question is whether this activity is causally related to learning. One clue in support of the idea that these signals may underlie learning comes from the lesion studies showing that various lesions of the medial temporal lobe produce a significant impairment in the ability of animals to learn new location–scene associations.[22–27] If this hypothesis is correct, we further predicted that some of the hippocampal cells should change their firing rate either at the same time or slightly before behavioral learning is expressed, at a time when this activity could drive the changes in behavior underlying learning. Changes in neural activity that occurred after behavioral learning is expressed would be consistent with a role in the strengthening of the newly formed association. To address this question, for each cell that changed for a particular condition, we estimated the trial number of learning as well as the trial number of neural change. FIGURE 4 shows a scatter plot of this comparison for all changing cells in the hippocampus. This plot shows that while about half of the changing cells changed before or at the same time as learning, the remaining half change after learning. These early changing cells suggest that the hippocampus is among the earliest brain structures to signal or drive new associative learning. Other recent studies have implicated other brain areas in new conditional motor association learning including the caudate,[34,35] prefrontal,[34,36] as well as premotor areas.[35] It will be important to direct future studies at examining how these different brain areas interact during the associative learning process.

## CONCLUSIONS AND IMPLICATIONS FOR AGING RESEARCH

We have shown that many hippocampal neurons signal learning with dramatic changes in their stimulus-selective response properties. While some neurons increase their activity (and stimulus selectivity) with learning, others decrease their activity (and stimulus selectivity) with learning suggesting that these changes represent an overall tuning of the hippocampal network. The observation that these changes can occur before behavioral learning is expressed, taken together with the findings of the detrimental effects of medial temporal lobe lesions on tasks requiring new associative learning, suggest that the hippocampal changing cells may drive the behavioral changes underlying learning. We have also shown similar changes in hemodynamic responses in the hippocampus and other related medial temporal lobe structures in a recent human fMRI study using a variant of our location–scene association task.[37] These findings suggest that associative learning signals can be studied in parallel in both human and nonhuman primate systems.

What are the implications of these basic neuroscience findings for the study of human aging and Alzheimer's disease? Given that forming new associations in memory is highly sensitive to medial temporal lobe damage and this brain region is also targeted in both aging and Alzheimer's disease, this suggests that monitoring brain activity during the location–scene learning task may be a powerful way of probing and delineating the specific deficits in signaling new associative learning that are present in both animal models of aging as well as in both aged and Alzheimer's patients. More generally, this strategy illustrates the critical interplay between clinical research efforts and basic experimental approaches that can provide novel paradigms or hypotheses to test both in animal models as well as in various patient populations. As we more fully define the patterns of normal neural activity seen during associative memory acquisition not only in the hippocampus proper, but throughout other key medial temporal lobe structures important for memory, this will provide an important framework against which we can compare deficits (or lack thereof) seen in the neurophysiological profiles of aged animals or the fMRI profiles of aged subjects or patients with Alzheimer's disease. This experimental approach suggested by our neurophysiological findings illustrates the point that our best hope for eventually understanding the specific memory deficits in aging and Alzheimer's disease is to keep the channels between basic research and clinic studies wide open and flowing.

# REFERENCES

1. SCOVILLE, W.B. & B. MILNER. 1957. Loss of recent memory after bilateral hippocampal lesions. J. Neurol. Neurosurg. Psych. **20:** 11–21.
2. SQUIRE, L.R., R.E. CLARK & P.J. BAILEY. 2004. Medial temporal lobe function and memory. In The Cognitive Neruosciences III. M. GAZZANIGA, Ed.: 691–708. The MIT Press. Cambridge, MA.
3. EICHENBAUM, H., P. DUDCHENKO, E. WOOD, et al. 1999. The hippocampus, memory, and place cells: is it spatial memory or a memory space? Neuron 23: 209–226.
4. ZOLA, S.M. & L.R. SQUIRE. 2005. The medial temporal lobe and the hippocampus. In The Oxford Handbook of Memory. E. TULVING, F.I. CRAIK, Eds.Oxford University Press, New York.
5. SUZUKI, W.A., S. ZOLA-MORGAN, L.R. SQUIRE & D.G. AMARAL. 1993. Lesions of the perirhinal and parahippocampal cortices in the monkey produce long-lasting memory impairment in the visual and tactual modalities. J. Neurosci. **13:** 2430–2451.
6. ZOLA-MORGAN, S. & L.R. SQUIRE. 1990. The neuropsychology of memory. Parallel findings in humans and nonhuman primates. Ann. N. Y. Acad. Sci. **608:** 434–450; discussion.
7. MISHKIN, M.. 1978. Memory in monkeys severely impaired by combined but not by separate removal of amygdala and hippocampus. Nature **273:** 297–298.
8. FORTIN, N.J., K.L. AGSTER & H.B. EICHENBAUM. 2002. Critical role of the hippocampus in memory for sequences of events. Nat. Neurosci. **5:** 458–462.
9. BUNSEY, M. & H. EICHENBAUM. 1996. Conservation of hippocampal memory functions in rats and humans. Nature **379:** 255–257.
10. BUNSEY, M. & H. EICHENBAUM. 1995. Selective damage to the hippocampal region blocks long term retention of a natural and nonspatial stimulus-stimulus association. Hippocampus **5:** 546–556.
11. BUNSEY, M. & H. EICHENBAUM. 1993. Critical role of the parahippocampal region for paired-associate learning in rats. Behav. Neurosci. **107:** 740–747.
12. BURWELL, R.D., & D.G. AMARAL. 1998a. Cortical afferents of the perirhinal, postrhinal and entorhinal cortices. J. Comp. Neurol. **398:** 179–205.
13. BURWELL, R.D. & D.G. AMARAL. 1998b. Perirhinal and postrhinal cortices of the rat: interconnectivity and connections with the entorhinal cortex. J. Comp Neurol. **391:** 293–321.

14. SUZUKI, W.A. & D.G. AMARAL. 1994a. Perirhinal and parahippocampal cortices of the macaque monkey: cortical afferents. J. Comp. Neurol. **350:** 497–533.
15. SUZUKI, W.A. & D.G. AMARAL. 1994b. Topographic organization of the reciprocal connections between monkey entorhinal cortex and the perirhinal and parahippocampal cortices. J. Neurosci. **14:** 1856–1877.
16. STARK, C.E. & L.R. SQUIRE. 2003. Hippocampal damage equally impairs memory for single items and memory for conjunctions. Hippocampus **13:** 281–292.
17. STARK, C.E., P.J. BAYLEY & L.R. SQUIRE. 2002. Recognition memory for single items and for associations is similarly impaired following damage to the hippocampal region. Learn. Mem. **9:** 238–242.
18. BAYLEY, P.J. & L.R. SQUIRE. 2002. Medial temporal lobe amnesia: gradual acquisition of factual information by nondeclarative memory. J. Neurosci. **22:** 5741–5748.
19. VARGHA-KHADEM, F., D.G. GADIAN, K.E. WATKINS, et al. 1997. Differential effects of early hippocampal pathology on episodic and semantic memory. Science **277:** 376–380.
20. EICHENBAUM, H. & N.J. COHEN. 2001. From Conditioning to Conscious Recollection. Oxford University Press, New York.
21. WIRTH, S., M. YANIKE, L.M. FRANK, et al. 2003. Single neurons in the monkey hippocampus and learning of new associations. Science **300:** 1578–1581.
22. BRASTED, P.J., T.J. BUSSEY, E.A. MURRAY & S.P. WISE. 2003. Role of the hippocampal system in associative learning beyond the spatial domain. Brain **126:** 1202–1223.
23. BRASTED, P.J., T.J. BUSSEY, E.A. MURRAY & S.P. WISE. 2002. Fornix transection impairs conditional visuomotor learning in tasks involving nonspatially differentiated responses. J. Neurophysiol. **87:** 631–633.
24. MURRAY, E.A., T.J. BUSSEY & S.P. WISE. 2000. Role of prefrontal cortex in a network for arbitrary visuomotor mapping. Exp. Br. Res. **133:** 114–129.
25. WISE, S.P. & E.A. MURRAY. 1999. Role of the hippocampal system in conditional motor learning: mapping antecedents to action. Hippocampus **9:** 101–117.
26. MURRAY, E.A. & S.P. WISE. 1996. Role of the hippocampus plus subjacent cortex but not amygdala in visuomotor conditional learning in rhesus monkeys. Behav. Neurosci. **110:** 1261–1270.
27. RUPNIAK, N.M., & D. GAFFAN. 1987. Monkey hippocampus and learning about spatially directed movements. J. Neurosci. **7:** 2331–2337.
28. VON BONIN, G. & P. BAILEY. 1947. The Neocortex of Macaca Mulatta. University of Illinois Press Urbana, IL.
29. SAKAI, K., & Y. MIYASHITA. 1991. Neural organization for the long-term memory of paired associates. Nature **354:** 152–155.
30. MESSINGER, A., L.R. SQUIRE, S.M. ZOLA & T.D. ALBRIGHT. 2001. Neuronal representations of stimulus associations develop in the temporal lobe during learning. Proc. Natl. Acad. Sci. **98:** 12239–12244.
31. ERICKSON, C.A., B. JAGADEESH & R. DESIMONE. 2000. Clustering of perirhinal neurons with similar properties following visual experience in adult monkeys. Nature Neurosci. **3:** 1143–1148.
32. ERICKSON, C.A., & R. DESIMONE. 1999. Responses of macaque perirhinal neurons during and after visual stimulus association learning. J. Neurosci. **19:** 10404–10416.
33. MOODY, S.L., S.P. WISE, G. DI PELLEGRINO & D.A. ZIPSER. 1998. A model that accounts for activity in primate frontal cortex during a delayed matching to sample task. J. Neurosci. **18:** 399–410.

34. PASUPATHY, A. & E.K. MILLER. 2005. Different time courses of learning-related activity in the prefrontal cortex and striatum. Nature **433:** 873–876.
35. BRASTED, P.J., & S .P. WISE. 2004. Comparison of learning-related neuronal activity in the dorsal premotor cortex and striatum. Eur. J. Neurosci. **19:** 721–740.
36. ASAAD, W.F., G. RAINER & E.K. MILLER. 1998. Neural activity in the primate prefrontal cortex during associative learning. Neuron **21:** 1399–1407.
37. LAW, J.R., M.A. FLANERY, S. WIRTH, *et al.* 2005. Functional magnetic resonance imaging activity during the gradual acquisition and expression of paired-associate memory. J. Neurosci. **25:** 5720–5729.

# Anatomical and Functional Phenotyping of Mice Models of Alzheimer's Disease by MR Microscopy

HELENE BENVENISTE,[a,b] YU MA,[b] JASBEER DHAWAN,[a] ANDREW GIFFORD,[a] S. DAVID SMITH,[a] IGOR FEINSTEIN,[a] CONGWU DU,[a,b] SAMUEL C. GRANT,[c,d] AND PATRICK R. HOF[e]

[a]Medical Department, Brookhaven National Laboratory, Upton, New York, USA

[b]Department of Anesthesiology, Stony Brook University, New York, New York, USA

[c]Department of Chemistry and Biomedical Engineering, The Florida State University, Tallahassee, Florida, USA

[d]The National High Magnetic Field Laboratory, Tallahassee, Florida, USA

[e]Department of Neuroscience, Mount Sinai School of Medicine, New York, New York, USA

ABSTRACT: The wide variety of transgenic mouse models of Alzheimer's disease (AD) reflects the search for specific genes that influence AD pathology and the drive to create a clinically relevant animal model. An ideal AD mouse model must display hallmark AD pathology such as amyloid plaques, neurofibrillary tangles, reactive gliosis, dystrophic neurites, neuron and synapse loss, and brain atrophy and in parallel behaviorally mimic the cognitive decline observed in humans. Magnetic resonance (MR) microscopy (MRM) can detect amyloid plaque load, development of brain atrophy, and acute neurodegeneration. MRM examples of AD pathology will be presented and discussed. What has lagged behind in preclinical research using transgenic AD mouse models is functional phenotyping of the brain; in other words, the ability to correlate a specific genotype with potential aberrant brain activation patterns. This lack of information is caused by the technical challenges involved in performing functional MRI (fMRI) in mice including the effects of anesthetic agents and the lack of relevant "cognitive" paradigms. An alternative approach to classical fMRI using external stimuli as triggers of brain activation in rodents is to electrically or pharmacologically stimulate regions directly while simultaneously locally tracking the activated interconnected regions of rodents using, for example, the

Address for correspondence: Helene Benveniste, M.D., Ph.D., Brookhaven National Laboratory, Medical Department, Bldg. 490, 30 Bell Avenue, Upton, NY 11973. Voice: 631-344-7006; fax: 631-344-5260.

benveniste@bnl.gov

Ann. N.Y. Acad. Sci. 1097: 12–29 (2007). © 2007 New York Academy of Sciences.
doi: 10.1196/annals.1379.006

manganese-enhanced MRI (MEMRI) technique. Finally, transgenic mouse models, MRM, and future AD research would be strengthened by the ability to screen for AD-like pathology in other non-AD transgenic mouse models. For example, molecular biologists may focus on cardiac or pulmonary pathologies in transgenic mice models and as an incidental finding discover behavioral AD phenotypes. We will present MRM data of brain and cardiac phenotyping in transgenic mouse models with behavioral deficits.

KEYWORDS: MR microscopy; phenotyping; imaging; mice; Alzheimer's disease; model

## IMAGING IN MULTIPLE PHYSICAL DIMENSIONS

Imaging of living matter is now possible across a wide range of spatial, temporal, and functional scales *in vitro* and *in vivo* using technological approaches ranging from MRI and computerized X-ray tomography to synchrotron Fourier transfer infrared micro-spectroscopy and low-energy electron microscopy (FIG. 1). MRI can resolve anatomically structures down to a spatial resolution of 3.0 $\mu M^{31}$ and functionally capture blood flow and tissue oxygenation changes induced by neuronal activation with a 1–3 sec temporal resolution.[2,3] Optical imaging and techniques that capture electrical activity or changes in the local magnetic field associated with neuronal firing (e.g., electroencephalography and magnetoencephalography) have less spatial resolution compared to MRI but operate in the millisecond time domain.[4,5] Positron emission tomography (PET) uses radiolabeled chemical compounds to capture neurochemical synaptic events occurring during execution of cognitive and behavioral paradigms or in response to a pharmacological challenge.[6] The ability to combine these techniques for *in vivo* studies is becoming technologically possible,[7] increasing the "bandwidth" of physical parameters acquired in a given scan session. This information ultimately enhances our capability to characterize, interpret, and understand molecular, chemical, and pathophysiological processes in diseased tissue.

## AD PATHOLOGY AND IMAGING IN THE HUMAN BRAIN

The hallmark pathological features of Alzheimer's disease (AD) in the human brain comprise amyloid deposits in the form of extracellularly located beta-amyloid ($A\beta$) positive plaques (neuritic plaques), diffuse amyloid deposits, amyloid angiopathy of the capillaries, arteries, and veins, intracellular neurofibrillary tangles, neuronal loss, and synaptic depletion, which presumably all lead to another key pathological feature: brain atrophy.[8] In the human brain, development of atrophy in certain highly vulnerable brain regions such as the hippocampus, entorhinal cortex, superior temporal cortex, and parts of the

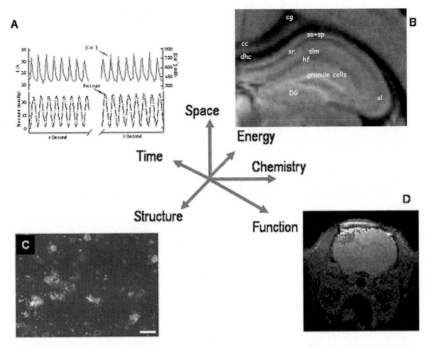

**FIGURE 1.** Imaging in different physical dimensions: (**A**) Optical diffusion fluorescence spectroscopy of the beating mouse heart demonstrating intracellular calcium transients in synchrony with the pressure gradient at a time resolution <10 msec (courtesy Du *et al.*); (**B**) High resolution MRM image at a spatial resolution of 0.0001 mm$^3$ from a perfusion-fixed mouse brain demonstrating anatomical structures of the dorsal hippocampus (cc = corpus callosum; dhc = dorsal hippocampal commisure; sr = stratum radiatum; slm = stratum lacunosum moleculare; dg = dentate ganule cells; so = stratum oriens; hf = hippocampal fissue); (**C**) Fourier transfer infrared micro-spectroscopy images of a human AD tissue specimen acquired at a spatial resolution of 10 μM demonstrating β-sheet protein (blue), Zn (red); images overlaid on a thioflavin stain; courtesy Miller *et al.*. (**D**) Functional MRI image of a rat brain acquired during forepaw activation using BOLD contrast showing activation in red in the area of somatosensory cortex.

dorsolateral prefrontal cortex[9] of subjects diagnosed with minimal cognitive impairment (MCI) are detectable using MRI, and tracking of subtle volumetric changes in these regions can be used to discriminate between normal subjects and subjects with MCI who later convert to AD.[10] It is also well known that the corpus callosum in AD subjects shrinks in certain parts, which is probably related to specific loss of corticocortical projecting neurons.[11,12] Other studies have performed more complex mathematical and statistical three-dimensional (3D) MRI brain data analysis and demonstrated characteristic increases in sulcal asymmetry in AD subjects compared to age-matched controls[13,14]

Individual Aβ plaques have not been identified in the human brain *in vivo* by MRI. Instead monoclonal antibodies to Aβ have been developed as well as a range of radiolabeled analogues of Congo red and thioflavin suitable for PET studies.[15] Two such compounds ([18]F-FDDNP, 6-dialkylamino-2-naphthylidene and [11]CPIP a derivative of thioflavin) have been tested in human subjects afflicted with AD and have demonstrated different retention times of the radiolabeled compound in certain brain areas such as the frontal and temporal cortex. However, there is debate on the clinical relevance of using this approach to assess the Aβ burden in humans given the fact that the tracers only label the insoluble, aggregated portion.

## AD TRANSGENIC MOUSE MODELS

Transgenic mouse models of AD have become essential biosystems for developing and defining optimal imaging approaches to visualize AD pathology *in vivo* as well as for understanding the genotype–phenotype interaction in this disease. There are multiple AD mouse models and some emphasize only one hallmark pathological AD feature while double- or triple-transgenic models develop more clinically relevant pathology (for overview see http://www.alzforum.org/res/com/tra/app/default.asp). For example, Aβ neuritic plaques develop in human amyloid precursor protein V717F (PDAPP)[16,17] and APP London V717I [18] mice. Tau pathology is found in the P201S tau transgenic mouse model[19]; the most clinically relevant models (at least from the point of view of human AD pathology) is the double and triple crossed models such as the mouse model that display tau hyperphosphorylation in hippocampal neurons and atrophy,[20] the APP/Tau mouse that develops amyloid deposits, NFT, and neuronal loss, and the recently developed 3xTg-AD mouse model (APP/Tau/PS1) that develops both neuritic Aβ plaques and tangles.[21,22]

To accelerate the formation of amyloid plaque formation as well as to investigate the role of ApoE in the maintenance of synapses and dendrites, the ApoE knockout and ApoE 4/4 mice models were created and have been applied in a number of imaging studies to be discussed below.[23]

## MR MICROSCOPY AND IMAGING
## OF TRANSGENIC MOUSE MODELS

MR imaging performed at a spatial resolution of at least 100 μM in one dimension is referred to as "MR microscopy" (MRM).[24] The high spatial resolution is achieved using higher magnetic field instruments with imaging capabilities ($>7T$, with 9.4T now achievable at the human scale and increasing as the magnet bore decreases; 21T is now available for large rodents), strong magnetic field gradients, and specialized radio frequency (RF) coils (for further review of technical requirements see Ref. 24). MRM can be performed *in vivo* or *in vitro* on excised tissue samples. *In vivo* studies of transgenic mouse models typically require anesthesia, physiological monitoring, and motion control during imaging, and for longitudinal studies it is advantageous that the scan time be optimized to be as short as possible to reduce anesthesia exposure and thus the morbidity and mortality of the mice.

## MRM AND DETECTION OF AMYLOID

MRM was first used to characterize AD pathology in human tissue by Huesgen et al. in 1993[25] who used formalin-fixed tissue samples and demonstrated atrophy of the hippocampus but not other AD pathology such as plaques or tangles. In a later study tissue samples from humans diagnosed with AD at different Braak and Braak stages (i.e., III–VI [26]) were imaged at a range of spatial resolutions and with different MR contrast parameters on a 7.0-T MR system.[27] By comparison with histology, plaques were detected in vitro at a spatial resolution of $5.9 \times 10^{-5}$ mm$^3$ using gradient echo imaging and T2* contrast.[27] It was hypothesized that the dark-appearing Aβ deposits on the high resolution T2* images were visible due to differences in local magnetic susceptibility between the plaque itself and the surrounding matrix.[27] This MR susceptibility phenomenon might occur if the Aβ plaques contained metals. Several studies in the past have demonstrated that amyloid deposits in the human brain also can contain metals. A recent imaging study using synchrotron Fourier transfer infrared microspectroscopy of human tissue samples from AD subjects was performed at a spatial resolution of 5–10 μM and confirmed this notion directly.[28] Specifically, accumulations of Zn, Cu, and Fe were found to be colocalized with Aβ deposits.[28] Interestingly, it also was shown that Zn and Cu were the most abundant and that the metal accumulations were not uniform and varied from plaque to plaque.[28]

The in vitro MRM study demonstrating amyloid in the human tissue samples by T2* contrast was challenged due to the lack of coregistration with histological evidence of iron deposits.[29] This information potentially confounded the data interpretation because the human tissue samples were not perfusion-fixed and contained blood-filled vessels. However, several recent MR studies performed in vivo as well as in vitro using various AD mouse models (for which tissue preparation can be controlled) have confirmed that (i) Aβ plaques can be visualized at high spatial resolution with T2-weighted contrast and (ii) the contrast between plaques and normal-appearing adjacent brain tissue is presumably related to the iron that resides within most plaques.[30–32] Thus, on T2-weighted MR images the plaques appear dark, which is most likely attributable to the T2-shortening effect induced by the paramagnetic iron itself. Thus T2 may be more sensitive to Aβ with fewer false positives (this would occur if the Fe contained in the plaque is in a paramagnetic form instead of a ferromagnetic form).[30] Another approach to image Aβ plaques has been to label Aβ with specific MR contrast agents that cross the blood–brain barrier.[33]

## DETECTION OF BRAIN ATROPHY IN THE MOUSE BRAIN

Development of selective brain atrophy in the hippocampus, entorhinal cortex, and other structures such as the corpus callosum is one of the key morphological features of preclinical AD and can, as previously pointed out, be observed in subjects that later convert from MCI to AD.[10] Thus this atrophy is an important feature to mimic in AD animal models, not only because of its clinical relevance but also due to the impact of amyloid deposits, tangles, and amyloid cerebral angiopathy in the later development of neuronal injury, cell death, and ensuing atrophy.

The challenge of accurately tracking the development of regional brain atrophy in 30–50 g mice has to be emphasized in light of the 3,000-fold difference between the human brain with a volume of ∼1,500 mL versus that of the mouse brain of only ∼0.5 mL. Thus in the human brain the voxel size required to resolve the anatomical structures of interest (typically human scans are acquired using a T1-weighted sequence using a voxel size of 1–1.5 $mm^3$) is sufficiently "large" from the point of view of proton signal and/or signal to noise. Furthermore, excellent MR image contrast exists in the human brain between white and gray matter or other such structures of interest necessary to define the tissue boundaries. However, such optimal conditions for anatomical resolution by MRI are not all met in the rodent brain. First, in the rodent brain gray and white matter contrast differs from that of the human brain probably related to the fact that the MR relaxation parameters T1 and T2 are (*a*) different in the two species and (*b*) dependent on the main magnet field strength. For example, when measured at 3.0 T, T1 values measured for gray and white matter in the normal human brain are reported as 1,331 and 832 msec[34] whereas T1 values in mouse brain gray and white matter measured at 9.4T are 1,789 and 2,100 msec.[35] Thus on T1-weighted MRIs of the mouse brain acquired at high field the delineation of tissue boundaries are not as clear as those of the human brain and MR contrast parameters have to be optimized for anatomical resolution (FIG. 2). Second, the voxel size necessary to resolve smaller volume structures like the hippocampus or amygdala in the mouse brain, which is in the range of 0.01–0.05 mL,[36] must be minute (on the order of 0.001 $mm^3$) necessitating MR scan acquisitions with high signal-to-noise ratios (SNR) involving optimized MR hardware (e.g., RF coils, gradients, shims), pulse sequences, and physiological-based gating of animal motion during *in vivo* scans.

For MRM scans acquired *in vivo* there are many anatomical regions that can only be partially defined due to the lack of adequate tissue contrast. For example, the border between the dorsal hippocampus and neocortex were not visible using diffusion contrast in a study tracking brain volume changes in normal and ApoE-deficient mice before and after cerebral ischemia.[37] FIGURE 3 shows diffusion scans of an ApoE-deficient mouse before and 42 days following exposure to transient cerebral ischemia and demonstrates the lack of well-defined borders between the dorsal hippocampus and adjacent

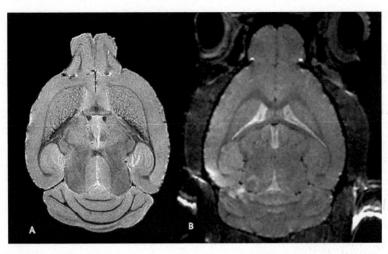

**FIGURE 2.** (**A**) MRM image of a C57BL6/J mouse brain formalin-fixed and excised from the skull acquired on a 17.6T MR instrument using T2* contrast and a spatial resolution of 0.0001 mm³. (**B**) MRM image of a C57BL6/J mouse brain acquired in vivo on a 9.4T instrument using T2 contrast and a spatial resolution of 0.001 mm³ (image courtesy Dr. Yu Ma).

neocortex as well as evidence of brain atrophy (enlargement of lateral ventricles) in the postischemic scan.[37] Due to lack of adequately defined anatomical borders, it also was not possible to quantify volume changes in other areas such as the caudate-putamen, globus pallidus, or cerebral cortex. Previous *in vivo* studies of mouse models of human diseases have used T2diffusion- or proton-weighted density MR contrast for anatomical brain scans with a manual segmentation approach for analysis and rather limited anatomical information has been extracted. Only obvious morphological structure variations such as differences in forebrain, ventricular, or cerebellar volumes have been reported[38–41] while information of more subtle differences such as subregional atrophy or geometrical differences have been sparse.[42] The latter would require more complex analysis procedures (e.g., multiple anatomical landmarks, alignment of samples, warping, etc.), more solid statistics demanding a larger number of animals, and minimal error on anatomical segmentation procedures. These requirements have been satisfied partially by the generation of rodent brain 3D atlas templates that can be used to guide segmentation in a semiautomated manner.[36,43,44]

## ATLAS TEMPLATES FOR SEGMENTATION OF THE MOUSE BRAIN

Segmentation accuracy is obviously dependent on the MR image quality (i.e., can anatomical areas of interest be visualized? If so, can all adjacent

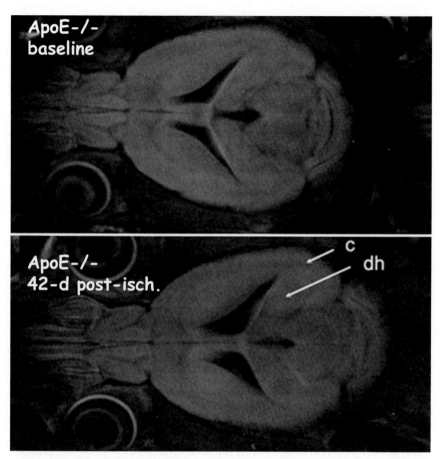

**FIGURE 3.** Tracking brain atrophy in ApoE-deficient mice following transient cerebral ischemia using MRM. The same ApoE-deficient mouse was scanned at baseline (left) and 42 days following a 5-min transient cerebral ischemic episode using diffusion-weighted contrast.[37] C = neocortex; dh = dorsal hippocampus.

tissue borders be defined clearly?) and on the computational strategies applied. MRI data analysis for human morphometric studies has developed rapidly over the last decade. A wide range of computational and mathematical strategies have been developed largely due to a concerted, international research effort focused on designing appropriate brain atlas templates and probabilistic atlases including sophisticated software suitable to detect subtle quantitative regional volumetric, surface, or structural shape changes in the diseased brains compared to a normal population.[45–49] For the rodent brain such tools also have been developed in parallel and now investigators can access 3D digital rat and mouse brain atlas templates created using different imaging modalities, contrast, and histological staining procedures.[36,43,50] We recently developed a digital brain atlas database from 10 normal C57BL6/J mouse brains excised from the skull after formalin fixation.[36] The brains were scanned on a 17.6-T instrument with a spatial resolution of $\tilde{0}.0001$ mm$^3$ using T2* contrast. The high contrast-to-noise in the images allowed for 20 different anatomical brain regions to be defined and from the segmented MR templates several types of atlases were developed (probabilistic atlas, average deformation atlas, average brain atlas, single atlases) and stored in a web-based database (available from www.bnl.gov/ctn/mouse).

The atlas template can be used to assist in segmenting MR images acquired of mouse brains with similar contrast parameters. For example, we recently reported preliminary data from a mouse model of attention deficit hyperactivity disorder (ADHD) developed by Avale et al. [51] that involves neonatal disruption of the central dopaminergic pathways with 6-hydroxydopamine (6-OHDA) in CF-1 outbred male mice. In adolescence these mice exhibit clear behavioral characteristics of ADHD including hyperactivity.[51] To also investigate the role of the D4 receptor in ADHD behaviors, neonatal lesions in dopamine D4 receptor knock out (Drd4$^{-/-}$) mice known to not develop the hyperactive behavioral phenotype also were studied. The preliminary data analysis of the MRM scans revealed subtle volume reductions (5–12%) in several brain regions [52] known to be reduced in humans diagnosed with ADHD such as the cerebellum and caudate-putamen.[45] However, interestingly, both mouse strains (CF-1 and Drd4$^{(-/-)}$) exhibited a similar morphological phenotype in spite of the known difference in the behavioral phenotype.[52] We are in the process of collecting and analyzing more data to further verify these preliminary morphological phenotypic findings. In another recent study, a cerebellar folia-deficient mutant mouse known to develop cerebellar hypoplasia was neuroanatomically phenotyped by MRM and compared with the wild-type strain.[53] Using an average atlas statistical approach the expected cerebellar hypoplasia was documented as were two new and unexpected morphological phenotypes: 38% reduction of the inferior colliculi and 14% reduction of the olfactory bulbs in the mutant compared to the wild-type mouse.[53] These studies demonstrate the advantage and sensitivity of using 3D MRM-based brain atlases for detection of subtle volumetric variations in genetic mouse strains.

We previously have reported on the neuroanatomical phenotype of homozygous and heterozygous PDAPP mice using diffusion-weighted MRI acquired longitudinally over 22 months.[54] In this preliminary study, we only manually segmented the most clearly defined brain regions such as forebrain, ventricles, and the cerebellum and found that the ventricle volume in homozygous PDAPP mice were smaller than that of heterozygous PDAPP and control mice. There was no clear evidence of brain atrophy at a time when amyloid plaques are known to develop (9 months of age). We are in the process of reevaluating this data sample using our 3D mouse brain atlas template to characterize more subtle changes in the entire brain. FIGURE 4 shows the previous quantitative

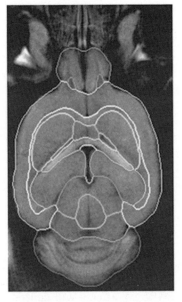
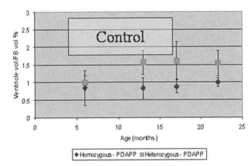

**FIGURE 4.** Longitudinal changes in the ventricular volume of the *in vivo* PDAPP mouse brain. Error bars display ± one standard deviation. An example *in vivo* image is displayed overlaid with the *in vitro* mouse brain template[36] to help delineate structural areas that will be analyzed in more detail to determine the full extent of morphological changes of this time course.

data of ventricular volume change (in percent of total forebrain volume) and an image of a PDAPP mouse brain with the digital segmented atlas template overlaid. Although not all tissue borders are present on the *in vivo* image (acquired at a spatial resolution of $59 \times 59 \times 467$ μM$^3$) the *in vitro* template can be overlaid and used as a guide when defining tissue borders *in vivo*.

## FUNCTIONAL MRI

Neurons in the central nervous system exhibit spontaneous electrical activity that changes with behavioral tasks (e.g., attention, learning, and conditioned place preference paradigms). Electrophysiological studies using multiunit electrode recordings have provided information on neuronal activity within a given neuronal population. It is now known that activity within a neuronal population with most stimuli will result in changes in the baseline and mean peak firing rate ("mean" referring to the neuronal population spike average), although the changes vary with the stimulus.[55–57] For example, in awake macaques monkeys with electrodes implanted in the inferotemporal cortex, the average spike count at baseline was found to be approximately 14 Hz and increased to 18 Hz during video watching.[58] Importantly, for a given stimulus the activation itself may not be associated with large increases in the *mean* neuronal spiking activity (i.e., more action potentials) because of the differences in individual neurons' spontaneous firing rates. For example, in rats implanted with multielectrode arrays 71% of neurons in striatum increased their firing rate during running and 29% decreased their firing rate; in the motor cortex 77% of the neurons increased their firing rate during movement while 23% decreased their firing rate.[59] In other words, for certain stimuli the population of neurons increasing their firing rate upon stimulation may not be much larger than the neuronal population that decreases their firing rate; hence the lack of an increase in the mean spiking activity. This phenomenon has important implications for neuronal activity measured by indirect techniques such as fMRI because for certain stimuli (cognitive, behavioral) the net increase in the mean neuronal spike activity may not be large enough to elicit detectable blood flow or tissue oxygenation changes, which is the basis for the blood oxygen level dependent (BOLD) contrast.

A large number of fMRI studies have been performed in subjects with clinical signs of early AD as well as more advanced stages. As mentioned above, the activation pattern observed during a given fMRI experiment will depend on the number of activated neurons and ensuing hemodynamic/vascular response elicited. As a consequence, any cognitive, sensory, motor, or behavioral paradigm will have to be carefully developed because the fMRI response depends on the task demands and increases with parametric changes in task difficulty. Furthermore, in subjects with AD the task needs to be tailored so that the subjects can perform it during imaging. Most fMRI studies involving memory tasks demonstrate deficient hippocampal activation in subjects with manifest AD.[60-63] Similar results have been obtained for attention tasks and several hypotheses explaining the activation patterns observed have been put forward.

## FUNCTIONAL MRI IN RODENTS

Functional MRI studies in small animals such as rats and mice are made difficult by the fact that most cognitive or behavioral stimuli used in humans cannot be applied and further by the fact that most studies are performed in anesthetized animals, which obviously interferes with neuronal activation.[64] This predicament has been demonstrated in a recent pharmacological fMRI study with a new nicotinic agonist that was found to elicit dose-dependent cerebral blood volume (CBV) responses in awake animals trained to lie still during scanning while in α-chloralose anesthetized rats, the same dose of the nicotinic agonist did not elicit a response.[65] fMRI studies in rodents typically use simple sensory or motor tasks such as paw, whisker, olfactory, and auditory paradigms that can be applied "passively" in the anesthetized rodent. FIGURE 5

Sagittal (lateral to medial)

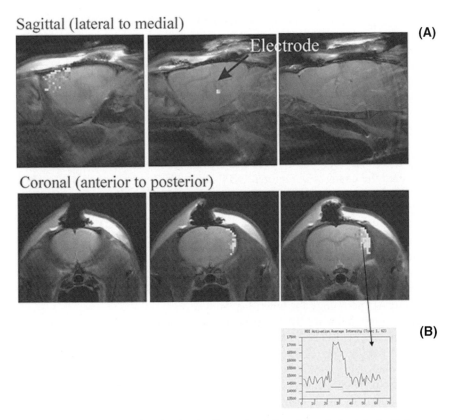

**(A)**

Coronal (anterior to posterior)

**(B)**

FIGURE 5. (A) Functional activation from stimulation via an electrode in the thalamus. BOLD signal is observed in the ipsilateral cortex. (B) ROI intensity plot taken from the cortical activation in coronal slice 3.

shows fMRI activation patterns in a rat anesthetized with α-chloralose during electrical forepaw stimulation (2 mA, 3 Hz) obtained using echoplanar imaging on a 9.4T system. To obtain reliable fMRI activation during such studies, it is extremely important to maintain physiological stability ($pCO_2$, blood pressure, body temperature) as well as to obtain an anesthetic state that does not interfere with the response. Several different anesthetics have been used successfully besides α-chloralose such as isoflurane, propofol, and dexmedotomidine.

A novel and more interesting approach to fMRI studies in rodents is to stimulate directly neuronal pathways of interest (e.g., primarily dopaminergic, glutamatergic, or cholinergic pathways) directly or indirectly using implanted MR-compatible (carbon fiber) electrodes that are activated during the fMRI acquisition (FIG. 5). This approach allows for a more direct examination of functionally relevant of neuronal circuits in normal and diseased conditions (e.g., reward systems in drug addiction models as well as cholinergic or glutamatergic pathways in AD models) and also can potentially have wide applications in understanding the genetic and environmental effects of involvement in neurocircuitry plasticity in transgenic mouse models. So far this approach has only been applied in the rat [66,67] and has to be adapted to the much smaller mouse brain.

Mouse studies are notoriously more difficult due to the difference in size and the challenge involved in reaching a stable anesthesia level and physiological state during the study often requiring intubation and mechanical ventilation. Only a few fMRI studies in mice have been reported.[68,69] Using APP23 transgenic mice that were anesthetized and mechanically ventilated, a recent study examined the changes in regional CBV after intravenous injection of an MR contrast agent and demonstrated that the activation in somatosensory cortex during stimulation of the hindpaw was less in amplitude (for certain electrical intensities) in 13- and 25-month-old APP23 transgenic mice compared to control mice.[68] The diminished CBV response in the APP23 transgenic mice could be due to loss of neuronal activation resulting from neuronal loss secondary to the disease process (e.g., Aβ deposits). More information in other transgenic mouse models would be required, however, to fully understand the effect of AD pathology for functional activation.

There are functional MRM approaches developed that indirectly circumvent the problem of anesthesia in a fashion similar to that done using radiolabeled fluoro-deoxyglucose (FDG) and PET, for which the stimulus is administered at the time of injection of the radioactive tracer while the subject is awake and cognitively challenged; 30–40 min later when the tracer has been trapped intracellularly the PET scan is performed while the subject is either awake or anesthetized. For example, it is possible to preload the mouse or rat brain with paramagnetic manganese (called Mn-enhanced MRI or MEMRI) prior to the experiment and then expose the unanesthetized animal to a given stimulus.[70–73] Subsequent scanning of the anesthetized animal using T1-contrast [73] displays signal enhancement due to Mn ions that enter synaptically activated neurons through voltage-gated calcium channels. The FDG-PET or MEMRI approach, of course, necessitates that the stimulus is "constant," prolonged, or repeated during the FDG- or Mn-uptake period and therefore, the brain activation pattern observed is an integration of the activity seen during this uptake interval, which can be longer than 24 h.[73]

## STUDIES OF BRAIN AND OTHER FUNCTIONAL PHENOTYPES

We are going to conclude this presentation with a new study approach that widens the functional phenotyping concept of transgenic mouse models exhibiting behavioral defects (e.g., hyperactivity, memory deficits, or other task specific deficiencies believed to be associated with brain abnormalities). We emphasize the importance of not only studying the brain in such studies but also linking potential neuroanatomical deficits to functional deficits in other body organs such as the heart, lungs, or immune system. In a collaborative study, we have recently begun characterizing the cerebral and cardiac phenotype of vasoactive intestinal peptide (VIP) deficient mice.[74] Preliminary MRM data from this study demonstrates a heterogenous distribution of abnormal anatomy (from subtle enlargement of lateral ventricles to fulminant hydrocephalus and lack of optical nerves) among the female VIP-deficient mice (that carries the same genotype). In addition, the cardiac functional phenotype also is variable with some mice displaying profound right ventricular enlargement and associated enlarged liver while others do not. We are in the process of linking the severity of the cerebral phenotype with that of the cardiac status and gender to further understand the interaction of these to systems in this particular genetic defect. Undoubtedly, such future studies will lead to novel, unexpected associations between genotype–phenotype in models of human disease.

## ACKNOWLEDGMENTS

The authors would like to acknowledge the financial support of the NIH through grants R01 EB 00233-04 and P41 RR16105 and the National High Magnetic Field Laboratory. MRI data were obtained at the Advanced Magnetic Resonance Imaging and Spectroscopy (AMRIS) facility in the McKnight Brain Institute of the University of Florida in addition to the SBU/BNL 9.4T microMRI facility at Brookhaven National Laboratory. We also would like to thank Dr. S. J. Blackband for valuable discussions in regards to this manuscript.

## REFERENCES

1. CIOBANU, L., D.A. SEEBER & C.H. PENNINGTON. 2002. 3D MR microscopy with resolution 3.7 microm by 3.3 microm by 3.3 microm. J. Magn. Reson. **158:** 178–182.
2. BOYNTON, G.M. *et al.* 1996. Linear systems analysis of functional magnetic resonance imaging in human V1. J. Neurosci. **16:** 4207–4221.
3. FRISTON, K.J. *et al.* 1995. Analysis of fMRI time-series revisited. Neuroimage **2:** 45–53.
4. CHANCE, B. 1993. NMR and time-resolved optical studies of brain imaging. Adv. Exp. Med. Biol. **333:** 1–7.
5. VILLRINGER, A. & B. CHANCE. 1997. Non-invasive optical spectroscopy and imaging of human brain function. Trends Neurosci. **20:** 435–442.
6. FOWLER, J.S. *et al.* 2004. 2-deoxy-2-[18F]fluoro-D-glucose and alternative radiotracers for positron emission tomography imaging using the human brain as a model. Semin. Nucl. Med. **34:** 112–121.
7. PICHLER, B.J. *et al.* 2006. Performance test of an LSO-APD detector in a 7-T MRI scanner for simultaneous PET/MRI. J. Nucl. Med. **47:** 639–647.

8. ESIRI, M.M. *et al.* 1997. Ageing and dementia. *In* Greenfield's Neuropathology, Vol. 2. D.I. Graham, & P.L. Lantos, Eds.: 153–213. Arnold. London.

9. HOF, P.R. & J.H. MORRISON. 2004. The aging brain: morphomolecular senescence of cortical circuits. Trends Neurosci. **27:** 607–613.

10. KILLIANY, R.J. *et al.* 2000. Use of structural magnetic resonance imaging to predict who will get Alzheimer's disease. Ann. Neurol. **47:** 430–439.

11. TEIPEL, S.J. *et al.* 2002. Progression of corpus callosum atrophy in Alzheimer disease. Arch. Neurol. **59:** 243–248.

12. TEIPEL, S.J. *et al.* 1998. Dissociation between corpus callosum atrophy and white matter pathology in Alzheimer's disease. Neurology **51:** 1381–1385.

13. THOMPSON, P.M. *et al.* 2003. Dynamics of gray matter loss in Alzheimer's disease. J. Neurosci. **23:** 994–1005.

14. THOMPSON, P.M. *et al.* 1998. Cortical variability and asymmetry in normal aging and Alzheimer's disease. Cereb. Cortex **8:** 492–509.

15. NORDBERG, A. 2004. PET imaging of amyloid in Alzheimer's disease. Lancet Neurol. **3:** 519–527.

16. GAMES, D. *et al.* 1995. Alzheimer-type neuropathology in transgenic mice over-expressing V717F beta-amyloid precursor protein. Nature **373:** 523–527.

17. HSIAO, K. *et al.* 1996. Correlative memory deficits, Abeta elevation, and amyloid plaques in transgenic mice. Science **274:** 99–102.

18. MOECHARS, D. *et al.* 1999. Early phenotypic changes in transgenic mice that over-express different mutants of amyloid precursor protein in brain. J. Biol. Chem. **274:** 6483–6492.

19. SANTACRUZ, K. *et al.* 2005. Tau suppression in a neurodegenerative mouse model improves memory function. Science **309:** 476–481.

20. ECHEVERRIA, V. *et al.* 2004. Rat transgenic models with a phenotype of intracellular Abeta accumulation in hippocampus and cortex. J. Alzheimers Dis. **6:** 209–219.

21. ODDO, S. *et al.* 2003. Amyloid deposition precedes tangle formation in a triple transgenic model of Alzheimer's disease. Neurobiol. Aging **24:** 1063–1070.

22. ODDO, S. *et al.* 2003. Triple-transgenic model of Alzheimer's disease with plaques and tangles: intracellular Abeta and synaptic dysfunction. Neuron **39:** 409–421.

23. POPKO, B. *et al.* 1993. Nerve regeneration occurs in the absence of apolipoprotein E in mice. J. Neurochem. **60:** 1155–1158.

24. BENVENISTE, H. & S. BLACKBAND. 2002. MR microscopy and high resolution small animal MRI: applications in neuroscience research. Prog. Neurobiol. **67:** 393–420.

25. HUESGEN, C.T. *et al.* 1993. *In vitro* MR microscopy of the hippocampus in Alzheimer's disease. Neurology **43:** 145–152.

26. BRAAK, H. & E. BRAAK. 1991. Neuropathological stageing of Alzheimer-related changes. Acta Neuropathol. (Berl.) **82:** 239–259.

27. BENVENISTE, H. *et al.* 1999. Detection of neuritic plaques in Alzheimer's disease by magnetic resonance microscopy. Proc. Natl. Acad. Sci. USA **96:** 14079–14084.

28. MILLER, L.M. *et al.* 2006. Synchrotron-based infrared and X-ray imaging shows focalized accumulation of Cu and Zn co-localized with beta-amyloid deposits in Alzheimer's disease. J. Struct. Biol. **155:** 30–37.

29. DHENAIN, M. *et al.* 2002. Senile plaques do not induce susceptibility effects in $T2^*$-weighted MR microscopic images. NMR Biomed. **15:** 197–203.

30. JACK, C.R. JR. *et al.* 2004. *In vivo* visualization of Alzheimer's amyloid plaques by magnetic resonance imaging in transgenic mice without a contrast agent. Magn. Reson. Med. **52:** 1263–1271.

31. JACK, C.R. JR., *et al.* 2005. *In vivo* magnetic resonance microimaging of individual amyloid plaques in Alzheimer's transgenic mice. J. Neurosci. **25:** 10041–10048.

32. VANHOUTTE, G. *et al.* 2005. Noninvasive *In vivo* MRI detection of neuritic plaques associated with iron in APP[V717I] transgenic mice, a model for Alzheimer's disease. Magn. Reson. Med. **53:** 607–613.

33. PODUSLO, J.F. *et al.* 2002. Molecular targeting of Alzheimer's amyloid plaques for contrast-enhanced magnetic resonance imaging. Neurobiol. Dis. **11:** 315–329.

34. WANSAPURA, J.P. *et al.* 1999. NMR relaxation times in the human brain at 3.0 tesla. J. Magn. Reson. Imaging **9:** 531–538.

35. KUO, Y.T. *et al.* 2005. *In vivo* measurements of T1 relaxation times in mouse brain associated with different modes of systemic administration of manganese chloride. J. Magn. Reson. Imaging **21:** 334–339.

36. MA, Y. *et al.* 2005. A three-dimensional digital atlas database of the adult C57BL/6J mouse brain by magnetic resonance microscopy. Neuroscience **135:** 1203–1215.

37. MCDANIEL, B. *et al.* 2001. Tracking brain volume changes in C57BL/6J and ApoE-deficient mice in a model of neurodegeneration: a 5-week longitudinal micro-MRI study. Neuroimage **14:** 1244–1255.

38. DUNN, J.F. & Y. ZAIM-WADGHIRI. 1999. Quantitative magnetic resonance imaging of the mdx mouse model of Duchenne muscular dystrophy. Muscle Nerve **22:** 1367–1371.

39. UTRIAINEN, A. *et al.* 2004. Structurally altered basement membranes and hydrocephalus in a type XVIII collagen deficient mouse line. Hum. Mol. Genet. **13:** 2089–2099.

40. TEN, V.S. *et al.* 2004. Late measures of brain injury after neonatal hypoxia-ischemia in mice. Stroke **35:** 2183–2188.

41. WAINWRIGHT, M.S. *et al.* 2004. Increased susceptibility of S100B transgenic mice to perinatal hypoxia-ischemia. Ann. Neurol. **56:** 61–67.

42. CYR, M. *et al.* 2005. Magnetic resonance imaging at microscopic resolution reveals subtle morphological changes in a mouse model of dopaminergic hyperfunction. Neuroimage **26:** 83–90.

43. DHENAIN, M., S.W. RUFFINS & R.E. JACOBS. 2001. Three-dimensional digital mouse atlas using high-resolution MRI. Dev. Biol. **232:** 458–470.

44. KOVACEVIC, N. *et al.* 2005. A three-dimensional MRI atlas of the mouse brain with estimates of the average and variability. Cereb. Cortex **15:** 639–645.

45. SOWELL, E.R. *et al.* 2003. Cortical abnormalities in children and adolescents with attention-deficit hyperactivity disorder. Lancet **362:** 1699–1707.

46. MAZZIOTTA, J.C. *et al.* 1995. Digital brain atlases. Trends Neurosci. **18:** 210–211.

47. THOMPSON, P.M. *et al.* 1997. Detection and mapping of abnormal brain structure with a probabilistic atlas of cortical surfaces. J. Comput. Assist. Tomogr. **21:** 567–581.

48. TOGA, A.W. *et al.* 1996. Informatics and computational neuroanatomy. Proc. AMIA Annu. Fall Symp. 299–303.

49. WOODS, R.P. *et al.* 1999. Creation and use of a Talairach-compatible atlas for accurate, automated, nonlinear intersubject registration, and analysis of functional imaging data. Hum. Brain Mapp. **8:** 73–79.

50. TOGA, A.W. *et al.* 1995. A 3D digital map of rat brain. Brain Res. Bull. **38:** 77–85.

51. AVALE, M.E. *et al.* 2004. The dopamine D4 receptor is essential for hyperactivity and impaired behavioral inhibition in a mouse model of attention deficit/hyperactivity disorder. Mol. Psychiatry. **9:** 718–726.

52. MA, Y. *et al.* 2006. Magnetic Resonance Microscopy of a Mouse Model of Attention-Deficit-Hyperactivity Disorder: Role of D4 dopamine receptors. 14th International Society for Magnetic Resonance in Medicine, Seattle, WA.

53. BOCK, N.A. *et al.* 2006. *In vivo* magnetic resonance imaging and semiautomated image analysis extend the brain phenotype for cdf/cdf mice. J. Neurosci. **26:** 4455–4459.

54. BENVENISTE, H. & S.J. BLACKBAND. 2006. Translational neuroscience and magnetic-resonance microscopy. Lancet Neurol. **5:** 536–544.

55. LAURITZEN, M. 2005. Reading vascular changes in brain imaging: is dendritic calcium the key? Nat. Rev. Neurosci. **6:** 77–85.

56. SCANNELL, J.W. *et al.* 1996. Visual motion processing in the anterior ectosylvian sulcus of the cat. J. Neurophysiol. **76:** 895–907.

57. SCANNELL, J.W. & M.P. YOUNG. 1999. Neuronal population activity and functional imaging. Proc. Biol. Sci. **266:** 875–881.

58. BADDELEY, R. *et al.* 1997. Responses of neurons in primary and inferior temporal visual cortices to natural scenes. Proc. Biol. Sci. **264:** 1775–1783.

59. COSTA, R.M., D. COHEN & M.A. NICOLELIS. 2004. Differential corticostriatal plasticity during fast and slow motor skill learning in mice. Curr. Biol. **14:** 1124–1134.

60. MUELLER, S.G. *et al.* 2005. The Alzheimer's disease neuroimaging initiative. Neuroimaging Clin. N. Am. **15:** 869–877, xi–xii.

61. POULIN, P. & K.K. ZAKZANIS. 2002. *In vivo* neuroanatomy of Alzheimer's disease: evidence from structural and functional brain imaging. Brain Cogn. **49:** 220–225.

62. PRVULOVIC, D. *et al.* 2005. Functional activation imaging in aging and dementia. Psychiatry Res. **140:** 97–113.

63. ROMBOUTS, S. & P. SCHELTENS. 2005. Functional connectivity in elderly controls and AD patients using resting state fMRI: a pilot study. Curr. Alzheimer Res. **2:** 115–116.

64. AUSTIN, V.C. *et al.* 2005. Confounding effects of anesthesia on functional activation in rodent brain: a study of halothane and alpha-chloralose anesthesia. Neuroimage **24:** 92–100.

65. SKOUBIS, P.D. *et al.* 2006. Mapping brain activity following administration of a nicotinic acetylcholine receptor agonist, ABT-594, using functional magnetic resonance imaging in awake rats. Neuroscience **137:** 583–591.

66. SHYU, B.C. *et al.* 2004. BOLD response to direct thalamic stimulation reveals a functional connection between the medial thalamus and the anterior cingulate cortex in the rat. Magn. Reson. Med. **52:** 47–55.

67. SHYU, B.C. *et al.* 2004. A method for direct thalamic stimulation in fMRI studies using a glass-coated carbon fiber electrode. J. Neurosci. Methods **137:** 123–131.

68. MUEGGLER, T. *et al.* 2003. Age-dependent impairment of somatosensory response in the amyloid precursor protein 23 transgenic mouse model of Alzheimer's disease. J. Neurosci. **23:** 8231–8236.

69. WEISS, C. *et al.* 2002. Impaired eyeblink conditioning and decreased hippocampal volume in PDAPP V717F mice. Neurobiol. Dis. **11:** 425–433.

70. PAUTLER, R.G. & A.P. KORETSKY. 2002. Tracing odor-induced activation in the olfactory bulbs of mice using manganese-enhanced magnetic resonance imaging. Neuroimage **16:** 441–448.

71. PAUTLER, R.G., A.C. SILVA & A.P. KORETSKY. 1998. *In vivo* neuronal tract tracing using manganese-enhanced magnetic resonance imaging. Magn. Reson. Med. **40:** 740–748.

72. WADGHIRI, Y.Z. *et al.* 2004. Manganese-enhanced magnetic resonance imaging (MEMRI) of mouse brain development. NMR Biomed. **17:** 613–619.

73. YU, X. *et al.* 2005. *In vivo* auditory brain mapping in mice with Mn-enhanced MRI. Nat. Neurosci. **8:** 961–968.

74. SZEMA, A.M. *et al.* 2006. Mice lacking the VIP gene show airway hyperresponsiveness and airway inflammation, partially reversible by VIP. Am. J. Physiol. Lung Cell Mol. Physiol. **291**(5): L880–L886.

# Various Dendritic Abnormalities Are Associated with Fibrillar Amyloid Deposits in Alzheimer's Disease

JAIME GRUTZENDLER,[a,b] KATHRYN HELMIN,[a] JULIA TSAI,[a] AND WEN-BIAO GAN[a]

[a] Skirball Institute of Biomolecular Medicine, Department of Physiology and Neuroscience, New York University School of Medicine, New York, New York, USA

[b] Current address: Northwestern University, Chicago, Illinois, USA

ABSTRACT: Dystrophic neurites are associated with fibrillar amyloid deposition in Alzheimer's disease (AD), but the frequency and types of changes in synaptic structures near amyloid deposits have not been well characterized. Using high-resolution confocal microscopy to image lipophilic dye-labeled dendrites and thioflavin-S-labeled amyloid plaques, we systematically analyzed the structural changes of dendrites associated with amyloid deposition in both a transgenic mouse model of AD (PSAPP) and in human postmortem brain. We found that in PSAPP mice, dendritic branches passing through or within 40 μm from amyloid deposits displayed various dendritic abnormalities such as loss of dendritic spines, shaft atrophy, bending, abrupt branch endings, varicosity formation, and sprouting. Similar structural alterations of dendrites were seen in postmortem human AD tissue, with spine loss as the most common abnormality in both PSAPP mice and human AD brains. These results demonstrate that fibrillar amyloid deposits and their surrounding microenvironment are toxic to dendrites and likely contribute to significant disruption of neuronal circuits in AD.

KEYWORDS: Alzheimer's disease, AD, amyloid plaques, dendrite

## INTRODUCTION

Alzheimer's disease (AD) is a progressive neurodegenerative disease that is pathologically characterized by the accumulation of amyloid-β peptide (Aβ) and neurofibrillary tangles in susceptible brain regions.[1-10] Many lines of

Address for correspondence: Wen-Biao Gan, New York University School of Medicine, 540 First Avenue, Skirball 5-4, New York, NY 10016. Voice: 212-263-2585; fax: 212-263-8214.
gan@saturn.med.nyu.edu

Ann. N.Y. Acad. Sci. 1097: 30–39 (2007). © 2007 New York Academy of Sciences.
doi: 10.1196/annals.1379.003

evidence suggest that synapse loss occurs early and progressively in the pathogenesis of AD and is closely associated with the duration and severity of cognitive impairment in AD patients.[11–17] The accumulation of both diffusible and fibrillar forms of Aβ has been linked to functional and structural synaptic alterations, contributing to the cognitive decline seen in AD. The presence of elevated levels of soluble Aβ peptides has been shown to lead to a reduction in long-term potentiation, as well as deficits in learning and memory that occur even before amyloid plaque formation.[18–25] In addition, the deposition of fibrillar amyloid has been associated with various morphological changes in synaptic structures. Electron microscopy studies in human AD tissue and transgenic mouse models have revealed dystrophic neurites surrounding the amyloid deposits,[26,27] while Golgi and immunocytochemical staining have shown aberrant neuritic sprouting near amyloid plaques.[28–31] Neuronal processes located near plaques exhibit increased curvature or tortuosity, and such distortion in neurite geometry has been implicated in the dysfunction of neuronal circuitry.[32–34] Recent studies in a mouse model of AD have shown that dendrites located near amyloid deposits exhibit local spine loss and shaft atrophy that may eventually lead to dendrite breakage, indicating that the deposition of fibrillar amyloid could contribute significantly to the progression of AD.[35]

In this study, we examined the frequency and types of dendritic structural abnormalities within and near amyloid deposits in a transgenic mouse (PSAPP) model of AD[36,37] as well as in human postmortem AD brain. We found several dendritic abnormalities, including spine loss, shaft atrophy and bending, branch breakage, and sprouting. In both PSAPP mice and human AD brain, dendritic spine loss was the most frequently seen structural abnormality in the vicinity of amyloid deposits. These results indicate that synaptic disruption is a prominent feature associated with fibrillar amyloid plaques and underscores the potential importance of therapies aimed at preventing or removing amyloid deposits in AD.

## METHODS

### Experimental Animals

Transgenic mice overexpressing mutant human amyloid precursor protein (Tg2576) and mutant human presenilin 1 (PS1$_{M146L}$) were obtained from Dr. Karen Duff at the Nathan Klein Institute at New York University.[38] Mice of 4 to 7 months of age were anesthetized with pentobarbital (80 mg/kg) and perfused transcardially with 40 mL of 4% paraformaldehyde. Brains were dissected out and postfixed for 10 min in 4% paraformaldehyde before slicing. Transversal slices (150–200 thick) at the level of the hippocampus were cut on a vibratome (Vibratome 1000, TPI Inc., St. Louis, MO) and were subjected to labeling.

## Postmortem Human Brain

The brains from two patients with a diagnosis of AD were obtained within 24 h postmortem. Small hippocampal and frontal lobe blocks were immediately placed in 4% paraformaldehyde for less than 12 h and then stored in PBS until the time of sectioning. Tissue slices of 200 μm were obtained with a vibratome prior to labeling.

## Labeling of Neurons

Neuronal structures were labeled with the DiOlistic technique as previously described.[39] Briefly, 3 mg of lipophilic dye DiI were dissolved in 100 μl of methylene chloride (Sigma, St. Louis, MO). The solution was used for coating a small amount (100 mg) of tungsten particles (1.5 μm diameter) (Bio-Rad, Hercules, CA) with the dye. Tungsten particles were introduced into Tefzel tubing (Bio-Rad cat 165-2441) for the preparation of "bullets." Dye-coated particles were delivered to the preparation using a commercially available biolistic device, a "gene gun" (Bio-Rad, Helios Gene Gun System). Tissues were protected from the air shock wave by interposing a membrane filter with a 3-μm pore size (Millipore cat TSTP04700) between the gun and the tissue. After particle delivery, the dye was allowed to diffuse for >24 h prior to mounting and imaging.

## Staining of Fibrillar Amyloid Deposits

Following lipophilic dye labeling, fibrillar amyloid deposits (neuritic plaques) were stained for 10 min in a solution of thioflavin-S (2 μg/mL, Sigma, cat T-1892) in 0.1 M PBS and then rinsed with 0.1 M PBS.

## Imaging of Neuronal Structures

Images of labeled neurons were acquired by a Zeiss LSM 510 confocal attached to an upright Zeiss Axioplan 2 microscope. Neurons were viewed under a 40X/1.30 oil immersion DIC Plan-Neuofluar objective. Neuronal structures labeled with DiI were sequentially scanned using the appropriate excitation lasers (458 nm for thioflavin S and 543 nm for DiI) combined with the appropriate emission filter (LP 560 for DiI and BP475-525 for thioflavin S). Stacks of images at 0.3–1.0-μm steps were acquired to generate a three-dimensional data set of imaged neurons.

## *Quantification of Spine Density, Dendritic Diameter, and Aβ Concentration*

Dendritic spine densities, dendritic diameters, and thioflavin-S labeling intensity profiles (a correlate of fibrillar Aβ deposit) were quantified with Metamorph software (Universal Imaging Corporation, Downingtown, PA) as described in Tsai *et al.*[35] Each dendrite was divided into 6-μm segments and spines were counted and diameters measured for each segment. Dendrites are considered exhibiting spine loss or shaft atrophy if they contain segments with more than 15% reduction in spine density or shaft diameter near amyloid deposits as compared to the adjacent segments of the same dendrites. Spine density was normalized to the spine density of segments in the same dendritic branch immediately adjacent to the segment passing through the amyloid deposit.

## RESULTS

We first examined the characteristics and frequency of structural dendritic alterations in a transgenic mouse model overexpressing mutant human amyloid precursor protein (APP) and mutant presenilin-1 (PS1) (PSAPP).[36,37] These mice begin to develop amyloid plaques at around 10 weeks of age and had large-scale deposition by 6 months of age.[38] Fixed hippocampal and cortical slices from PSAPP mice between 4 to 7 months of age were labeled by ballistic delivery of lipophilic dyes (DiOlistic technique), which labels neuronal dendrites in a Golgi-like manner (FIG. 1A).[39,40] Fibrillar amyloid deposits were labeled with thioflavin-S and dendrites in and around these deposits were visualized using high-resolution confocal microscopy.

We found that dendrites passing through or near fibrillar amyloid deposits showed various abnormalities including spine loss, dendritic shaft atrophy and bending, abrupt branch ending within and near deposits, branch sprouting, and varicosity formation (TABLE 1). Spine loss and shaft atrophy were observed, respectively, in 41% (101/244) and 24% (58/244) of dendrites passing through or within 40 μm of amyloid deposits (FIG. 1B, C; see METHODS). Overall, dendritic segments within amyloid deposits showed ~40% reduction in spine density and ~20% reduction in shaft diameter as compared to those outside deposits.[35] Consistent with previous studies,[20,41] we found that dendrites closely surrounding or inside fibrillar deposits were more likely to exhibit shaft bending (FIG. 1A-B). Within ~40 μm from the edge of deposits, over half of the dendrites curved around deposits as if being displaced from their original locations. Furthermore, 34% of dendrites (16/47) passing through deposits displayed single or multiple sharp bends (TABLE 1).

The fourth most frequently encountered dendritic abnormality was abrupt ending of dendrites near or within amyloid deposits (FIG. 1B; TABLE 1).[35] This

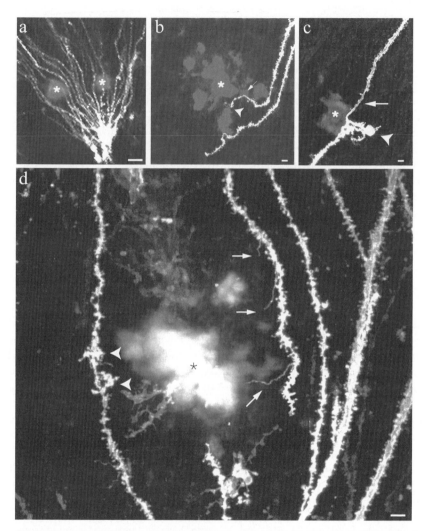

**FIGURE 1.** Dendritic structural abnormalities seen near fibrillar amyloid deposits in PSAPP mice labeled with the DiOlistic technique. **(A)** A cell with dendrites bending around amyloid deposits. **(B)** Dendrite abruptly ending inside an amyloid deposit (arrowhead), as well as spine loss and dendritic atrophy (*arrow*). **(C)** Dendritic varicosity near amyloid deposit (arrowhead) and spine loss and dendritic atrophy (*arrow*). **(D)** Dendritic sprouting near plaque (*arrows*), bending around plaque, and small varicosities (arrowheads). Amyloid deposits are marked with asterisks. Scale bars, 10 μm for A and 5 μm for B–D.

finding suggests that amyloid deposits may induce the breakage of nearby dendrites, consistent with previous results from *in vivo* imaging studies.[35] Occasionally, some dendritic shafts near deposits (5%; 12/244 dendrites) exhibited sprouting (unusually long, thin processes that do not resemble typical

TABLE 1. Frequency of dendritic abnormalities within 40 μm of fibrillar amyloid deposits in PSAPP mice[a]

| Abnormality | Frequency (number of dendrites) | Percentage of dendrites (%) |
|---|---|---|
| Spine loss | 101/244 | 41 |
| Sharp bending within plaques | 16/47 | 34 |
| Shaft atrophy | 58/244 | 24 |
| Abrupt ending | 31/244 | 13 |
| Sprouting | 12/244 | 5 |
| Varicosities | 3/244 | 1 |

[a]$n = 4$ animals.

*Note:* A total of 244 dendrites from 4 PSAPP animals were examined for various dendritic abnormalities. In the case of sharp bending within plaques, only those dendrites passing through plaques ($n = 47$ dendrites, 4 PSAPP animals) were used.

dendritic spines; FIG. 1D). Sprouting dendrites were found concurrently with other abnormalities, such as abruptly ending dendrites, suggesting that sprouting could occur as a compensatory mechanism following dendritic breakage.

A rare but occasional amyloid deposit-associated abnormality was the presence of dendritic varicosities (1%; 3/244 dendrites; FIG. 1C), which in contrast are seen very frequently in axons near amyloid plaques.[35] Axonal varicosities have been shown to contain large numbers of clustered vesicles that can be labeled by antibodies against presynaptic proteins.[42] Lack of synaptic vesicles could explain why dendrites are much less prone to varicosity formation.

To determine whether fibrillar amyloid deposits in human AD brain are associated with similar dendritic abnormalities as those in PSAPP transgenic mice, we analyzed dendrites in slices obtained post mortem from the frontal cortices and hippocampi of two elderly patients with a diagnosis of AD. Confocal microscopy of lipophilic dye-labeled dendrites passing through thioflavin-S positive amyloid deposits revealed several dendritic abnormalities similar to those seen in transgenic PSAPP mice. On average, we observed a 23% reduction in dendritic spine density ($n = 120$ dendrites near 52 plaques; $P < 0.05$) on segments passing through or up to 15 μm from the thioflavin-S-positive plaques when compared to the immediately adjacent dendritic segments from the same dendritic branch outside of the plaque (FIG. 2A–C). Approximately 35% of these dendritic segments displayed at least a 15% reduction in spine density. Because of the large variability in spine density in different dendrites and regions in human tissue, we did not quantify spine density in dendritic branches that were not in the vicinity of plaques. In addition to spine loss, dendritic varicosities and sprouting were also occasionally (1–2% of dendrites) seen near plaques (FIG. 2C). However, in contrast to PDAPP mice, no obvious dendritic shaft atrophy or breakage was seen in the 120 dendrites observed (FIG. 2D).

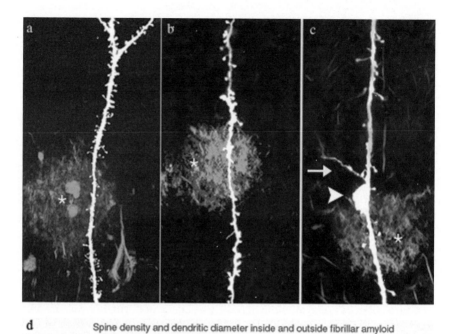

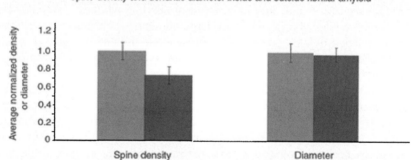

**FIGURE 2.** Dendritic structural abnormalities seen near fibrillar amyloid deposits in postmortem human AD brain. **(A–B)** Lipophilic dye-labeled dendrites passing through thioflavin-S-positive amyloid plaques show decreased spine density inside amyloid deposits. **(C)** Varicosity (*arrowhead*) and sprouting (*arrow*) on a dendrite passing through an amyloid plaque. **(D)** A 23% decrease in spine density is seen on dendritic segments passing through amyloid deposits (*dark gray bars*) when compared to adjacent segments on the same dendrite but outside the amyloid plaque (*light gray bars*); no significant difference in dendrite diameter is seen. Amyloid deposits are marked with asterisks.

## DISCUSSION

The accumulation of amyloid-β peptide in susceptible brain regions is one of the pathological hallmarks of Alzheimer's disease.[1–10] To better understand the impact of amyloid deposition on the process of neuronal circuit disruption in

AD, we examined the type and frequency of dendritic structural abnormalities in a transgenic mouse model of AD (PSAPP) and in postmortem human AD tissue. Spine loss, shaft atrophy, and dendritic bending were the most common abnormalities seen in PSAPP mice, with abnormalities such as dendritic breakage, sprouting, and varicosities seen less frequently. In the human AD brain, spine loss was the most common abnormality, but sprouting and varicosities were also occasionally seen.

Overall dendritic structural changes are much more marked in PSAPP mice than in the human brain. These differences may be due to the fact that amyloid deposition in mice is likely to accumulate much more rapidly. Despite the lower degree of dendritic toxicity in humans, the detrimental effect of amyloid deposition could last over the much longer life span of a human and therefore may have a large cumulative effect on neuronal circuit disruption.

These studies demonstrate that fibrillar amyloid deposits and/or the microenvironment that surrounds them have a toxic effect on dendrites leading to the elimination of spines. This effect is highly local, suggesting that signals derived either from the amyloid deposits and/or the surrounding glial cells are responsible for the damage. Accumulation of soluble amyloid peptides could be the primary event in generating various dendritic abnormalities. Alternatively, fibrillar Aβ may activate surrounding astrocytes and microglia to produce substances that lead to neuritic structural changes in AD.[43] A combination of cellular and molecular mechanisms could be involved in generating the various dendritic abnormalities we observed here. Because the amyloid burden could be extremely high in certain susceptible brain regions, synaptic pathology associated with amyloid deposition could lead to a large-scale and permanent disruption in neuronal circuitry. It is therefore important in the future to develop treatment strategies to prevent and/or alleviate synaptic pathology associated with amyloid deposition.

## ACKNOWLEDGMENTS

This work was supported by the NIH grants to WBG.

## REFERENCES

1. ALZHEIMER, A. 1907. Uber eine eigenartige Erkyankung der Hirnrinde. Algermeine Z Psychiatrie 146–148.
2. TERRY, R.D. & R. KATZMAN. 1983. Senile dementia of the Alzheimer type. Ann. Neurol. **14:** 497–506.
3. TERRY, R.D. 1997. The pathology of Alzheimer's disease: numbers count. Ann. Neurol. **41:** 7.
4. YANKNER, B.A. 1996. Mechanisms of neuronal degeneration in Alzheimer's disease. Neuron **16:** 921–932.

5. LaFerla, F.M. & S. Oddo. 2005. Alzheimer's disease: abeta, tau and synaptic dysfunction. Trends Mol. Med. **11:** 170–176.
6. Armstrong, R.A. 2006. Plaques and tangles and the pathogenesis of Alzheimer's disease. Folia Neuropathol. **44:** 1–11.
7. Mott, R.T. & C.M. Hulette. 2005. Neuropathology of Alzheimer's disease. Neuroimag. Clin. N. Am. **15:** 755–765, ix.
8. Bouras, C. *et al.* 1994. Regional distribution of neurofibrillary tangles and senile plaques in the cerebral cortex of elderly patients: a quantitative evaluation of a one-year autopsy population from a geriatric hospital. Cereb. Cortex. **4:** 138–150.
9. Lewis, D.A. *et al.* 1987. Laminar and regional distributions of neurofibrillary tangles and neuritic plaques in Alzheimer's disease: a quantitative study of visual and auditory cortices. J. Neurosci. **7:** 1799–1808.
10. Wegiel, J. *et al.* 2001. Shift from fibrillar to nonfibrillar Abeta deposits in the neocortex of subjects with Alzheimer disease. J. Alzheimer's Dis. **3:** 49–57.
11. Masliah, E., A. Miller & R.D. Terry. 1993. The synaptic organization of the neocortex in Alzheimer's disease. Med. Hypotheses **41:** 334–40.
12. Scheff, S.W. & D.A. Price. 1993. Synapse loss in the temporal lobe in Alzheimer's disease. Ann. Neurol. **33:** 190–199.
13. Gomez-Isla, T. *et al.* 1997. Neuronal loss correlates with but exceeds neurofibrillary tangles in Alzheimer's disease. Ann. Neurol. **41:** 17–24.
14. Terry, R.D. *et al.* 1991. Physical basis of cognitive alterations in Alzheimer's disease: synapse loss is the major correlate of cognitive impairment. Ann. Neurol. **30:** 572–580.
15. Masliah, E. *et al.* 1993. Quantitative synaptic alterations in the human neocortex during normal aging. Neurology **43:** 192–197.
16. Terry, R.D. 2000. Cell death or synaptic loss in Alzheimer disease. J. Neuropathol. Exp. Neurol. **59:** 1118–1119.
17. Selkoe, D.J. 2002. Alzheimer's disease is a synaptic failure. Science **298:** 789–791.
18. Kamenetz, F. *et al.* 2003. APP processing and synaptic function. Neuron. **37:** 925–937.
19. Walsh, D.M. *et al.* 2002. Naturally secreted oligomers of amyloid beta protein potently inhibit hippocampal long-term potentiation *in vivo*. Nature **416:** 535–539.
20. D'Amore, J.D. *et al.* 2003. *In vivo* multiphoton imaging of a transgenic mouse model of Alzheimer disease reveals marked thioflavine-S-associated alterations in neurite trajectories. J. Neuropathol. Exp. Neurol. **62:** 137–145.
21. Mucke, L. *et al.* 2000. High-level neuronal expression of abeta 1-42 in wild-type human amyloid protein precursor transgenic mice: synaptotoxicity without plaque formation. J. Neurosci. **20:** 4050–4058.
22. Lindner, M.D. *et al.* 2006. Soluble Abeta and cognitive function in aged F-344 rats and Tg2576 mice. Behav. Brain Res. **173:** 62–75.
23. Dodart, J.C., C. Mathis & A. Ungerer. 2000. The beta-amyloid precursor protein and its derivatives: from biology to learning and memory processes. Rev. Neurosci. **11:** 75–93.
24. Koistinaho, M. *et al.* 2001. Specific spatial learning deficits become severe with age in beta -amyloid precursor protein transgenic mice that harbor diffuse beta -amyloid deposits but do not form plaques. Proc. Natl. Acad. Sci. USA. **98:** 14675–14680.

25. SHEMER, I. *et al.* 2006. Non-fibrillar beta-amyloid abates spike-timing-dependent synaptic potentiation at excitatory synapses in layer 2/3 of the neocortex by targeting postsynaptic AMPA receptors. Eur. J. Neurosci. **23:** 2035–2047.

26. KURT, M.A. *et al.* 2001. Neurodegenerative changes associated with beta-amyloid deposition in the brains of mice carrying mutant amyloid precursor protein and mutant presenilin-1 transgenes. Exp. Neurol. **171:** 59–71.

27. MASLIAH, E. *et al.* 1996. Comparison of neurodegenerative pathology in transgenic mice overexpressing V717F beta-amyloid precursor protein and Alzheimer's disease. J. Neurosci. **16:** 5795–5811.

28. SCHEIBEL, A.B. & U. TOMIYASU. 1978. Dendritic sprouting in Alzheimer's presenile dementia. Exp. Neurol. **60:** 1–8.

29. PROBST, A. *et al.* 1983. Neuritic plaques in senile dementia of Alzheimer type: a Golgi analysis in the hippocampal region. Brain Res. **268:** 249–254.

30. MASLIAH, E. *et al.* 1991. Patterns of aberrant sprouting in Alzheimer's disease. Neuron **6:** 729–739.

31. PHINNEY, A.L. *et al.* 1999. Cerebral amyloid induces aberrant axonal sprouting and ectopic terminal formation in amyloid precursor protein transgenic mice. J. Neurosci. **19:** 8552–8559.

32. KNOWLES, R.B. *et al.* 1999. Plaque-induced neurite abnormalities: implications for disruption of neural networks in Alzheimer's disease. Proc. Natl. Acad. Sci. USA. **96:** 5274–5279.

33. LE, R. *et al.* 2001. Plaque-induced abnormalities in neurite geometry in transgenic models of Alzheimer disease: implications for neural system disruption. J. Neuropathol. Exp. Neurol. **60:** 753–758.

34. BACSKAI, B.J. *et al.* 2003. Four-dimensional multiphoton imaging of brain entry, amyloid binding, and clearance of an amyloid-beta ligand in transgenic mice. Proc. Natl. Acad. Sci. USA. **100:** 12462–12467.

35. TSAI, J. *et al.* 2004. Fibrillar amyloid deposition leads to local synaptic abnormalities and breakage of neuronal branches. Nat. Neurosci. **7:** 1181–1183.

36. DUFF, K. *et al.* 1996. Increased amyloid-beta42(43) in brains of mice expressing mutant presenilin 1. Nature **383:** 710–713.

37. HSIAO, K. *et al.* 1996. Correlative memory deficits, Abeta elevation, and amyloid plaques in transgenic mice. Science **274:** 99–102.

38. HOLCOMB, L. *et al.* 1998. Accelerated Alzheimer-type phenotype in transgenic mice carrying both mutant amyloid precursor protein and presenilin 1 transgenes. Nat. Med. **4:** 97–100.

39. GAN, W.B. *et al.* 2000. Multicolor "DiOlistic" labeling of the nervous system using lipophilic dye combinations. Neuron **27:** 219–225.

40. GRUTZENDLER, J., J. TSAI & W.B. GAN. 2003. Rapid labeling of neuronal populations by ballistic delivery of fluorescent dyes. Methods **30:** 79–85.

41. SPIRES, T.L. *et al.* 2005. Dendritic spine abnormalities in amyloid precursor protein transgenic mice demonstrated by gene transfer and intravital multiphoton microscopy. J. Neurosci. **25:** 7278–7287.

42. BRENDZA, R.P. *et al.* 2003. PDAPP; YFP double transgenic mice: a tool to study amyloid-beta associated changes in axonal, dendritic, and synaptic structures. J. Comp. Neurol. **456:** 375–383.

43. EIKELENBOOM, P. *et al.* 2002. Neuroinflammation in Alzheimer's disease and prion disease. Glia **40:** 232–239.

# Two-Photon Imaging of Astrocytic Ca²⁺ Signaling and the Microvasculature in Experimental Mice Models of Alzheimer's Disease

TAKAHIRO TAKANO,[a] XIAONING HAN,[a] RASHID DEANE,[b] BERISLAV ZLOKOVIC,[b] AND MAIKEN NEDERGAARD[a]

[a]*Department of Neurosurgery, Center for Aging and Developmental Biology, University of Rochester Medical Center, Rochester, New York, USA*

[b]*Frank P. Smith Laboratories for Neuroscience and Neurosurgical Research, University of Rochester Medical School, Rochester, New York, USA*

ABSTRACT: The sequence of events leading to neurodegeneration in Alzheimer's disease (AD) remains poorly understood. One prominent hypothesis is that neurovascular dysfunction contributes to both disease initiation and progression. Histologic analysis has supported this idea by demonstrating that vascular abnormalities are present early in the disease and most often perivascular amyloid deposits in the microvasculature. Two-photon *in vivo* imaging of mouse models of AD represents a unique approach to studying microvascular dysfunction in intact animals. We report here that a subpopulation of mice in early stages of AD (2–4 months) displays instability of vascular tone. Some, but not all animals exhibited oscillatory changes in arteriole diameter and poor vasodilation in response to sensory stimulation. An increased frequency of spontaneous astrocytic Ca²⁺ increases was noted in animals with unstable vasculature. Because astrocytes recently have been shown to control local microcirculation and contribute to functional hyperemia, we suggest that abnormal astrocytic activity may contribute to vascular instability in AD and thereby to neuronal demise.

KEYWORDS: Alzheimer's disease; astrocytes; vasodilation

## INTRODUCTION

Several independent lines of evidence suggest that neurovascular dysfunction contributes to Alzheimer's disease. Epidemiologic studies have shown

Address for correspondence to: Takahiro Takano, Department of Neurosurgery, Center for Aging and Developmental Biology, University of Rochester Medical Center, 601 Elmwood Ave, Box 645, Rochester, NY 14642. Voice: 585-275-3720; fax: 585-273-5561.
Takahiro_Takano@URMC.rochester.edu

Ann. N.Y. Acad. Sci. 1097: 40–50 (2007). © 2007 New York Academy of Sciences.
doi: 10.1196/annals.1379.004

that cognitive impairment correlates with amyloid angiopathy.[1] Cerebrovascular dysfunction or impairment of activity-induced vasodilation precedes neuronal degeneration in patients at early stages of Alzheimer's disease and similar defects have been noted in experimental mouse models of AD.[2,3] One of the hallmarks of AD is increased accumulation of amyloid beta peptide (Aβ) in the brain. Aβ is in itself a vasoconstrictor and mice overexpressing Aβ exhibit reduced endothelial cell-dependent vasorelaxation.[1] Although larger vessels display thinning of the vessel wall, the primary site of pathological disturbances is in the capillary network.[2] The amyloid deposits are associated with endothelial wall degeneration,[4] local inflammatory responses, and activation of microglial cells as well as astrocytes.[1] In this regard, it is of interest that new studies have found that astrocytes are in control of local microcirculation.[5,6] We will describe here our analysis of microvascular dysfunction in several transgenic models of AD using two-photon *in vivo* imaging in triple transgenic 3XTg-AD mice,[7] transgenic mice expressing Dutch/Iowa mutations,[8,9] and commercially available transgenic mice APPSWE(Tg2576).[10] All animals included in the study were 2–4 months old.

## ASTROCYTES ARE INVOLVED IN SEVERAL ASPECTS OF BRAIN FUNCTION

In addition to their supportive roles, astrocytes also express neurotransmitter receptors and respond to neuronal activity by increases in cytosolic $Ca^{2+}$.[11] The ability of astrocytes to sense neuronal activity and respond with increases in cytosolic $Ca^{2+}$, has been a topic of intense research in the last couple of years.[12] Astrocytes display two distinct types of $Ca^{2+}$ signaling modalities: $Ca^{2+}$ oscillations and propagating $Ca^{2+}$ waves.[13–15] Astrocytic $Ca^{2+}$ oscillations and $Ca^{2+}$ waves are associated with the release of gliotransmitters, including glutamate, ATP/adenosine, and $PGE_2$. Several lines of work have shown that gliotransmitters modulate synaptic transmission by both pre- and postsynaptic mechanisms,[16] microglial cell activation, [17,18] and local microcirculation (see below).

## ASTROCYTES IN CONTROL OF LOCAL MICROCIRCULATION

Given that cerebral microvessels are extensively ensheathed by astrocytic processes[19,20] thereby physically linking the intraparenchymal vasculature with synapses, it is tempting to speculate that astrocytes are involved in activity-induced hyperemia. Two studies in slice preparations were the first to show that astrocytes can regulate vascular tone.[5,6] Carmignoto and coworkers found that electric stimulation of cortical slices was linked to vasodilation, which was inhibited by metabotropic glutamate (mGlu) receptor antagonists and indomethacin.[5] It was proposed that astrocytes released a vasoactive agent, possibly $PGE_2$, which mediated arterial relaxation. However, another publication using hippocampal slices showed similar convincing data suggesting that astrocytes mediate vasoconstriction.[6] It is difficult to reconcile these two sets of observations. One experimental problem linked to studying blood flow regulation in slices is the absence of blood flow. Possibly, the lack of perfusion pressure, the poor tolerance of endothelial cells to slice preparation, artificial increases in $O_2$ tension, and damage of serotonergic vascular innervation initiate signaling pathways not active in the intact animal with normal perfusion. To overcome the inherent problems associated with studies in slice preparations, we recently adapted two-photon laser-scanning microscopy for the study of microvasculature control in adult mice. We showed that photolysis of caged $Ca^{2+}$ in astrocytic endfeet invariably was associated with vasodilation.[21] Vasodilation averaged 18%, corresponding to an almost 40% increase in local perfusion. A specific COX-1 inhibitor SC-560, as well as indomethacin, attenuated astrocyte-induced vasodilation, suggesting that astrocytes by the release of COX-1 metabolic products mediate vasodilation. This notion was supported by the strong COX-1 immunoreactivity around penetrating cortical arteries, which colocalized with astrocytic endfeet.[21]

## EXPERIMENTAL APPROACH TO STUDY OF MICROCIRCULATION IN ALZHEIMER'S DISEASE

Cortex is ideally suited for two-photon imaging of live adult mice. Technically, a cranial window is prepared in anesthetized adult animals. A femoral artery is cannulated for continuous monitoring of mean arterial blood pressure and analysis of blood gases. Body temperature is kept at 37°C by a temperature-controlled heating blanket. The exposed cortex is loaded with $Ca^{2+}$ indicators (fluo-4 AM), or sulforhodamine 101 (SR101) and the cranial window is closed by a coverslip. To minimize brain swelling, cortex is covered by agarose before mounting the coverslip (FIG. 1).

Use of transgenic mice expressing GFP or its spectral variant YFP under the astrocyte specific promoter, GFAP,[22] or the neuronal specific promoter, Thy1,[23] allows easy cell identification in live intact brain. An advantage of these transgenic mice is that both GFP and YFP are highly fluorescent using two-photon imaging (FIG. 2). Double-loading with the astrocyte-specific indicator, SR101 and $Ca^{2+}$ indicator, fluo-4 AM indicated that astrocytes are the only cell type in the intact cortex of live animals that take up fluo-4 AM when using surface loading (FIG. 3). To outline the vasculature, we administered tetramethylrhodamine isothiocyanate-dextran (TRITC-dextran, MW 160K) intravenously prior to imaging.

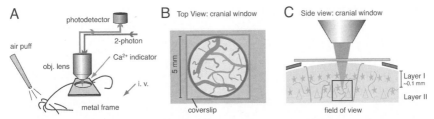

**FIGURE 1.** Experimental setup. (**A**). Two-photon laser scanning microscopy with ketamine/xylazine-anesthetized mouse. A metal frame was attached to the skull and a cranial window was made over the barrel cortex. The exposed cortex after the removal of dura matter was loaded with a calcium indicator dye fluo-4 AM and the vasculature was visualized by i.v. administration of TRITC-dextran (MW 160 K). The whiskers were stimulated by air puffs delivered by a Picospritzer controlled by Master-8.[27] (**B**). A top view of the cranial window. The opening was covered by a coverslip to suppress brain pulsation. Pial arteries and veins were identified under bright field microscopy and penetrating arteries were traced from surface by two-photon imaging. (**C**). A side view of the cranial window. Layers I and II (40–150 μM deep) are accessible to two-photon imaging. Note: A color version of the figure appears in the online version of the article.

In our initial experiments we focused on early abnormalities of transgenic models of AD. We have chosen to evaluate astrocytic $Ca^{2+}$ signaling and microvasculature control in three models: 3XTg-AD,[7] Dutch/Iowa,[9] and APP-SWE(Tg2576).[10] All animals were 2–4 months of age or at a time point prior to extracellular amyloid deposits, neuronal degeneration, and increase in GFAP expression.[24,25] The first abnormality noted was that the unloaded cortex often contained fluorescent aggregates of variable sizes (FIG. 4). These autofluorescent aggregates did not colocalize with Aβ intraneuronal or extracellular immunostaining in vibratome sections prepared from the same animals

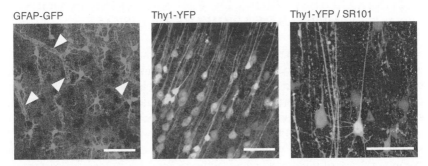

**FIGURE 2.** Identifying live astrocytes and neurons. Transgenic mice expressing GFP under the astrocyte specific promoter GFAP (GFAP-GFP, left panel, white arrows point to astrocyte endfeet around small vessels), or YFP under the neuronal specific promoter, Thy1 (Thy1-YFP, middle panel), and the Thy1-YFP mice labeled with the astrocyte-specific marker sulforhodamine 101 (right panel). Scale bar, 100 μM. Note: A color version of the figure appears in the online version of the article.

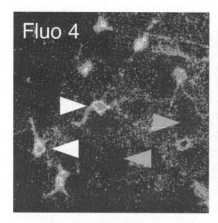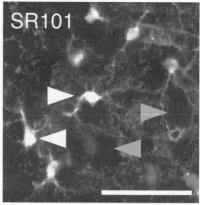

**FIGURE 3.** Cortical astrocytes located 150 μM below the pial surface (cortical layer II). The exposed cortex was double-labeled with fluo-4 AM and an astrocyte-specific marker Sulforhodamine 101. Astrocytic cell bodies (white arrowhead), major processes, and vascular endfeet load with both Fluo-4 and sulforhodamine 101. Neurons do not load with either dyes and appear as black holes (green arrowhead). Scale bar, 80 μM. Note: A color version of the figure appears in the online version of the article.

(FIG. 4). Furthermore, littermate controls display a similar degree of accumulation of fluorescent aggregates. It is therefore questionable that the autofluorescent aggregates relate to accumulation of Aβ. Autofluorescent plaques have not been observed in wild-type mice of several different strains, including FVB/NJ and SJL. We suspect that the autofluorescent aggregates in transgenic mice models of AD may result from years of inbreeding.

## SPONTANEOUS ASTROCYTIC Ca²⁺ SIGNALING IN MOUSE MODELS OF ALZHEIMER'S DISEASE

Our previous studies have shown that spontaneous $Ca^{2+}$ increases are rare in anesthetized adult mice. Cytosolic $Ca^{2+}$ remains stable during prolonged observation periods in astrocytic cell bodies, whereas astrocytic processes display spontaneous, but short-lasting and infrequent $Ca^{2+}$ transients. Physiologic stimulation such as whisker stimulation evoked prompt increases in $Ca^{2+}$ in astrocytes in barrel cortex. Pharmacologic analysis revealed that astrocytic $Ca^{2+}$ signaling in response to whisker stimulation is mediated predominantly by synaptic release of glutamate, which activates mGlu receptor in astrocytes. In turn, intracellular stores of $Ca^{2+}$ are mobilized in a G-protein-coupled process.

In contrast to the low $Ca^{2+}$ signaling activity in unstimulated control mice (0.4 ± 0.1 /min with $N = 3$ animals), we found that astrocytes in APP-SWE mice exhibited a higher frequency of spontaneous $Ca^{2+}$ oscillations with 2.3 ± 0.6 /min (FIG. 5A,B). 3XTg mice (2–4 months) exhibited mixed results.

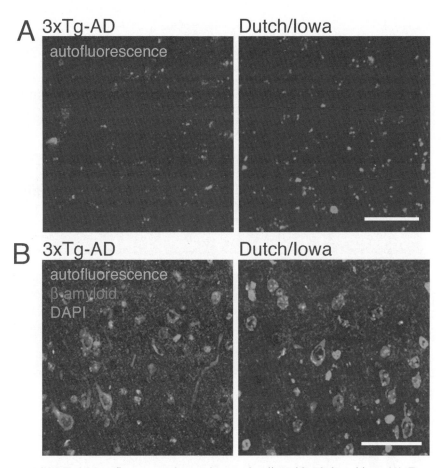

**FIGURE 4.** Autofluorescent plaques do not colocalize with Aβ depositions. (**A**). Two-photon images of autofluorescence in live intact cortex in mouse models of AD. Images are projected from serial images of cortex obtained from 70–130 μM (steps, 10 μM). Scale bar, 50 μM. (**B**). Immunostaining for human Aβ (red), autofluorescence signal (green), and nuclei (DAPI, blue). Images were collected from cortical coronal sections by confocal microscopy. Autofluorescence and Aβimmunoreactivity do not colocalize. Scale bar, 50 μM. Note: A color version of the figure appears in the online version of the article.

While mostly quiet (0.9 ± 0.0 /min), we have also encountered an unusually high frequency of spontaneous $Ca^{2+}$ oscillations (3.5 ± 0.1 /min) (FIG. 5A,B). In contrast, spontaneous $Ca^{2+}$ activity in Dutch/Iowa mice (2–4 months) was low and indistinguishable from controls in all animals studied (0.7 ± 0.1 /min) (FIG. 5A,B). Interestingly, i.v. administration of Aβ40 peptide (0.4 mg/kg) was associated with a significant increase in the frequency of $Ca^{2+}$ oscillation in Dutch/Iowa mice. For example, in one Dutch/Iowa mouse, we counted as many as 3.6 /min major $Ca^{2+}$ increase and ∼50 /min minor increase at 50 min after

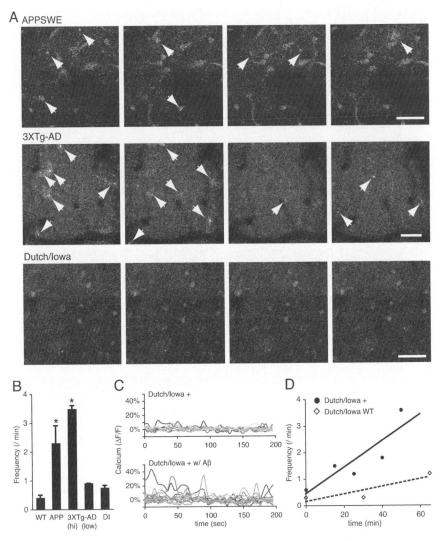

**FIGURE 5.** (**A**). Two-photon images of spontaneous astrocytic $Ca^{2+}$ oscillations in APPSWE, 3XTg-AD, and Dutch/Iowa mice. White arrows indicate spontaneous $Ca^{2+}$ increase. Scale bars, 50 μM. (**B**). Summary histogram of spontaneous $Ca^{2+}$ oscillations in wild-type (WT), APPSWE (APP), two distinct patterns in 3XTg-AD (high and low), and Dutch/Iowa (DI) mice. The $Ca^{2+}$ event is counted when the fluorescence increase is greater than twice the standard deviation of overall fluctuations. Mean + SEM *, $P < 0.01$, Dunnett test compared with WT. (**C**). Spontaneous $Ca^{2+}$ oscillations before and 50 min after the administration of Aβ40 (0.4 mg/kg mouse). (**D**). Spontaneous $Ca^{2+}$ oscillations plotted frequency as a function of time after Aβ40 injection. Note: A color version of the figure appears in the online version of the article.

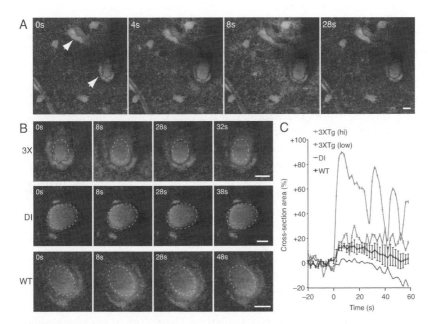

**FIGURE 6. (A).** Whisker-induced astrocytic $Ca^{2+}$ increases (green) and arterial va-sodilation (red) in barrel cortex. Cortical layer I was imaged 40 μM below the surface. Ar-rows indicate the cross-sectional view of arteries surrounded by astrocytic endfeet. Scale bar, 10 μM. **(B).** Various vascular responses to whisker stimulation in 3XTg-AD, Dutch/Iowa +, and Dutch/Iowa wild-type mice. At the first frame right before the whisker stimulation, the basal cross-section size of arteries was shown. The second frame shows the vascular re-sponse after the stimulation, where vasodilation was induced in 3XTg and WT mice, while DI remained unaffected. At third frame the vasodilation of 3XTg was reduced to nearly basal size while WT stayed dilated. At the last frame the artery of 3XTg re-dilated while WT showed the gradual recovery to the basal size. DI remained in the basal size throughout. Scale bars, 10 μM. **(C).** Time-course changes in arterial cross-section area in a 3XTg-AD mouse with an abnormally high frequency and amplitude of spontaneous $Ca^{2+}$ oscillations, a 3XTg-AD mouse with low $Ca^{2+}$ oscillations, a Dutch/Iowa+ mouse with reduced $Ca^{2+}$ oscillations, and wild-type mice (mean ± SEM of 4 animals). Note: A color version of the figure appears in the online version of the article.

the administration of Aβ40 (Fig. 5C). Aβ40 peptide caused only a moderate increase of oscillations in a wild-type littermate control (1.2 /min major $Ca^{2+}$ increase and ~15 /min minor increase at 65 min after the administration). The frequency of astrocytic $Ca^{2+}$ oscillations increased as a function of time after the injection of Aβ in both Dutch/Iowa and controls (FIG. 5D).

## VASCULAR DYSFUNCTION

Aβ and amyloid deposition is often perivascular and is primarily accumu-lated in walls of smaller vessels. Two-photon imaging represents, therefore, a unique approach to studying vascular dysfunction in mouse models of AD. A viable approach to evaluating neurovascular function is analysis of functional hyperemia evoked by sensory stimulation. Neuronal activity is in normal brain coupled to a rapid 30–80% increase in local perfusion. We find that whisker stimulation (5 Hz, 1 min) consistently triggered vasodilation in the barrel cortex of mice (FIG. 6A). In control wild-type mice, whisker stimulation evoked within 1–2 sec with a 22.3 ± 1.7% peak increase in vessel cross-section area of arterioles in barrel cortex ($N = 4$ animals). In mouse models of AD, abnormalities were observed in some, but not all animals. One 3XTg-AD mouse displayed an abnormally large vasodilation (93.0 ± 10.0%, $n = 6$) increase in peak dilation (FIG. 6B,C). In addition, the dilation was not sustained, but exhibited repetitive cycles of dilation followed by constriction (FIG. 6B,C). Interestingly, this mouse also exhibited high spontaneous $Ca^{2+}$ activity (FIG. 5A), suggesting a possible link between astrocytic $Ca^{2+}$ activity and vascular control. The other 3XTg-AD mice displayed normal peak amplitude of 22.9 ± 6.2%, ($N = 3$), but the vessel dilations were unstable (FIG. 6C). Two out of three Dutch/Iowa mice, on the other hand, exhibited a significant reduction of vasodilation (6.2 ± 1.5%, $N = 3$ animals) (FIG. 6B,C). On the other hand, the average vasodilation in APPSWE mice was somewhat decreased, with 17.3 ± 5.4% ($N = 3$ animals) peak dilation. The abnormal vascular responses to whisker stimulation could be divided into two major groups: (1) abnormally large or unstable vascular responses to sensory stimulation. In a single animal, oscillatory changes in vessel diameter even occurred in the absence of sensory stimulation; (2) reduced or absent vasodilation in response to whisker stimulation. Additional studies will be needed to identify the mediators of the abnormal regulation of the microvasculature in AD models and to establish the contributory roles of astrocytes versus vascular smooth muscle cells in the pial and small penetrating arteries[26] in regulating the flow to the brain in response to brain activation.

## CONCLUSION

Two-photon *in vivo* imaging of astrocytic $Ca^{2+}$ signaling, as well as intact vasculature revealed abnormalities of both astrocytes and microvascular control in three different experimental mouse models of AD. Some, but not all animals studied exhibited an increase in spontaneous astrocytic $Ca^{2+}$ signaling. Animals with abnormal astrocytic activity also displayed instability of the vascular tone with oscillatory cycles of relaxation/constriction of small arteries. Aβ administration increased the frequency of spontaneous astrocytic $Ca^{2+}$ increases. Our study provides functional data supporting the notion that reactive changes of astrocytes and abnormalities of the microcirculation occur in early stages of the disease preceding amyloid deposition and neuronal loss.

# REFERENCES

1. ZLOKOVIC, B.V. 2005. Neurovascular mechanisms of Alzheimer's neurodegeneration. Trends Neurosci. **28:** 202–208.
2. FARKAS, E., & P.G. LUITEN. 2001. Cerebral microvascular pathology in aging and Alzheimer's disease. Prog. Neurobiol. **64:** 575–611.
3. IADECOLA, C. 2004. Neurovascular regulation in the normal brain and in Alzheimer's disease. Nat. Rev. Neurosci. **5:** 347–360.
4. WU, Z., H. GUO, N. CHOW, *et al.* 2005. Role of *MEOX2* homeobox gene in neurovascular dysfunction in Alzheimer disease. Nature Med. **11:** 959–965.
5. ZONTA, M., M.C. ANGULO, S. GOBBO, *et al.* 2003. Neuron-to-astrocyte signaling is central to the dynamic control of brain microcirculation. Nat. Neurosci. **6:** 43–50.
6. MULLIGAN, S.J., & B.A. MACVICAR. 2004. Calcium transients in astrocyte endfeet cause cerebrovascular constrictions. Nature **431:** 195–199.
7. ODDO, S., A. CACCAMO, J.D. SHEPHERD, *et al.* 2003. Triple-transgenic model of Alzheimer's disease with plaques and tangles: intracellular Abeta and synaptic dysfunction. Neuron **39:** 409–421.
8. VAN NOSTRAND, W.E., J.P. MELCHOR, H.S. CHO, *et al.* 2001. Pathogenic effects of D23N Iowa mutant amyloid beta-protein. J. Biol. Chem. **276:** 32860–32866.
9. DAVIS, J., F. XU, R. DEANE, *et al.* 2004. Early-onset and robust cerebral microvascular accumulation of amyloid beta-protein in transgenic mice expressing low levels of a vasculotropic Dutch/Iowa mutant form of amyloid beta-protein precursor. J. Biol. Chem. **279:** 20296–20306.
10. HSIAO, K., P. CHAPMAN, S. NILSEN, *et al.* 1996. Correlative memory deficits, Abeta elevation, and amyloid plaques in transgenic mice. Science **274:** 99–102.
11. VERKHRATSKY, A., R.K. ORKAND, & H. KETTENMANN. 1998. Glial calcium: homeostasis and signaling function. Physiol. Rev. **78:** 99–141.
12. VOLTERRA, A. & J. MELDOLESI. 2005. Astrocytes, from brain glue to communication elements: the revolution continues. Nat. Rev. Neurosci. **6:** 626–640.
13. CORNELL-BELL, A.H., S.M. FINKBEINER, M.S. COOPER, & S.J. SMITH. 1990. Glutamate induces calcium waves in cultured astrocytes: long range glial signaling. Science **247:** 470–474.
14. CORNELL-BELL, A.H., & S.M. FINKBEINER. 1991. $Ca^{2+}$ waves in astrocytes. Cell Calcium **12:** 185–204.
15. SANDERSON, M. 1995. Intercellular calcium waves mediated by inositol trisphosphate. Ciba. Found. Symp. **188:** 175–194.
16. ARAQUE, A., V. PARPURA, R.P. SANZGIRI, & P.G. HAYDON. 1999. Tripartite synapses: glia, the unacknowledged partner. Trends Neurosci. **22:** 208–215.
17. DAVALOS, D., J. GRUTZENDLER, G. YANG, *et al.* 2005. ATP mediates rapid microglial response to local brain injury in vivo. Nat. Neurosci. **8:** 752–758.
18. NIMMERJAHN, A., F. KIRCHHOFF, & F. HELMCHEN. 2005. Resting microglial cells are highly dynamic surveillants of brain parenchyma *in vivo.* Science. **308:** 1314–1318.
19. SIMARD, M., G. ARCUINO, T. TAKANO, *et al.* 2003. Signaling at the gliovascular interface. J. Neurosci. **23:** 9254–9262.
20. ANDERSON, C.M. & M. NEDERGAARD. 2003. Astrocyte-mediated control of cerebral microcirculation. Trends Neurosci. **26:** 340–344; author reply 344–345.
21. TAKANO, T., G.F. TIAN, W. PENG, *et al.* 2006. Astrocyte-mediated control of cerebral blood flow. Nat. Neurosci. **9:** 260–267.

22. ZHUO, L., B. SUN, C.L. ZHANG, et al. 1997. Live astrocytes visualized by green fluorescent protein in transgenic mice. Dev. Biol. **187:** 36–42.
23. FENG, G., R.H. MELLOR, M. BERNSTEIN, et al. 2000. Imaging neuronal subsets in transgenic mice expressing multiple spectral variants of GFP. Neuron **28:** 41–51.
24. UJIIE, M., D.L. DICKSTEIN, D.A. CARLOW, & W.A. JEFFERIES. 2003. Blood-brain barrier permeability precedes senile plaque formation in an Alzheimer disease model. Microcirculation **10:** 463–470.
25. BAILEY, T.L., C.B. RIVARA, A.B. ROCHER, & P.R. HOF. 2004. The nature and effects of cortical microvascular pathology in aging and Alzheimer's disease. Neurol. Res. **26:** 573–578.
26. CHOW, N., R.D. BELL, R. DEANE, et al. 2007. Serum response factor and myocardin mediate cerebral arterial hypercontractility and blood flow dysregulation in Alzheimer's phenotype. Proc. Natl. Acad. Sci. USA (In press).
27. WANG, X., N. LOU, Q. XU, et al. 2006. Astrocytic Ca(2+) signaling evoked by sensory stimulation in vivo. Nat. Neurosci. **9:** 816–823.

# Synaptic and Mitochondrial Morphometry Provides Structural Correlates of Successful Brain Aging

CARLO BERTONI-FREDDARI,[a] PATRIZIA FATTORETTI,[a]
BELINDA GIORGETTI,[a] YESSICA GROSSI,[a] MARTA BALIETTI,[a]
TIZIANA CASOLI,[a] GIUSEPPINA DI STEFANO,[a]
AND GEMMA PERRETTA[b]

[a]Neurobiology of Aging Laboratory, INRCA Research Department, Ancona, Italy

[b]Istituto di Neurobiologia e Medicina Molecolare-CNR, Roma, Italy

ABSTRACT: Average synaptic size (S), synaptic numeric density (Nv) and
surface density (Sv), average mitochondrial volume, mitochondrial numeric density, and mitochondrial volume density were measured by morphometry in the frontal (FC) and temporal (TC) cortex from adult and
old monkeys (Macaca fascicularis). In relation to aging, Sv did not change,
while Nv was significantly decreased in TC, but not in FC. S was significantly increased in FC and TC. No significant difference due to age
was found with regard to mitochondrial ultrastructure. Considering the
functional significance of the above parameters, their substantial age-
related constancy suggests that they may reasonably represent structural
correlates of successful brain aging.

KEYWORDS: synaptic pathology; Macaca fascicularis; synaptic morphometry; synaptic plasticity; mitochondrial morphometry; synaptic
mitochondria; age-related synaptic deterioration; mitochondrial structural dynamics; mitochondrial volume homeostasis

## INTRODUCTION

As morphological correlates of brain performances, synaptic junctions play
a primary role in signal transduction and information processing between nerve
cells; in this respect, the age-related derangements in cell-to-cell communication might be due to a progressive deterioration of synaptic ultrastructural

Address for correspondence: Carlo Bertoni-Freddari, Ph.D., Neurobiology of Aging Laboratory,
INRCA Research Department, Via Birarelli 8, 60121 Ancona, Italy. Voice: +39-071-800-4163; fax:
+39-071-206791.
c.bertoni@inrca.it

Ann. N.Y. Acad. Sci. 1097: 51–53 (2007). © 2007 New York Academy of Sciences.
doi: 10.1196/annals.1379.019

features and/or to a decline of their adaptive plastic potential to respond to environmental challenges.[1] To seek precocious age-dependent signs of synaptic pathology as alterations predisposing to functional impairments, we carried out a computer-assisted morphometric study on synapses and synaptic mitochondria in the frontal (FC) and temporal (TC) brain cortex from adult and old monkeys (*Macaca fascicularis*). The average synaptic size (S), the synaptic numeric density (Nv: number of contacts/$\mu$m$^3$ of tissue) and the synaptic surface density (Sv: overall area of the synaptic contact zones/$\mu$m$^3$ of tissue), the average mitochondrial volume (V), the number of mitochondria/$\mu$m$^3$ of tissue (Nvm: numeric density), and the overall volume covered by mitochondria/$\mu$m$^3$ of tissue (Vv: volume density) were the parameters taken into account. The results of our study are shown in TABLE 1. No significant age-related difference in Sv was found either in FC and TC, while Nv of old monkeys was significantly decreased in TC, but did not change in FC. S was significantly increased both in TC and FC of old animals. Either in FC and TC no significant differences due to age were revealed for any of the above-mentioned mitochondrial parameters. Tenable interpretations of the present findings need to take into account the well-documented potential for plastic rearrangement of both synapses and mitochondria[2]; this can be estimated by morphometric procedures, which enable the measurement of selected parameters, closely related to the functional capacities of the neuronal connecting network.[3,4] In this context, the parameters analyzed in this study appear as reliable markers of nerve cell structural dynamics; the substantially unchanged ultrastructural

TABLE 1. Computer-assisted morphometry in the brain of adult and old monkeys

| | Synapses | | | |
|---|---|---|---|---|
| | Sv ($\mu$m$^2$/$\mu$m$^3$) | Nv (N.Syn/$\mu$m$^3$) | S ($\mu$m$^2$) | N.Syn/Neur |
| Frontal cortex | | | | |
| Adult | $0.079 \pm 0.005$ | $0.870 \pm 0.047$ | $0.138 \pm 0.001$ | $1925.650 \pm 48.687$ |
| Old | $0.090 \pm 0.005$ | $0.800 \pm 0.025$ | $0.171 \pm 0.004^*$ | $2073.62 \pm 100.842$ |
| Temporal cortex | | | | |
| Adult | $0.084 \pm 0.001$ | $0.869 \pm 0.012$ | $0.152 \pm 0.004$ | $2111.470 \pm 125.223$ |
| Old | $0.091 \pm 0.005$ | $0.762 \pm 0.021$ | $0.189 \pm 0.011^*$ | $1812.920 \pm 118.543$ |
| | Synaptic mitochondria | | | |
| | Vv ($\mu$m$^3$/$\mu$m$^3$) | Nv (N.Mito/$\mu$m$^3$) | V ($\mu$m$^3$) | Fmax ($\mu$m) |
| Frontal cortex | | | | |
| Adult | $0.074 \pm 0.001$ | $0.521 \pm 0.052$ | $0.192 \pm 0.02$ | $0.581 \pm 0.016$ |
| Old | $0.072 \pm 0.003$ | $0.490 \pm 0.048$ | $0.200 \pm 0.028$ | $0.596 \pm 0.017$ |
| Temporal cortex | | | | |
| Adult | $0.067 \pm 0.008$ | $0.453 \pm 0.036$ | $0.207 \pm 0.039$ | $0.584 \pm 0.037$ |
| Old | $0.072 \pm 0.007$ | $0.488 \pm 0.012$ | $0.192 \pm 0.022$ | $0.592 \pm 0.018$ |

$^*P < 0.05$ vs. the adult value.

pattern of the synaptic junctional zones in adult and old monkeys, associated with the constancy of the mitochondrial morphology, suggests that the present data might represent structural correlates of successful brain aging.

## REFERENCES

1. BERTONI-FREDDARI, C., P. FATTORETTI, T. CASOLI & G. DI STEFANO. 2006. Neurobiology of the aging brain. *In* Handbook of Models for the Study of Human Aging. M. Conn, Ed.: 485–506. Elsevier. San Diego, CA.
2. BEREITER-HAHN, J. & M. VOTH. 1994. Dynamics of mitochondria in living cells: shape changes, dislocation, fusion and fission of mitochondria. Microsc. Res. Tech. **27:** 198–219.
3. COGGESHAL, R.E. & H.A. LEKAN. 1996. Methods for determining number of cells and synapses: a case for more uniform standard review. J. Comp. Neurol. **364:** 6–15.
4. ARENDT, T. 2001. Disturbance of neuronal plasticity is a critical pathogenetic event in Alzheimer's disease. Int. J. Devl. Neurosi. **19:** 231–245.

# Impaired Recognition Memory and Decreased Prefrontal Cortex Spine Density in Aged Female Rats

MAUREEN WALLACE,[a] MAYA FRANKFURT,[b] ADOLFO ARELLANOS,[a] TOMOKO INAGAKI,[a] AND VICTORIA LUINE[a]

[a]Department of Psychology, Hunter College of CUNY, New York, New York, USA

[b]Department of Physiology/Pharmacology, CUNY Medical School, New York, New York, USA

ABSTRACT: Aged F344 female rats (21 months) showed decreased performance, as compared to young rats (4 months), on an object recognition memory task. Golgi impregnation measured dendritic spine density of pyramidal neurons in the prefrontal cortex (layer II–III), a brain area important for recognition memory. Densities of spines in aged rats were 16% lower in tertiary, apical dendrites, but not significantly different in secondary basal dendrites. Concurrent measures of memory and spine density in the young and aged subjects show that age-related declines in recognition memory are associated with decreased cortical spine density.

KEYWORDS: aging; memory; golgi; dendritic spine density; prefrontal cortex

## INTRODUCTION

Aging results in a decline of some cognitive abilities in rats and also influences the morphology of brain structures.[1] In females, aging changes may be further exacerbated by the loss of gonadal hormones, but few studies have used female rodents. The effects of aging are especially important because life expectancy is continuously rising and females live longer than males. Therefore, young and aged female rats were examined for performance of the recognition memory task, object recognition. Following testing, dendritic spine density in the prefrontal cortex, a brain structure known to have a role in recognition memory, was measured.

Address for correspondence: Maureen Wallace, Department of Psychology, Hunter College of CUNY, 695 Park Ave., New York, NY 10021. Voice: 212-772-4234; fax: 212-772-5620.
mauwllc@aol.com

Ann. N.Y. Acad. Sci. 1097: 54–57 (2007). © 2007 New York Academy of Sciences.
doi: 10.1196/annals.1379.026

Ten Fischer 344 rats aged 19 months and eight rats aged 2 months on arrival were used. All animals were tested on a recognition task (object recognition). In the sample trial, subjects explored two identical objects. An intertrial delay was given, and then in the recognition–retention trial, the old (original) and a new object were presented and time exploring each was recorded. Gradually increasing intertrial delays were given until the rats could no longer discriminate (i.e., remember) old and new objects. Subjects were then sacrificed and brains were removed for Golgi impregnation to measure dendritic spine density of pyramidal cells in the prefrontal cortex, a brain structure known to have a role in memory function.[2] Impregnation was by the FD Rapid GolgiStain kit (FD NeuroTechnologies, Inc., Ellicott City, MD). Dendritic spine density of pyramidal neurons in the prefrontal cortex (layer II–III) was measured using the Spot Advanced program, version 3.5 for Windows (© Diagnostic ¨Instruments, Inc., 1997–2002, Sterling Heights, MI) and a Nikon Eclipse E400 microscope. For each animal entered into the data, six tertiary apical dendrites and six secondary basal dendrites were selected for counting according to previously established methods for the prefrontal cortex.[3]

In object recognition testing, young and aged subjects significantly discriminated between old and new objects at 10-min intertrial delays (data not shown). At a 1-h intertrial delay, aged rats no longer significantly discriminated between the objects (FIG. 1). Analysis by a two-way ANOVA (group × object) showed a group × object interaction at a 1-h intertrial delay

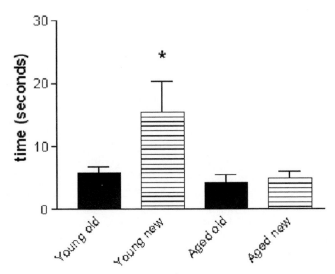

**FIGURE 1.** Object recognition test. Mean exploration time in seconds ± SEM of old (*solid bar*) and new (*striped bar*) objects for young ($n = 8$) and aged ($n = 10$) rats. $T$-test indicates young animals could discriminate between old and new objects ($p < 0.04$) while aged animals could not ($p < 0.3$).

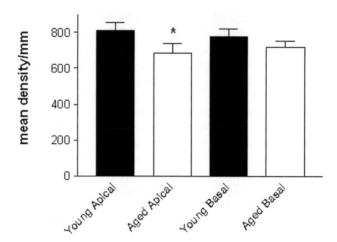

**FIGURE 2.** Prefrontal cortex pyramidal neuron spine density. Bars represent the mean number of spines/mm ±SEM on pyramidal cells in the prefrontal cortex for tertiary apical dendritic branches and secondary basal dendritic branches in young (*black bars*) and aged (*white bars*) rats ($n$ = 6/group). $T$-test indicates aged rats had a significant decrease in spine density relative to young rats on tertiary apical dendritic branches ($p < 0.04$) but not secondary basal dendritic branches ($p < 0.15$).

($F(1,28) = 4.9, p < 0.04$), with paired $t$-test indicating that the young animals could significantly discriminate between old and new objects ($p < 0.04$) while the aged animals could not make this discrimination ($p < 0.3$).

Spine density was 16% lower in aged than young rats for tertiary, apical dendrites of prefrontal cortex pyramidal neurons ($t$-test, $p < 0.04$; FIG. 2). Spine density was not different between the groups on secondary basal dendrites in this area ($p < 0.15$).

Current findings show that aging is associated with a decrease in performance of a recognition memory task. Further, the aged subjects also showed a small, but significant decrease in dendritic spine density in the prefrontal cortex. This age-related decline in memory confirms previous studies in female rats using spatial memory tasks.[4] Decreases in prefrontal cortex spine density are novel findings in rats. Moreover, previous studies have generally not examined both morphology and behavior in the same subjects. Thus, these results suggest that aging is associated with a decline in memory function that may be mediated by morphological changes in brain areas important for cognition.

**ACKNOWLEDGMENT**

This research was supported by NIH grants R25 GM60665 and S06 GM60654 with supplement from NIA.

# REFERENCES

1. TANG, Y., W. JANSSEN, J. HAO, *et al.* 2004. Estrogen replacement increases spino philin-immunoreactive spine number in the prefrontal cortex of female rhesus monkeys. Cereb. Cortex **14:** 215–223.
2. ENNACEUR, A., N. NEAVE & J.P. AGGLETON. 1997. Spontaneous object recognition and object location memory in rats: the effects of lesions in the cingulate cortices, the medial prefrontal cortex, the cingulum bundle and the fornix. Exp. Brain Res. **113:** 509–519.
3. WELLMAN, C. 2001. Dendritic reorganization of pyramidal neurons in medial pre-frontal cortex after chronic corticosterone administration. J. Neurobiol. **49:** 245–253.
4. MARKAM, J., J. PYCH & J. JURASKA. 2002. Ovarian hormone replacement to aged ovariectomized female rats benefits acquisition of the morris water maze. Horm. Behav. **42:** 284–293.

# Alzheimer Amyloid β-Peptide A-β$_{25-35}$ Blocks Adenylate Cyclase-Mediated Forms of Hippocampal Long-Term Potentiation

BLAINE E. BISEL,[a] KRISTEN M. HENKINS,[b] AND KAREN D. PARFITT[a,b]

[a]Program in Molecular Biology, Pomona College, Claremont, California, USA

[b]Program in Neuroscience and Department of Biology, Pomona College, Claremont, California, USA

ABSTRACT: Progressive memory loss and deposition of amyloid β (Aβ) peptides throughout cortical regions are hallmarks of Alzheimer's disease (AD). Several studies in mice and rats have shown that overexpression of amyloid precursor protein (APP) or pretreatment with Aβ peptide fragments results in the inhibition of hippocampal long-term potentiation (LTP) as well as impairments in learning and memory of hippocampal-dependent tasks. For these studies we have investigated the effects of the Aβ$_{25-35}$ peptide fragment on LTP induced by adenylate cyclase stimulation followed immediately by application of Mg$^{++}$-free acSF ("chemLTP"). Treatment of young adult slices with the Aβ$_{25-35}$ peptide had no significant effect on basal synaptic transmission in area CA1, but treatment with the peptide for 20 min before inducing chemLTP with isoproterenol (ISO; 1 μM) or forskolin (FSK;10 μM) + Mg$^{++}$-free acSF resulted in complete blockade of LTP. In contrast, normal ISO-chemLTP was observed after treatment with the control peptide Aβ$_{35-25}$. The ability of the Aβ$_{25-35}$ peptide fragment to block this and other forms of synaptic plasticity may help elucidate the mechanisms underlying hippocampal deficits observed in animal models of AD and/or AD individuals.

KEYWORDS: β-amyloid peptide; Aβ$_{25-35}$; long-term potentiation; hippocampus; adenylate cyclase

## INTRODUCTION

The cAMP signaling pathway appears to be essential in rodents for triggering sustained enhancement of synaptic transmission and for consolidation

Address for correspondence: Karen D. Parfitt, Ph. D., Department of Biology, Pomona College, 175 W. Sixth St., Claremont, CA 91711. Voice: 909-621-8604; fax: 909-621-8878.
kparfitt@pomona.edu

Ann. N.Y. Acad. Sci. 1097: 58–63 (2007). © 2007 New York Academy of Sciences.
doi: 10.1196/annals.1379.020

of spatial information into long-term storage. We and others have observed changes with aging in forms of hippocampal long-term potentiation (LTP) that are mediated by the cAMP signal transduction pathway. These include age-related changes in late-phase LTP,[1] changes in "AC-LTP"[2] and "chemLTP"[3] induced by adenylate cyclase stimulation followed immediately by application of $Mg^{++}$-free artificial cerebrospinal fluid (aCSF). ChemLTP, first characterized by Mahkinson *et al.*,[4] requires the concomitant activation of the cAMP pathway and NMDA receptors, whereas either signaling pathway alone fails to produce persistent potentiation.[2] In hippocampal slices prepared from young adult rats, chemLTP is robust and long-lasting, whereas it is significantly attenuated in slices from aged rats.[3,5] Thus, nonpathological aging results in significant changes in synaptic plasticity.

Alzheimer's Disease (AD) is characterized by the accumulation of senile plaques and neurofibrillary tangles in affected brain regions, particularly the hippocampus. The senile plaques are composed largely of β-amyloid peptide (Aβ), a 39-42 amino acid peptide cleaved from amyloid precursor protein (APP) by the action of β- and γ-secretases. $A\beta_{25-35}$ is the shortest fragment of $A\beta_{1-42}$ needed for amyloid formation.[6] At low (nM) concentrations, it has been shown to inhibit tetanus-induced LTP both *in vivo*[7,8] and *in vitro*.[8,9] The Aβ disruption of synaptic plasticity may be due to alterations in calcium homeostasis,[10-12] the PKA/CREB pathway,[13] or other signaling pathways. In this study, we have examined the effects of $A\beta_{25-35}$ on chem LTP produced by β-adrenergic receptor or adenylate cyclase stimulation, followed immediately by application of $Mg^{++}$-free aCSF. $A\beta_{25-35}$ was applied for a short time (20 min) at a concentration (200 nM) that affects synaptic function in the absence of neurotoxicity.[6]

## METHODS

Fischer 344 rats were obtained from Simonsen Laboratories and hippocampal slices from young (6-week-old) adult male rats were prepared as previously described.[14] A single slice was placed in a recording chamber, where it was submerged and superfused continuously at a rate of 3–4 mL/min with artificial cerebrospinal fluid (ACSF) containing (in mM): NaCl, 119; KCl, 2.5; $MgCl_2$, 1.3; $CaCl_2$, 2.5; $NaH_2PO_4$, 1.0; $NaHCO_3$, 26.2; and glucose, 11. This solution was gassed with 95% $O_2$/5%$CO_2$, bringing it to pH 7.4. To induce LTP,[4] magnesium was not added to the ACSF and $CaCl_2$ was increased to 10 mM. Extracellular recording electrodes were placed in stratum radiatum, and stimulating pulses (0.1 msec duration) were delivered to the Schaffer collateral-commissural fibers via concentric tungsten electrodes. Signals were amplified, filtered, and measured as described by Reis *et al.*[2] In all experiments, manipulations were made only after stable responses had been obtained for at least 20 min. LTP was induced by applying isoproterenol (ISO; 1 μM) or

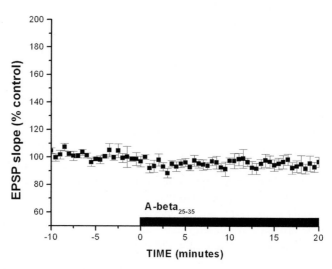

**FIGURE 1.** $A\beta_{25-35}$ does not affect basal synaptic transmission. Perfusion of $A\beta_{25-35}$ (200 nM) for 20 min did not significantly change the initial slope of the EPSPs ($n = 6$).

forskolin (FSK; 10 $\mu$M) to the bathing medium for 10 min, followed by treatment with $0Mg^{++}/$ 10 mM $Ca^{++}$ $aCSF^1$; these protocols are referred to as ISO-chemLTP and FSK-chem LTP, respectively. ISO and FSK were obtained from Sigma-Aldrich; $A\beta_{25-35}$ and $A\beta_{35-25}$ (applied at 200 nM) were obtained from Bachem. Changes in synaptic strength were compared in $A\beta_{25-35}$-treated versus $A\beta_{35-25}$-treated or untreated slices, using repeated measures analysis of variance (ANOVA), with EPSP slope over time as the repeated measure and $\beta$ amyloid treatment as a factor. Where stated, $n$ represents the number of slices used in each experiment. Results are reported as the mean $\pm$SE.

## RESULTS AND DISCUSSION

To determine whether $A\beta_{25-35}$ had any effect on basal synaptic transmission, we compared the initial slopes of extracellular excitatory postsynaptic potentials (EPSPs) before and after the perfusion of $A\beta_{25-35}$(FIG. 1). This application did not have any significant effect on the observed responses (101.2 $\pm$ 2.9% without peptide, 95.6 $\pm$ 4.4% 15–20 min after peptide treatment; $P >$ 0.05). Similarly, the reverse (control) peptide $A\beta_{35-25}$ had no effect on basal synaptic transmission (FIG. 2). We also examined the effects of $A\beta_{25-35}$ and $A\beta_{35-25}$ on ISO-chemLTP. In the presence of the reverse $A\beta_{35-25}$ peptide, we observed a persistent increase in the EPSP slope that was more than twofold greater than the baseline (pre-ISO) responses (FIG. 2). In contrast, pretreatment with $A\beta_{25-35}$ completely blocked ISO-chemLTP; as in the control experiments, there was a robust increase in EPSP slope following treatment with

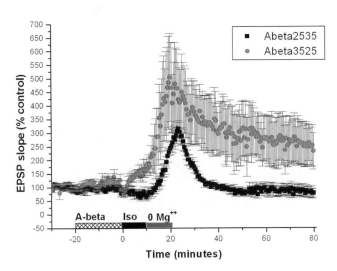

**FIGURE 2.** ISO-chem LTP was induced in the presence of the reverse peptide $A\beta_{35-25}$, but not in the presence of $A\beta_{25-35}$. $A\beta_{35-25}$ or $A\beta_{25-35}$ were perfused for 20 min, followed by perfusion of the $\beta$-adrenergic receptor agonist ISO (1 $\mu$M, 10 min) and then 0 $Mg^{++}$/10mM $Ca^{++}$ aCSF (10 min). Persisting potentiation was not observed following treatment with the forward peptide, and the differences in EPSP slope between slices treated with the forward versus reverse peptides were significant 55–60 min following the switch to normal aCSF ($P < 0.01$). Mean potentiation at this time was 83.2 $\pm$ 19.5% of baseline for $A\beta_{25-35}$-treated slices ($n = 3$) and 258.5 $\pm$ 77.2% of baseline for $A\beta_{35-25}$ –treated slices ($n = 5$).

$0Mg^{++}$/ 10 mM $Ca^{++}$ aCSF, but this increase did not persist (FIG. 2). Similarly, we failed to observe FSK-chemLTP in the presence of $A\beta_{25-35}$, whereas in its absence FSK-chem LTP is significantly greater and very stable for at least 1 h (FIG. 3) or more following the switch from 0 $Mg^{++}$/ 10mMCa$^{++}$ to normal aCSF.

These results show that $A\beta_{25-35}$ disrupts a cAMP-mediated form of LTP. This may be due to inhibition of protein kinase A (PKA) activity by $A\beta_{25-35}$, as shown by Vitolo and colleagues[13] with $A\beta_{1-42}$; this may involve the persistence of the regulatory subunit of PKA, RII$\alpha$.[13] Alternatively or in addition, the inhibition of chemLTP may be due to the ability of $A\beta_{25-35}$ to alter calcium dynamics,[8,10,11] calcineurin activity,[12] and/or NMDA receptor function[12] in the postsynaptic cells. The chemical means of inducing LTP here is advantageous in that the majority of synapses in a slice, rather than a small minority, are potentiated. This will allow us to further investigate the ways in which $A\beta_{25-35}$ and other $\beta$-amyloid peptides and nonpathological aging affect intracellular signals, such as second messenger levels and protein phosphorylation, which are necessary for synaptic plasticity and intact cognitive function.

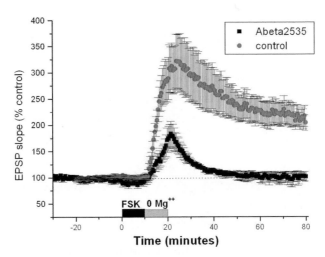

**FIGURE 3.** FSK-chem LTP was blocked by A$\beta_{25-35}$. In the absence of the $\beta$-amyloid peptide, LTP was induced by perfusing slices with the adenylate cyclase activator forskolin (10 $\mu$M, 10 min) followed by 0 Mg$^{++}$/10mM Ca$^{++}$ aCSF (10 min). Mean potentiation 55–60 min following the switch to normal aCSF was 212.8 $\pm$ 17.9% of baseline ($n = 10$); following treatment with A$\beta_{25-35}$ the EPSP slopes at this time were 101.3 $\pm$ 9.6% of baseline ($n = 3$), significantly different from responses in slices not treated with A$\beta_{25-35}$ ($P < 0.01$). The A$\beta_{25-35}$ peptide was applied at time –20 to 0 min.

# REFERENCES

1. BACH, M.E., M. BARAD, *et al.* 1999. Age-related defects in spatial memory are correlated with defects in the late phase of hippocampal long-term potentiation in vitro and are attenuated by drugs that enhance the cAMP signaling pathway. Proc. Natl. Acad. Sci. USA **96:** 5280–5285.
2. REIS, G.F., M.B. LEE, *et al.* 2005. Adenylate cyclase-mediated forms of synaptic potentiation in hippocampal area CA1 are reduced with aging. J. Neurophysiol. **93:** 3381–3389.
3. RASKIN, J.S. & K.D. PARFITT. 2002. Changes with Aging in an Adenylate Cyclase-Mediated Form of Long Term Potentiation in Hippocampal Area CA1. Program Number 444.12, 2002 Abstract Viewer/Itinerary Planner. Society for Neuroscience. Washington DC: CD ROM.
4. MAKHINSON, M., J.K. CHOTINER, *et al.* 1999. Adenylyl cyclase activation modulates activity-dependent changes in synaptic strength and Ca2+/calmodulin-dependent kinase II autophosphorylation. J. Neurosci. **19:** 2500–2510.
5. KUO, S.P., & K.D. PARFITT. 2004. Changes with aging in forskolin-stimulated and basal cyclic AMP in the hippocampus. Program No. 905.5. 2004 Abstract Viewer/Itinerary planner (online). Society for Neuroscience. Washington, DC.
6. PIKE, C.J., A.J. WALENCEWICZ-WASSERMAN, *et al.* 1995. Structure-activity analyses of beta-amyloid peptides: contributions of the beta 25-35 region to aggregation and neurotoxicity. J. Neurochem. **64:** 253–265.

7. FREIR, D.B., C. HOLSCHER & C.E. HERRON. 2001. Blockade of long-term potentiation by beta-amyloid peptides in the CA1 region of the rat hippocampus *in vivo*. J. Neurophysiol. **85:** 708–713.

8. FREIR, D.B., D.A. COSTELLO & C.E. HERRON. 2003. A-beta25-35-induced depression of long-term potentiation in area CA1 in vivo and in vitro is attenuated by verapamil. J. Neurophysiol. **89:** 3061–3069.

9. CHEN, Q.S., B.L. KAGAN, *et al.* 2000. Impairment of hippocampal long-term potentiation by Alzheimer amyloid beta-peptides. J. Neurosci. Res. **60:** 65–72.

10. MATTSON, M.P., S.W. BARGER, *et al.* 1993. Beta-amyloid precursor protein metabolites and loss of neuronal Ca2+ homeostasis in Alzheimer's disease. Trends Neurosci. **16:** 409–414.

11. UEDA, K., S. SHINOHARA, *et al.* 1997. Amyloid β protein potentiates calcium influx through L-type calcium channels: a possible involvement of free radicals. J. Neurochem. **68:** 265–271.

12. CHEN, Q.S., W.Z. WEI, T. SHIMAHARA & C.W. XIE. 2002. Alzheimer amyloid beta-peptide inhibits the late phase of long-term potentiation through calcineurin-dependent mechanisms in the hippocampal dentate gyrus. Neurobiol. Learn. Mem. **77:** 354–371.

13. VITOLO, O.V., A. SANT'ANGELO, V. COSTANZO, *et al.* Amyloid beta–peptide inhibition of the PKA/CREB pathway and long-term potentiation: reversibility by drugs that enhance cAMP signaling. Proc. Natl. Acad. Sci. USA **99:** 13217–13221.

14. MADISON, D.V. & R.A. NICOLL. 1986. Actions of noradrenaline recorded intracellularly in rat hippocampal CA1 pyramidal neurones, in vitro. J. Physiol. **372:** 221–244.

# Age-Related Changes in Neuronal Susceptibility to Damage

## Comparison of the Retinal Ganglion Cells of Young and Old Mice Before and After Optic Nerve Crush

AI LING WANG, MING YUAN, AND ARTHUR H. NEUFELD

*Laboratory for the Investigation of the Aging Retina, Department of Ophthalmology, Northwestern University School of Medicine, Chicago, Illinois, USA*

ABSTRACT: To investigate whether or not the aging phenotype has increased vulnerability to axonal injury *in vivo*, we quantitated the loss of retinal ganglion cells (RGCs) after optic nerve crush. After crush, young animals lost 20% in 3 days and 50% of their RGCs in 7 days; however, old animals lost 40% in 3 days and 70% of their RGCs in 7 days. Our results showed that the time course in the loss of RGCs after crush in old mice is faster than that in young mice. Thus, old age increases susceptibility for the loss of RGCs following axonal damage.

KEYWORDS: retinal ganglion cell; optic nerve crush; fluoro-gold; age

## INTRODUCTION

Age as a risk factor for neuronal damage suggests intrinsic changes in neurons, in their supporting cells, or both, which make neurons more susceptible to injury.[1] Vulnerable neurons are typically large with axons that extend relatively long distances, from one region of the central nervous system (CNS) to another or from the CNS to peripheral targets.[2] There are several reasons why long projection neurons might be particularly vulnerable to aging, including a high energy requirement, reliance on axonal transport, a large cell surface area, and a significant requirement for support from nonneural cells.[3]

Address for correspondence: Arthur H. Neufeld, Ph.D., Laboratory for the Investigation of the Aging Retina, Department of Ophthalmology, Northwestern University School of Medicine, Tarry 13-753, 303 E. Chicago Avenue, Chicago, IL 60611. Voice: 312-503-1079; fax: 312-503-1210.
a-neufeld@northwestern.edu

Ann. N.Y. Acad. Sci. 1097: 64–66 (2007). © 2007 New York Academy of Sciences.
doi: 10.1196/annals.1379.027

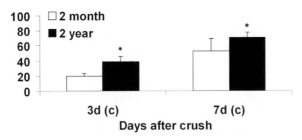

**FIGURE 1.** Old age increases susceptibility for the loss of RGCs following axonal damage.

We have used retinal ganglion cells (RGCs) to model age as a risk factor for neuronal injury. We have asked whether or not the aging phenotype has increased vulnerability to axonal injury *in vivo*. The spatial separation of the parts of the RGC, cell body in the retina, axon in the optic nerve and terminals in the superior colliculus, and the ability to retrogradely label and then specifically count only this type of cell body in the retina, make the RGC ideal for definitively addressing the fate of the neuronal cell body in young and old mice. We hypothesized that if the aging phenotype has any increased susceptibility to axonal damage, retrograde degeneration of RGCs in old mice should be much faster than that in young mice after optic nerve crush.

To quantitate the loss of RGCs after crush, fluoro-gold, a retrograde tracer, was injected into the superior colliculus 3 days before crush. The axons of the optic nerve were then crushed with fine forceps for 10 sec, 1 mm posterior to the globe, under direct visualization. Interruption of the RGC axons was judged to be a separation of the proximal and distal optic nerve ends within an intact meningeal sheath. At 3 and 7 days after the crush, RGC bodies were counted in retinal flatmounts of old and young mice.[4] Counting of RGCs was performed in four quadrants (one field/quadrant) of central retina/eye (approximately 0.5 mm from optic nerve head) and in four quadrants (two fields/quadrant) of peripheral retina/eye (approximately 1 mm from the optic nerve head) at 200 × magnification using fluorescence microscopy (Olympus AX70, Japan). We estimate that we counted approximately 25% of the total number of RGCs in the mouse retina.

Young animals lost approximately 20% of their RGCs in 3 days and 50% of their RGCs in 7 days after optic nerve crush in the peripheral retina and in the central retina. However, old animals lost approximately 40% of their RGCs in 3 days and 70% of their RGCs in 7 days after optic nerve crush in the peripheral retina and in the central retina (FIG. 1).

With age, there were changes in the glia supporting RGCs in the retina. Old mice lost approximately 40% of their astrocytes compared with the young mice. Aging has a differential impact on astrocytes near vessels versus away from vessels. Astrocytes near vessels were retained in old animals. Astrocytes away from the vessels in old retinas were lost. Muller cells, specialized glia in the retina, project irregularly thick and thin processes to the outer-limiting membrane and to the inner-limiting membrane in both old and young mice. In the inner-limiting membrane, surrounding the RGCs, the endfeet of Muller cells were thicker with vacuoles in old mice, compared with young mice. Thus, with age the changes in the glia supporting the RGCs may impact the survival of the RGC following injury.

Our results show that the time course in the loss of fluoro-gold containing RGC bodies after crush in old mice is much faster than that in young mice. Thus, compared to young mice, old age increases susceptibility for the loss of RGCs following damage.

## REFERENCES

1. KAWAI, S.I., S. VORA, S. DAS, et al. 2001. Modeling of risk factors for the degeneration of retinal ganglion cells after ischemia/reperfusion in rats: effects of age, caloric restriction, diabetes, pigmentation, and glaucoma. FASEB J. **15:** 1285–1287.
2. MATTSON, P.M & T. MAGNUS. 2006. Ageing and neuronal vulnerability. Nat. Rev. Neurosci. **7:** 278–294.
3. SIERADZAN, K.A. & D.M. MANN. 2001. The selective vulnerability of nerve cells in Huntington's disease. Neuropathol. Appl. Neurobiol. **27:** 1–21.
4. NEUFELD, A.H. & E.N. GACHIE. 2003. The inherent, age-dependent loss of retinal ganglion cells is related to the lifespan of the species. Neurobiol. Aging **24:** 167–172.

# Top-Down Modulation and Normal Aging

ADAM GAZZALEY[a,b] AND MARK D'ESPOSITO[b]

[a]Department of Neurology and Physiology, Keck Center of Integrative Neuroscience, University of California, San Francisco, California, USA

[b]Helen Wills Neuroscience Institute and Department of Psychology, University of California, Berkeley, California, USA

ABSTRACT: Normal aging is characterized by cognitive deficits that cross multiple domains and impair the ability of some older individuals to lead productive, high-quality lives. One of the primary goals of research in our laboratories is to study age-related alterations in neural mechanisms that underlie a wide range of cognitive processes so that we may generate a unifying principle of cognitive aging. Top-down modulation is the mechanism by which we enhance neural activity associated with relevant information and suppress activity for irrelevant information, thus establishing a foundation for both attention and memory processes. We use three converging technologies of human neurophysiology to study top-down modulation in aging: functional magnetic resonance imaging (fMRI), electroencephalography (EEG), and transcranial magnetic stimulation (TMS). Using these tools we have discovered that healthy older adults exhibit a selective inability to effectively suppress neural activity associated with distracting information and that this top-down suppression deficit is correlated with their memory impairment. We are now further characterizing the basis of these age-related alterations in top-down modulation and investigating interventions to remedy them.

KEYWORDS: aging; top-down modulation; fMRI; ERP; EEG; attention; working memory

Individuals over 65 years of age currently make up more than 13% of the American population. Over the next 30 years, this percentage will double and the number of senior adults is expected to swell to 70 million *(U.S. Census Bureau, Decennial Census Data, and Population Projections, 2000)*. This dramatic increase in the size of the older population will have far-reaching societal consequences. Although neuroscience research has largely focused on severe forms of age-related intellectual deterioration seen in dementia, cognitive decline in nondemented seniors, or *cognitive aging*, is pervasive and can severely

Address for correspondence: Adam Gazzaley, M.D., Ph.D., University of California, 1700 4th Street, Room 102 C, San Francisco, CA 94143-2522. Voice: 415-476-2162; fax: 415-514-4451.
adam.gazzaley@ucsf.edu

Ann. N.Y. Acad. Sci. 1097: 67–83 (2007). © 2007 New York Academy of Sciences.
doi: 10.1196/annals.1379.010

constrain an otherwise productive life. Cognitive deficits are a cause of great distress to many older adults who feel that their ability to lead a high-quality life is negatively impacted by this decline and it is often considered the most debilitating aspect of aging.[1] Exploring the neural impairments that underlie cognitive deficits, as well as the compensatory changes that allow many older adults to remain cognitively intact, is an important step in alleviating this burden and delaying or preventing the debilitating functional decline of dementia.

Insidious impairments in the cognitive abilities of many older adults is a well-documented phenomenon and a substantial body of research has revealed performance deficits in multiple cognitive domains, such as working memory (WM), episodic memory, and attention.[2,3] Despite heterogeneity in the nature and severity of decline between older individuals, common features have been observed on neuropsychological testing, for example, decreases in processing speed on many different tests.[4] In an attempt to account for common features, several hypotheses have been proposed. Three frequently cited hypotheses in the aging literature are: (1) *the processing speed hypothesis* in which performance deficits are attributed to generalized slowing of processing speed,[4] (2) *the executive deficit (frontal aging) hypothesis*, which proposes that executive abilities dependent on frontal lobe integrity are affected earlier and to a greater magnitude than other processes,[5] and (3) *the inhibitory deficit hypothesis*, which suggests a reduction in the efficiency of inhibitory mechanisms.[6] It is important to note that these hypotheses are largely based on neuropsychological data. We are now attempting to generate a parsimonious principle of cognitive aging by exploring alterations in *neural mechanisms* associated with aging.

The search for alterations in the brain that produce cognitive deficits has involved a variety of experimental approaches, including neurophysiological, neurochemical, and neuroanatomical methodologies. Although anatomical studies have revealed subtle age-related structural changes, such as alterations in dendritic arborization and spine count,[7,8] many studies have revealed no such changes, including preservation of neuronal number with aging.[9–14] Despite the lack of overwhelming evidence for structural alterations, there has been a steady accumulation of studies revealing physiological changes[15–19] and changes in neurotransmitter levels with aging.[20,21] These observations have led to an emerging view that changes in neural signaling, rather than structural alterations, account for age-related cognitive deficits. This principle has been a guiding force for the application of the more recently applied technologies of functional brain imaging to study age-related brain alterations. Functional neuroimaging techniques, such as positron emission tomography (PET), functional magnetic resonance imaging (fMRI), and electroencephalography (EEG), allow us to record correlates of brain activity in human research subjects during the performance of cognitive tasks and is thus particularly well suited to explore the neural basis of cognitive aging in humans.[22]

# NEURAL MEASURES OF TOP–DOWN MODULATION

The experiments that we describe in this article review our recent attempt to generate unifying aging principles based on our view that neural alterations are likely not limited to localized brain regions, but rather in the functional connections between brain regions. This is consistent with the manner in which the brain generates higher-order cognitive abilities; cognition is an emergent process subserved by the integration of signals across distributed brain regions, or *neural networks*, rather than a product of independently functioning isolated brain regions.[23] By evaluating changes that occur in neural networks, we hope to identify an underlying cause of the diverse cognitive deficits associated with normal aging. To accomplish this, our experimental focus has been on the neural process of *top-down modulation*, selected both because it serves as a foundation for many cognitive abilities, such as attention, WM, and episodic memory, all of which are vulnerable in aging, and its very basis has been attributed to functional interactions between distant brain regions.

How we perceive stimuli in our environment involves an integration of two distinct influences: externally and internally driven attention. Sensory input from our surroundings often demand attention based on stimulus characteristics, such as novelty or salience *(bottom-up processing),* but we are also capable of directing attention toward or away from encountered stimuli based on our goals *(top-down modulation).*[24–26] Top-down modulation underlies our essential ability to focus on what is task relevant and ignore irrelevant distractions by differentially *enhancing* and/or *suppressing* neural activity in sensory cortical regions depending on the relevance of the information to our goals. This modulation is achieved by neural connections subserving dynamic interactions between widely distributed brain regions at the "top" (prefrontal cortex [PFC]) and the "bottom" (visual association cortex [VAC]);[27–29,30] and has been described to occur both when a stimulus is present and when a stimulus is absent. Thus, it serves as a neural mechanism that underlies the processes of selective attention and memory encoding when a stimulus is present[25,31–33] and mental imagery, WM maintenance and anticipation when a stimulus is absent.[34–37] Although numerous functional imaging studies have examined age-related changes in neural activity associated with attention and memory,[22,38] our research is directed at specifically exploring alterations in top-down modulation with aging.

Our first goal to explore alterations in top-down modulation in aging was to define reliable measures of both top-down enhancement and suppression of neural activity in young adults. We chose to do this in the context of a visual WM task when information is presented that must be held in mind for a short period of time. In a commonly used task to study WM, the delayed-recognition task, a subject is first required to remember a stimulus presented during a "cue" period and then maintain this information for a brief "delay" interval when the stimulus is absent. Lastly, the subject responds to a "probe" stimulus to determine

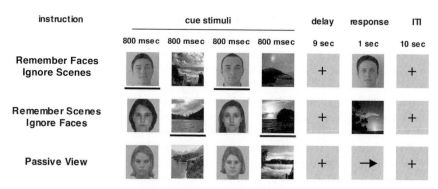

**FIGURE 1.** Experimental design of the selective WM task. Tasks differed in the instructions given at the beginning of each run and in the response requirements. Participants were instructed to (1) Remember Faces and Ignore Scenes, (2) Remember Scenes and Ignore Faces, and (3) Passively View both Faces and Scenes—with no attempt to remember or evaluate them. In the memory trials response period, a face or scene stimulus was presented (depending upon the condition), and participants were required to report with a button press whether the stimulus matched one of the previously presented stimuli. During the response period of the Passive View task, an *arrow* was presented and participants were required to make a button press indicating the direction of the *arrow*. (Adapted from Gazzaley et al.[39])

whether the information was successfully retained. Thus, the cognitive stages are segregated in time and can be investigated in relative isolation by recording during these distinct stages with microelectrodes in animals and event-related fMRI and EEG in human research subjects. We modified the classic delayed-recognition task to generate a *selective* WM task so as to directly study the processes of enhancement and suppression. To identify distinct measures of top-down enhancement and suppression we developed a paradigm consisting of three delayed-recognition tasks in which aspects of visual information are held constant while the task demands are manipulated (FIG. 1).[39] During each trial, participants observe sequences of two faces and two natural scenes presented in a randomized order. The tasks differ in the instructions informing the participants how to process the stimuli: (1) *Remember Faces and Ignore Scenes*, (2) *Remember Scenes and Ignore Faces*, or (3) *Passively View* faces and scenes without attempting to remember them. In each task, the period in which the cue stimuli are presented is balanced for bottom-up visual information, thus allowing us to probe the influence of goal-directed behavior on neural activity (top-down modulation). In the two memory tasks, the encoding of the task-relevant stimuli requires selective attention and thus permits the dissociation of physiological measures of enhancement and suppression relative to the passive baseline. Specifically, neural activity measures recorded in VAC that are greater in magnitude for the memory tasks compared to the passive baseline reflect enhancement, while activity measures below passive baseline reflect suppression. In the memory tasks, following a 9-sec delay the participants are tested on their ability to recognize a probe stimulus as being one of the task-relevant cues, yielding a behavioral measure of WM performance. In addition, a postexperiment surprise recognition memory enables us to evaluate incidental long-term memory of the stimuli.

The experiments we performed using this paradigm employed both event-related fMRI and EEG on counterbalanced sessions to record correlates of neural activity while the subjects performed the task. This allowed us to capitalize on the high spatial resolution achievable with the fMRI blood oxygen level dependent (BOLD) signal and the high temporal resolution attained when recording electrical activity with EEG. Although both measures are thought to reflect cortical activity driven by local cortical processing and the summation of postsynaptic potentials on synchronously active, large ensembles of neurons,[40–42] changes in BOLD signal can be localized to cortical regions separated by millimeters and EEG can resolve activity changes in the millisecond range. Thus, these techniques offer complementary, but unique information to study the modulation of activity at the neuronal population level.

For fMRI, we used an independent functional localizer task to identify stimulus-selective regions in the VAC. This allowed us to assess the top-down modulation of activity in regions that are separable based on perceptual differences. We identified both face-selective regions and scene-selective regions in the fusiform gyrus and the parahippocampal/lingual gyrus, respectively,[43–45] and then used them as regions of interest to study activity modulation based on the goals of the task. For the purpose of this article, we will focus on the fMRI data from the left scene-selective region, since it yielded the most robust measures of top-down modulation. For EEG, we used a face-selective event-related potential (ERP), the N170, a component localized to posterior occipital electrodes and reflecting VAC activity with face specificity.[46]

Our fMRI and EEG data revealed that in young adults ($n = 17$, 19–30 years of age), top-down modulation of both activity magnitude (fMRI) and processing speed (ERP) occurs above and below the passive baseline depending on task instruction (FIG. 2). For the fMRI data, all younger subjects exhibited greater activity during the encoding period when attempting to remember scenes compared to ignoring scenes, despite viewing the same number of scenes in both conditions ($P < 10^{-5}$). In addition, 82% of the younger subjects enhanced activity above the passive view baseline when remembering scenes and 88% suppress activity below the passive view baseline when ignoring scenes (enhancement, $P < 0.005$; suppression, $P < 0.0005$). Comparable findings of significant enhancement and suppression were observed for the peak latency of the N170 component, revealing that top-down modulation occurs for both the magnitude of activity and the speed of cortical processing.[39] We thus established reliable measures of top-down enhancement and suppression that could then serve as functional biomarkers to study cognitive aging.

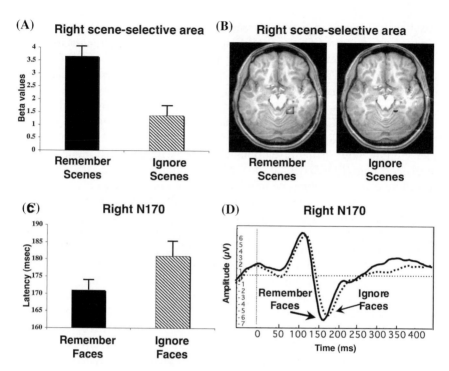

**FIGURE 2.** Activity data for *Remember* and *Ignore* conditions: fMRI and ERP. (**A**) Group data: Average beta values in the scene selective area revealing greater activity in Remember Scenes vs. Ignore Scenes condition. (**B**) A representative subject demonstrating the BOLD signal level within the masked scene selective in Remember Scenes vs. Ignore Scenes condition. (**C**) Group data: Average peak latency for the right N170 in PO8 electrode revealing earlier latency for Remember Faces vs. Ignore Faces. (**D**) Grand-averaged waveforms of the time-locked ERP to face stimuli revealing earlier latency for Remember Faces vs. Ignore Faces. *Error bars* indicate standard error of the mean. (Adapted from Gazzaley et al.[39])

## TOP–DOWN MODULATION IN AGING

To evaluate if these modulation indices change with aging we repeated the identical fMRI study on healthy older adults ($n = 16$, 60–77 years of age) (FIG. 3).[47] As we observed in the younger subjects, the older subjects exhibited greater activity in the scene-selective region when attempting to remember scenes versus ignore scenes ($P < 0.0005$), revealing they were capable of top-down modulation. However, while 88% of the older participants enhanced activity above the passive view baseline (enhancement, $P < 0.0005$), only 44% suppressed activity (suppression, $P = 0.72$), revealing the absence of significant suppression of task-irrelevant information in the older population. To compare across age groups, we calculated three

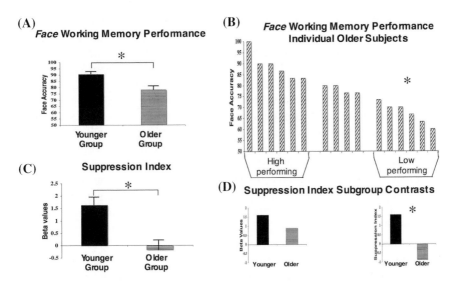

**FIGURE 3.** Relationship of suppression deficit and WM deficit. (**A** and **C**) Across-group comparisons of (**A**) Face WM accuracy (*$P = 0.001$) and (**C**) suppression indices (*$P < 0.005$). (**B**) Subgroups of the six high-performing and the six low-performing older individuals (*$P < 10^{-5}$) on the Remember Faces condition. (**D**) A significant suppression deficit is only present in the low-performing older subgroup (* $P < 0.05$). *Error bars* indicate standard error of the mean. (Adapted from Gazzaley et al.[47])

modulation indices: overall modulation index (Remember Scenes–Ignore Scenes), enhancement index (Remember Scenes–Passive View), and suppression index (Passive View–Ignore Scenes). The use of these indices enabled across-group comparisons to be performed without directly contrasting BOLD signal magnitude between populations that might have vascular responsivity differences.[48] This analysis revealed the presence of an age-related decrease in the degree of overall modulation ($P < 0.05$). Critically, this age-related decrease in modulation can be attributed to a selective decrease in the subcomponent process of suppression ($P < 0.005$) (FIG. 2 D), as there was no significant difference in the enhancement subcomponent ($P = 0.27$). We have also replicated this finding and confirmed that it is a neural change and not a blood flow change by identifying a similar selective suppression deficit of the N170 latency shift in an EEG experiment on older subjects.[49]

In addition to exhibiting a decrease in the suppression index during encoding, as a population the older participants were cognitively impaired on the WM tasks in terms of both reduced accuracy and a slower reaction time compared to the younger population.[47] We further determined that only the subpopulation of older adults with a significant WM deficit on the task had a significant suppression deficit. This subpopulation also rated the scenes that were viewed during the Ignore Scenes task as significantly more familiar than the younger participants rated them on the surprise postexperiment recognition test, revealing increased incidental long-term memory of distracting information and supporting our neural data that task-irrelevant scenes were not suppressed. To more directly evaluate the relationship between top-down modulation during encoding and subsequent WM recognition performance in the older subjects, we performed a Pearson's correlation between the suppression index and Remember Faces WM accuracy. The analysis revealed that the suppression index in older subjects significantly correlates with WM performance ($r = 0.53$, $P < 0.05$), such that the degree of top-down suppression during encoding predicts WM recognition accuracy, establishing the relationship between an age-related deficit in selective attention (specifically the suppression of task-irrelevant information), incidental long-term memory encoding, and interference during the WM task. Thus, while older adults are able to enhance sensory neural activity for relevant information, they are unable to sufficiently suppress neural activity for irrelevant information. The correlation between suppression indices and WM performance in the older adults implies that because of limited WM capacity, older individuals are overwhelmed by interference from failing to ignore distracting information, resulting in memory impairment.

The findings of these studies reveal that an age-related alteration in a basic neural process, such as top-down modulation, can influence multiple cognitive domains. In addition to revealing that an alteration in top-down modulation underlies cognitive aging deficits, our studies also contribute to the interpretation of an existing hypothesis of cognitive aging, the *inhibitory deficit hypothesis of aging*.[6] Behavioral evidence on the interaction between attention and WM processes in aging has suggested that age-related cognitive impairments are associated with increased sensitivity to interference from task-irrelevant information.[50,51] However, the premise that a specific deficit in attentional inhibitory processes negatively impacts WM performance has remained controversial due to the challenges in dissociating cognitive subcomponent processes, such as enhancement and suppression of neural activity, using behavioral measures alone.[52] Recent attempts at using physiological measures to evaluate inhibitory deficits in aging have supported the inhibitory hypothesis, but also failed to resolve the controversy by not establishing the specificity of an attention deficit to inhibition and not directly relating impaired attentional processing to WM deficits, which is necessary if this hypothesis truly reflects a unifying principle crossing cognitive domains.[19,53,54] Our findings serve to resolve controversy surrounding the inhibitory deficit hypothesis of aging by establishing specificity of an attentional deficit to the suppression of task-irrelevant information (i.e., a suppression deficit occurs in the setting of preserved enhancement) and directly relating this suppression deficit to WM impairment.

## ONGOING STUDIES

The older individuals that participated in our aging studies were healthy, well educated, and cognitively intact compared to age-matched controls on extensive neuropsychological testing, allowing us to generalize these findings as a hallmark of normal cognitive aging. Encouragingly, the deficits we reported at the population level do not seem to be a universal characteristic of aging, as a subgroup of the older population with preserved suppression abilities also exhibited intact WM performance, reflecting the variability of the aging process and highlighting the importance of top-down suppression in cognition. This variability of neural and cognitive measures in the older population led us to question what is normal and consider two possible interpretations: (1) The impaired group represents what occurs during the normal aging process independent of neuropathology and the intact individuals (one third of the group) are examples of successful aging or (2) The intact group reflects the normal aging process and the impaired individuals (one-third of the group) are exhibiting the earliest signs of pathological cognitive impairment. Thus, our study raises the important question: Is this suppression deficit a harbinger of impending dementia? We are pursuing an answer to this question by following these older adults longitudinally and planning future studies in which we couple our fMRI functional biomarkers with other markers of Alzheimer's disease: hippocampal volumes, as assessed by structural MRI, *in vivo* amyloid PET imaging, and *ApoE* genotyping. Additionally, we are evaluating if there are within group differences between the older individuals that participated in this study, which might supply a clue to the heterogeneity of the population. For example, leukoariosis—white matter lucencies identified on FLAIR MRI—might be disproportionally present in the impaired subgroup, supporting an age-related relationship between white matter connectivity impairment, alterations in top-down modulation, and cognitive deficits.

Aside from focusing on questions related to the heterogeneity of the older population, our laboratories are also interested in understanding the neural basis of the modulation alterations in older adults that exhibit WM impairment. To assess this, we have initiated studies to explore the neural processes that underlie top-down modulation, so that we may better understand the changes that occur with age. Our studies are guided by the view that complex cognitive processes are not localized to brain regions functioning in isolation, but rather are emergent properties of neural networks interactions.[23,55–57] Top-down modulation is not believed to be an intrinsic property of sensory cortices, but rather mediated by cortical projections from higher-order cortical regions, often thought to be located in multimodal association cortex, such as the PFC and parietal cortex.[30] The extensive reciprocal connections between the PFC and virtually all cortical and subcortical structures situate the PFC in a unique neuroanatomical position to monitor and manipulate diverse cognitive processes.[58,59] These anatomically defined networks establish the structural basis by which the PFC may exert top-down control, but there is also accumulating physiological evidence of PFC networks and their role in control processes. Neuronal recordings and neuroimaging data have revealed that top-down modulation of visual processing involves simultaneous activation of these regions.[37,60–63] In addition, we observe increased BOLD signal in PFC in the memory tasks of our paradigm relative to the passive view task, suggesting a role of these regions as a "top" in goal-directed VAC activity modulation. It is important to note that these studies, including our own data, reveal indirect evidence of functional interaction between these areas.[30,64] There are, however, two invasive studies in monkeys that support the PFC as a direct driving force of activity modulation in the VAC, where the visual information is represented and stored.[27,29] Additionally in humans, combined stroke–ERP studies have provided evidence of frontal cortex dependent top-down modulatory influences on VAC occurring in the first few hundred milliseconds of visual processing.[28]

Traditionally, most functional imaging studies have used univariate analyses, permitting only the independent assessment of activity within each brain region in isolation. However, there has been the steady development of multivariate approaches to analyzing neuroimaging data in a manner more directly in alignment with the network model of the cognition.[65–71] Multivariate analyses generate functional and effective connectivity maps of interacting brain regions, thus emphasizing the role of brain regions within the context of activity in other regions and the cognitive processes being performed. Several groups have begun to establish the presence of functional interactions between the PFC and posterior cortical regions during cognitive control processes, such as attention, WM, and visual imagery.[72–74] We have recently developed a new method to analyze event-related fMRI data sets in a multivariate manner.[67] We then applied this method to characterize the neural networks involved in maintaining a representation of an image in mind over a brief period of time (visual WM)[75] and the networks involved in incidental long-term memory.[76] We are now in the process of performing a functional connectivity analysis on the encoding phase of the selective WM task we have described. Preliminary evidence has revealed regions of robust functional connectivity between the PFC and VAC, further supporting the role of the PFC as a control region. We are also exploring age-related changes in these functional connections in an attempt to understand the basis of an age-related top-down suppression deficit.

The possibility that there is an impairment in PFC function with age and that this might be the underlying source of the top-down modulation deficit we identified in the older subjects is consistent with another well-established hypothesis of cognitive aging, *the frontal hypothesis*. Advocates of this hypothesis propose that early and prominent alterations in frontal lobe integrity underlie the cognitive deficits that occur with normal aging. However, as with the inhibitory deficit hypothesis, controversy surrounds this claim.[2] For example, structural MRI studies have reported atrophy limited to the medial temporal lobes and frontal cortex,[77] generalized atrophy with age,[78] and no atrophic changes.[79] Similarly, functional imaging studies have revealed decreases in PFC activity, while others have revealed increases.[22] It has thus been challenging to use neuroimaging techniques alone to parcel out the significance of structural and functional changes in the aging brain. In an attempt to resolve this controversy, we are now directly exploring the role of the PFC in top-down modulation by employing a unique coupling of fMRI, EEG, and a "reversible lesion" technique offered by repetitive transcranial magnetic stimulation (rTMS).

Although fMRI permits us to identify brain regions of interest, it is inherently limited in that it is a correlational technique and thus unable to assess causality, necessity, and the exact role of a region within a network for a cognitive operation. To accomplish this, we need to manipulate function in a brain region and observe the effects of perturbation on neural activity in distant brain regions, as well as cognitive performance. TMS allows us to do this by applying a focal magnetic pulse to a subject's scalp, resulting in a brief electric current in the underlying cortex and synchronous neural firing.[80] When applied in a repetitive manner at low frequency the stimulation results in a transient disruption of neural activity in a defined region of cortex that lasts for a brief period of time after the TMS is performed.[81–84] The recent development of this technology now enables us to perform "virtual lesion" experiments in a safe manner in human subjects.[85] We recently performed a pilot study using 1Hz rTMS to transiently disrupt PFC regions in young adults that were preidentified with fMRI and assessed the consequences on cognitive performance and top-down modulation in sensory regions using EEG. This experiment used the same selective WM paradigm we used in our recent aging study. Our goals are to determine if by selectively disrupting PFC pathways in young adults, both neural measures of top-down modulation and cognitive performance can be made to mimic the pattern seen in older adults. The pilot study performed on four subjects revealed encouraging preliminary results. Transient disruption of fMRI-identified regions in the middle frontal gyrus resulted in an alteration of distant neural measures of top-down modulation. Specifically, the increase in P300 amplitude that occurs in the remember condition versus the ignore condition was diminished, and additionally, there was a significant slowing of the response time on the WM memory task.[86] This pattern of a decrease in P300 for the relevant information and slower response time is identical to a finding that we observe in the older subjects performing this task without rTMS.[87] A full-scale study is now under way to directly evaluate the causal role of the PFC in goal-directed modulation of visual cortex activity.

In addition to our efforts at manipulating PFC function directly with rTMS, we are also modifying the task demands in young adults performing the selective WM task in a manner that taxes PFC function. There is an extensive literature on the role of the PFC in WM,[88] and so in an ongoing experiment we are assessing if having young subjects perform a nonverbal WM task concurrently with our visual WM task influences top-down modulation measures and differentially affects enhancement and suppression. To accomplish this, at the beginning of each trial, subjects are presented auditorily with six digits to memorize. On half of the trials the digit sequence was random (*high load*); on the other half the digit sequence was "1,2,3,4,5,6" (*low load*). After hearing the digits, the participants then performed the face/scene WM paradigm as previously described. Preliminary results revealed that the high digit load did not alter the participants' ability to enhance activity levels in the scene-selective region during the Remember Scenes task, but did result in increased BOLD signal associated with the irrelevant scenes in the Ignore Scenes task.[89] Thus, increasing the WM load in younger adults produced a selective suppression deficit identical to that seen in older adults performing the task without the increased load. This suggests that the age-related alteration in top-down modulation we recently documented may result from PFC changes in aging expressed as decreased WM resources with age. If further studies support that PFC alterations with aging underlie the top-down suppression deficit, this will serve to reconcile the *frontal* and *inhibitory deficit* hypotheses of aging.


## CONCLUSIONS

Coupling the many tools of human neuroimaging technology with our recently developed cognitive paradigm has allowed us to reveal an age-related alteration in top-down modulation, a neural mechanism that underlies the diverse cognitive processes affected by aging. Our recent studies exploring alterations in neural networks that underlie these modulation alterations point to changes in PFC as a potential etiology. This is suggested by preliminary studies that have replicated aging top-down modulation changes in healthy young adults by increasing WM load, presumably taxing PFC function, and by transiently disrupting activity in the PFC regions with rTMS. This association between a suppression deficit and alterations in PFC control in aging may serve to reconcile the *inhibitory* and *frontal* hypothesis of cognitive aging and propels us along on our ultimate goal of defining underlying principles of cognitive aging. More research is needed that integrates the various technologies of human neurophysiology to capitalize on their unique strengths. Future studies are now planned to use neural measures as functional biomarkers to explore the therapeutic role of cognitive training and pharmacological treatment in improving cognitive abilities in older adults.

# REFERENCES

1. BAYLES, K.A. & A.W. KASNIAK. 1987. Communication and Cognition in Normal Aging and Dementia. Little, Brown. Boston, MA.
2. GREENWOOD, P.M. 2000. The frontal aging hypothesis evaluated. J. Int. Neuropsychol. Soc. **6:** 705–726.
3. CRAIK, F.I. & T.A. SALTHOUSE. 2000. Handbook of Aging and Cognition II. Erlbaum. Mahwah, NJ.
4. SALTHOUSE, T.A. 1996. The processing-speed theory of adult age differences in cognition. Psychol. Rev. **103:** 403–428.
5. WEST, R.L. 1996. An application of prefrontal cortex function theory to cognitive aging. Psychol. Bull. **120:** 272–292.
6. HASHER, L. & R.T. ZACKS. 1988. Working memory, comprehension and aging: a review and a new view. In The Psychology of Learning and Motivation. G.H. Bower, Ed.: 193–225. Academic Press. New York.
7. ANDERSON, B. & V. RUTLEDGE. 1996. Age and hemisphere effects on dendritic structure. Brain **119**(Pt 6): 1983–1990.
8. DE BRABANDER, J.M., R.J. KRAMERS & H.B. UYLINGS. 1998. Layer-specific dendritic regression of pyramidal cells with ageing in the human prefrontal cortex. Eur. J. Neurosci. **10:** 1261–1269.
9. BENNETT, P.J. et al. 2001. The effects of aging on visual memory: evidence for functional reorganization of cortical networks. Acta Psychol. (Amst) **107:** 249–273.
10. GOMEZ-ISLA, T. et al. 1996. Profound loss of layer II entorhinal cortex neurons occurs in very mild Alzheimer's disease. J. Neurosci. **16:** 4491–4500.
11. GAZZALEY, A.H. et al. 1997. Preserved number of entorhinal cortex layer II neurons in aged macaque monkeys. Neurobiol. Aging **18:** 549–553.
12. WEST, M.J. et al. 1994. Differences in the pattern of hippocampal neuronal loss in normal ageing and Alzheimer's disease. Lancet **344:** 769–772.
13. MORRISON, J.H. & P.R. HOF. 1997. Life and death of neurons in the aging brain. Science **278:** 412–419.
14. PETERS, A. 2002. Structural changes in the normally aging cerebral cortex of primates. Prog. Brain Res. **136:** 455–465.
15. EBERLING, J.L. et al. 1997. Cerebral glucose metabolism and memory in aged rhesus macaques. Neurobiol. Aging **18:** 437–443.
16. ALMAGUER, W. et al. 2002. Aging impairs amygdala-hippocampus interactions involved in hippocampal LTP. Neurobiol. Aging **23:** 319–324.
17. SHANKAR, S., T.J. TEYLER & N. ROBBINS. 1998. Aging differentially alters forms of long-term potentiation in rat hippocampal area CA1. J. Neurophysiol. **79:** 334–341.
18. PELOSI, L. & L.D. BLUMHARDT. 1999. Effects of age on working memory: an event-related potential study. Brain Res. Cogn. Brain Res. **7:** 321–334.
19. CHAO, L.L. & R.T. KNIGHT. 1997. Prefrontal deficits in attention and inhibitory control with aging. Cereb. Cortex **7:** 63–69.
20. PEDIGO, N.W. JR. 1994. Neurotransmitter receptor plasticity in aging. Life Sci. **55:** 1985–1991.
21. GAZZALEY, A.H. et al. 1996. Circuit-specific alterations of N-methyl-D-aspartate receptor subunit 1 in the dentate gyrus of aged monkeys. Proc. Natl. Acad. Sci. USA **93:** 3121–3125.

22. GAZZALEY, A. & M. D'ESPOSITO. 2003. The contribution of functional brain imaging to our understanding of cognitive aging. Sci. Aging Knowledge Environ. **2003(4):** PE2.

23. GAZZALEY, A. & M. D'ESPOSITO. Neural networks: an empirical neuroscience approach toward understanding cognition. Cortex **42:** 1037–1040.

24. FRITH, C. 2001. A framework for studying the neural basis of attention. Neuropsychologia **39:** 1367–1371.

25. BAR, M. 2003. A cortical mechanism for triggering top-down facilitation in visual object recognition. J. Cogn. Neurosci. **15:** 600–609.

26. CORBETTA, M. & G.L. SHULMAN. 2002. Control of goal-directed and stimulus-driven attention in the brain. Nat. Rev. Neurosci. **3:** 201–215.

27. FUSTER, J.M., R.H. BAUER & J.P. JERVEY. 1985. Functional interactions between inferotemporal and prefrontal cortex in a cognitive task. Brain Res. **330:** 299–307.

28. BARCELO, F., S. SUWAZONO & R.T. KNIGHT. 2000. Prefrontal modulation of visual processing in humans. Nat. Neurosci. **3:** 399–403.

29. TOMITA, H. *et al.* 1999. Top-down signal from prefrontal cortex in executive control of memory retrieval. Nature **401:** 699–703.

30. GAZZALEY, A. & M. D'ESPOSITO. 2007. Unifying prefrontal cortex function: executive control, neural networks and top-down modulation. *In* The Human Frontal Lobes. J. Cummings & B. Miller, Eds. Psychology Press. New York.

31. TREUE, S. & J.C. MARTINEZ TRUJILLO. 1999. Feature-based attention influences motion processing gain in macaque visual cortex. Nature **399:** 575–579.

32. WOJCIULIK, E., N. KANWISHER & J. DRIVER. 1998. Covert visual attention modulates face-specific activity in the human fusiform gyrus: fMRI study. J. Neurophysiol. **79:** 1574–1578.

33. PESSOA, L., S. KASTNER & L.G. UNGERLEIDER. 2003. Neuroimaging studies of attention: from modulation of sensory processing to top-down control. J. Neurosci. **23:** 3990–3998.

34. ISHAI, A., J.V. HAXBY & L.G. UNGERLEIDER. 2002. Visual imagery of famous faces: effects of memory and attention revealed by fMRI. Neuroimage **17:** 1729–1741.

35. KASTNER, S. *et al.* 1999. Increased activity in human visual cortex during directed attention in the absence of visual stimulation. Neuron **22:** 751–761.

36. FUSTER, J.M. 1990. Inferotemporal units in selective visual attention and short-term memory. J. Neurophysiol. **64:** 681–697.

37. MILLER, E.K., L. LI & R. DESIMONE. 1993. Activity of neurons in anterior inferior temporal cortex during a short-term memory task. J. Neurosci. **13:** 1460–1478.

38. GRADY, C.L. 2000. Functional brain imaging and age-related changes in cognition. Biol. Psychol. **54:** 259–281.

39. GAZZALEY, A. *et al.* 2005. Top-down enhancement and suppression of the magnitude and speed of neural activity. J. Cogn. Neurosci. **17:** 507–517.

40. LOGOTHETIS, N.K. *et al.* 2001. Neurophysiological investigation of the basis of the fMRI signal. Nature **412:** 150–157.

41. SILVA, L.D. 1991. Neural mechanisms underlying brain waves: from neural membranes to networks. EEG Clin. Neurophysiol. **79:** 81–93.

42. CHAWLA, D., E.D. LUMER & K.J. FRISTON. 1999. The relationship between synchronization among neuronal populations and their mean activity levels. Neural Comput. **11:** 1389–1411.

43. PUCE, A. *et al.* 1995. Face-sensitive regions in human extrastriate cortex studied by functional MRI. J. Neurophysiol. **74:** 1192–1199.

44. KANWISHER, N., J. MCDERMOTT & M.M. CHUN. 1997. The fusiform face area: a module in human extrastriate cortex specialized for face perception. J. Neurosci. **17:** 4302–4311.
45. EPSTEIN, R. & N. KANWISHER. 1998. A cortical representation of the local visual environment. Nature **392:** 598–601.
46. BENTIN, S. *et al.* 1996. Electrophysiological studies of face perception in humans. J. Cogn. Neurosci. **8:** 551–565.
47. GAZZALEY, A. *et al.* 2005. Top-down suppression deficit underlies working memory impairment in normal aging. Nat. Neurosci. **8:** 1298–1300.
48. D'ESPOSITO, M., L.Y. DEOUELL & A. GAZZALEY. 2003. Alterations in the BOLD fMRI signal with ageing and disease: a challenge for neuroimaging. Nat. Rev. Neurosci. **4:** 863–872.
49. MCEVOY, L.K. *et al.* 2004. Age-related impairment in top-down modulation of visual processing: ERP evidence. Soc. Neurosci. Abstracts.
50. WEST, R. 1999. Visual distraction, working memory, and aging. Mem. Cognit. **27:** 1064–1072.
51. MAY, C.P., L. HASHER & M.J. KANE. 1999. The role of interference in memory span. Mem. Cognit. **27:** 759–767.
52. MCDOWD, J.M. 1997. Inhibition in attention and aging. J. Gerontol. B. Psychol. Sci. Soc. Sci. **52:** P265–P273.
53. ALAIN, C. & D.L. WOODS. 1999. Age-related changes in processing auditory stimuli during visual attention: evidence for deficits in inhibitory control and sensory memory. Psychol. Aging **14:** 507–519.
54. MILHAM, M.P. *et al.* 2002. Attentional control in the aging brain: insights from an fMRI study of the stroop task. Brain Cogn. **49:** 277–296.
55. MESULAM, M. 1981. A cortical network for directed attention and unilateral neglect. Ann. Neurol. **10:** 309–325.
56. FUSTER, J.M. Cortex and Mind: Unifying Cognition. 2003. Oxford University Press. New York.
57. MESULAM, M.M. 1990. Large-scale neurocognitive networks and distributed processing for attention, language, and memory. Ann. Neurol. **28:** 597–613.
58. BARBAS, H. 2000. Connections underlying the synthesis of cognition, memory, and emotion in primate prefrontal cortices. Brain Res. Bull. **52:** 319–330.
59. GOLDMAN-RAKIC, P.S. & H.R. FRIEDMAN. 1991. The circuitry of working memory revealed by anatomy and metabolic imaging. *In* Frontal Lobe Function and Dysfunction. H. Levin, H. Eisenberg & A. Benton, Eds.: 72–91. Oxford University Press. New York.
60. MORAN, J. & R. DESIMONE. 1985. Selective attention gates visual processing in the extrastriate cortex. Science **229:** 782–784.
61. UNGERLEIDER, L.G., S.M. COURTNEY & J.V. HAXBY. 1998. A neural system for human visual working memory. Proc. Natl. Acad. Sci. USA **95:** 883–890.
62. CORBETTA, M.. 1998. Frontoparietal cortical networks for directing attention and the eye to visual locations: identical, independent, or overlapping neural systems? Proc. Natl. Acad. Sci. USA **95:** 831–838.
63. D'ESPOSITO, M. *et al.* 1998. Functional MRI studies of spatial and nonspatial working memory. Brain Res. Cogn. Brain Res. **7:** 1–13.
64. MILLER, B.T. & M. D'ESPOSITO. 2005. Searching for "the top" in top-down control. Neuron **48:** 535–538.
65. MCINTOSH, A.R. 1998. Understanding neural interactions in learning and memory using functional neuroimaging. Ann. N. Y. Acad. Sci. **855:** 556–571.

66. FRISTON, K.J. *et al*. 1993. Functional connectivity: the principal-component analysis of large (PET) data sets. J. Cereb. Blood Flow Metab. **13:** 5–14.
67. RISSMAN, J., A. GAZZALEY & M. D'ESPOSITO. 2004. Measuring functional connectivity during distinct stages of a cognitive task. Neuroimage **23:** 752–763.
68. SUN, F.T., L.M. MILLER & M. D'ESPOSITO. 2004. Measuring interregional functional connectivity using coherence and partial coherence analyses of fMRI data. Neuroimage **21:** 647–658.
69. PENNY, W.D. *et al*. 2004. Comparing dynamic causal models. Neuroimage **22:** 1157–1172.
70. LIN, F.H. *et al*. 2003. Multivariate analysis of neuronal interactions in the generalized partial least squares framework: simulations and empirical studies. Neuroimage **20:** 625–642.
71. FRISTON, K. *et al*. 2000. Nonlinear PCA: characterizing interactions between modes of brain activity. Philos. Trans. R. Soc. Lond. B. Biol. Sci. **355:** 135–146.
72. ROWE, J. *et al*. 2002. Attention to action: specific modulation of corticocortical interactions in humans. Neuroimage **17:** 988.
73. MECHELLI, A. *et al*. 2004. Where bottom-up meets top-down: neuronal interactions during perception and imagery. Cereb. Cortex **14:** 1256–1265.
74. MCINTOSH, A.R. *et al*. 1996. Changes in limbic and prefrontal functional interactions in a working memory task for faces. Cereb. Cortex **6:** 571–584.
75. GAZZALEY, A., J. RISSMAN & M. DESPOSITO. 2004. Functional connectivity during working memory maintenance. Cogn. Affect. Behav. Neurosci. **4:** 580–599.
76. SEIBERT, T.M. *et al*. 2005. Top-down enhancement of hippocampal-visual association cortex interactions underlies incidental long-term memory. Soc. for Neurosci. Meet. Abstract.
77. RAZ, N. *et al*. 1997. Selective aging of the human cerebral cortex observed *in vivo*: differential vulnerability of the prefrontal gray matter. Cereb Cortex **7:** 268–282.
78. DECARLI, C. *et al*. 1995. The effect of white matter hyperintensity volume on brain structure, cognitive performance, and cerebral metabolism of glucose in 51 healthy adults. Neurology **45:** 2077–2084.
79. MUELLER, E.A. *et al*. 1998. Brain volume preserved in healthy elderly through the eleventh decade. Neurology **51:** 1555–1562.
80. HALLETT, M. 2000. Transcranial magnetic stimulation and the human brain. Nature **406:** 147–150.
81. PASCUAL-LEONE, A. *et al*. 1998. Study and modulation of human cortical excitability with transcranial magnetic stimulation. J. Clin. Neurophysiol. **15:** 333–343.
82. KOSSLYN, S.M. *et al*. 1999. The role of area 17 in visual imagery: convergent evidence from PET and rTMS. Science **284:** 167–170.
83. CHEN, R. *et al*. 1997. Depression of motor cortex excitability by low-frequency transcranial magnetic stimulation. Neurology **48:** 1398–1403.
84. BOROOJERDI, B. *et al*. 2000. Reduction of human visual cortex excitability using 1-Hz transcranial magnetic stimulation. Neurology **54:** 1529–1531.
85. WASSERMANN, E. 1998. Risk and safety of repetitive transcranial magnetic stimulation: report and suggested guidelines from the International Workshop on the Safety of Repetitive Transcranial Magnetic Stimulation. EEG Clin. Neurophysiol. **108:** 1–16.
86. MILLER, B.T. *et al*. 2005. Functional deactivation of the prefrontal cortex disrupts posterior physiological signals: joint TMS/EEG evidence for PFC-mediated top-down modulation. Soc. Neurosci. Abstracts.

87. KELLEY, J. *et al.* 2005. Top-down modulation deficit of the P300 in normal aging. Soc Neurosci. Abstracts.
88. COURTNEY, S.M. *et al.* 1998. The role of prefrontal cortex in working memory: examining the contents of consciousness. Philos. Trans. R. Soc. Lond. B. Biol. Sci. **353:** 1819–1828.
89. RISSMAN, J., A. GAZZALEY & M. D'ESPOSITO. 2005. The effect of phonological working memory load on top-down enhancement and suppression of visual processing. Soc. Neurosci. Abstracts.

# Brain Aging and Its Modifiers

## Insights from *in Vivo* Neuromorphometry and Susceptibility Weighted Imaging

NAFTALI RAZ,[a] KAREN M. RODRIGUE,[a] AND E. MARK HAACKE[b]

[a]*Institute of Gerontology and Department of Psychology, Wayne State University, Detroit, Michigan, USA*

[b]*Department of Radiology, Wayne State University School of Medicine, Detroit, Michigan, USA*

ABSTRACT: Aging is marked by individual differences and differential vulnerability of cognitive operations and their neural substrates. Cross-sectional studies of brain volume reveal greater age-related shrinkage of the prefrontal cortex (PFC) and the hippocampus than in the entorhinal and primary visual cortex. Longitudinal studies of regional brain shrinkage indicate that when individual differences are controlled, larger and broader shrinkage estimates are evident, with most polymodal cortices affected to the same extent. The mechanisms of age-related shrinkage are unclear. Vascular risk factors may exacerbate brain aging and account for some of the observed declines as both the PFC and the hippocampus show elevated vulnerability to hypertension. MRI techniques that are sensitive to small vessels function, tissue oxygenation, and perfusion may be especially well suited to study brain aging and its vascular modifiers. We present an example of one such technique, susceptibility weighted imaging (SWI), that allows direct measurement of $T2^*$ values that reflect deoxy- to oxyhemoglobin fraction in blood vessels and iron deposits in cerebral tissue. The $T2^*$ shortening is associated with advanced age, but the effect is significantly stronger in the PFC and the hippocampus than the entorhinal and visual cortices. Moreover, $T2^*$ is shorter in hypertensive participants than in their matched normotensive counterparts, and the difference is especially prominent in the hippocampus, thus mirroring the findings of the neuromorphometric studies. Future research on brain aging would benefit from combining structural and metabolic techniques in a longitudinal design, as such studies will allow examination of leading–trailing effects of those factors.

KEYWORDS: aging; MRI; brain; longitudinal; vascular risk; susceptibility weighted imaging; deoxyhemoglobin; iron

Address for correspondence: Naftali Raz, Ph. D., Institute of Gerontology, Wayne State University, 87 E Ferry St., 226 Knapp Bldg., Detroit, MI 48202. Voice: 313-577-2297; fax: 508-256-5689.
nraz@wayne.edu

Ann. N.Y. Acad. Sci. 1097: 84–93 (2007). © 2007 New York Academy of Sciences.
doi: 10.1196/annals.1379.018

# INTRODUCTION

Aging is marked by substantial variability across individual organisms, among organs and systems, and within organs' cellular elements. Postmortem (PM) studies reveal a plethora of age-related differences in human brain specimens: reduced brain size, expansion of cerebral ventricles and sulci, loss of myelin, region-specific loss of neuronal bodies, rarefication of cerebral vasculature, and reduced synaptic density.[1-3] However, PM methods preclude examination of longitudinal trajectories of aging and make study of cognitive correlates of brain differences rather difficult.

The advent of magnetic resonance imaging (MRI) created conditions for *in vivo* examination of brain structure and function in healthy behaving humans. Moreover, MRI methods enable longitudinal follow-up and afford an opportunity to gauge true trajectories of change in brain structure and function. Multiple questions of normal and pathological development in late adulthood can be addressed with the help of MRI, among them determining of brain changes in normal and successful aging, transition from normal aging to its pathological expressions, as well as studying the processes that modify the normal trajectory of aging and affect its cognitive expressions. Most current MRI methods still derive their indices from assessing states and vicissitudes of only one element, brain hydrogen. Nonetheless, they allow interrogation of a wide variety of brain structural and functional properties, including changes in volume, microstructure, hemodynamics, and metabolism. In this brief survey, we focus on two types of MRI-based assessment of the brain: regional volumetry (neuromorphometry) and evaluation of regional differences in resting state magnetic susceptibility.

In MRI-based neuromorphometry, there are multiple ways of measuring regional brain volumes. Significant effort and ingenuity are being devoted to the development of computerized and largely automated methods of image analysis that allow relatively fast processing of vast amounts of MRI data.[4-7] However, the neuroanatomic validity of those approaches has not been clearly established, especially when measures are conducted on less than ideal MRI scans from samples with a great range of individual differences. Thus, for the time being, algorithmic methods of neuromorphometry occupy a position of an initial search tool that generates a list of candidate regions, in a way similar to microarray technology in genomics that allows narrowing the list to candidate genes with expectation of a more customized and specific follow-up investigation.

Manual methods, the gold standard of neuromorphometry, have face validity and have a close conceptual link to classic methods of neuroanatomy, in which a visualized cerebral region demarcated by clearly defined landmarks is measured. With the right amount of training and knowledge of neuroanatomy, operators using those methods can attain high a degree of inter-rater reliability.[8] The hyperintense spots observed in the white matter on T2-weighted MRI scans appear in asymptomatic older adults at the fifth decade of life and reflect multiple neuropathological and benign causes, including altered myelin production cycle, expansion of perivascular spaces, and microinfarcts.[9] Besides calendar age, WMH is predicted by an assortment of vascular disease factors.[10] The volume of WMH can also be measured manually, separated by lobes and types of WMH.[22]

Neuromorphometric studies vary in methods of measurement, rules of region demarcation, and criteria for sample selection. However, general trends in findings across the extant literature are discernable, especially when quantitative information from multiple studies is pooled together. Such a general trend in cross-sectional studies of regional brain volumes vis-à-vis age suggests that although calendar age is associated with generalized reduction of brain volume, the polymodal (especially prefrontal) cortical regions are more significantly affected than the rest of the neocortex, with primary (but not secondary) visual cortices maintaining their integrity.[11] The hippocampus evidences a remarkably wide range of estimated age-related differences, from zero to large effects, with some studies showing nonlinear age-accelerated trends.[8,12,13] Although reasons for such inconsistency are unknown, it is plausible that they reflect the variability in sample admixture of preclinical pathology, vascular and Alzheimer's type.

Cross-sectional design has many advantages but its main weakness is inability to measure true change. Longitudinal studies that would allow measurement of true change and evaluation of individual variability of brain-aging trajectories are still rare. To date, most of the longitudinal investigations with a few notable exceptions[14-16] (see Ref. 11 for a review) evaluated global brain parameters, such as ventricular volume (relatively large, age accelerated expansion noted) and total brain volume (very modest decline observed), as well as change in WMH burden (modest expansion). As far as regional volumes are concerned, longitudinal follow-ups were by and large limited to the medial temporal structures and to the samples restricted to older adults. Such studies have typically reported hippocampal and sometimes, entorhinal shrinkage at a rate of 1–2% per annum (e.g., Ref. 17). Although longitudinal investigations confirmed many of the estimates based on cross-sectional studies, some notable discrepancies were found.

The advantages of the longitudinal approach can be illustrated by a recent study of 72 generally healthy adults (with exception of several individuals with controlled hypertension), who were assessed twice within a 5-year interval.[15] In that study, we found longitudinal change in the prefrontal cortex (PFC) and the hippocampus commensurate with the cross-sectional estimates. In contrast, inferior parietal lobule volumes that consistently appeared age-insensitive on cross-sectional measures[8,18] and revealed no age-related differences at baseline and follow-up alike, evidenced the same rate of longitudinal shrinkage as did the PFC.[15] The findings in that study are summarized in FIGURE 1. The observed discrepancy reinforces the need for longitudinal

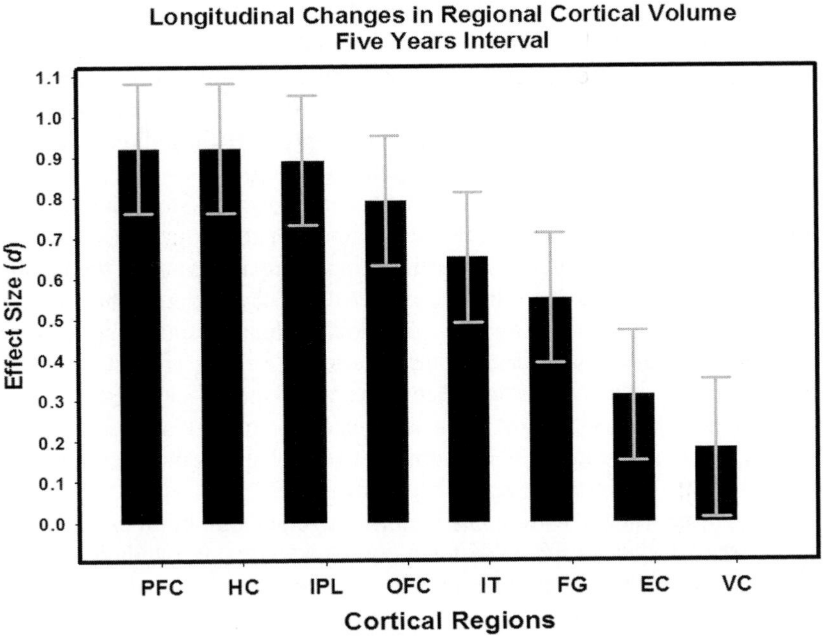

## Longitudinal Changes in Regional Cortical Volume
### Five Years Interval

**FIGURE 1.** Summary of 5-year changes in cortical regions (based on Raz *et al.*, 2005).[15] The effects size (Cohen's *d*) is the difference between the baseline and 5-year follow-up measures in standard deviation units. PFC = lateral prefrontal cortex; HC = hippocampus; IPL = inferior parietal lobule; OFC = orbitofrontal cortex; IT = inferior temporal cortex; FG = fusiform gyrus; EC = entorhinal cortex; VC = primary visual cortex. The *bars* indicate 95% confidence limits of *d*. Lack of overlap between the confidence limits indicated by the bars is tantamount to statistically significant difference at $P < 0.05$, two-tailed.

assessment and verification of age-related change estimates based on cross-sectional studies.

Despite inter-study discrepancies with respect to the estimated shrink-age rates, it is clear that even in healthy adults, the brain loses volume. Nonetheless, the biological meaning of such loss observed on MRI is unclear as are the mechanisms underlying the phenomenon. In all likelihood, multiple factors play significant and complementary roles in creating a pattern of preservation and decline of the aging brain. An important group of factors that probably shape and modify the trajectories of normal aging consists of various correlates of vascular disease and vascular risk. The brain's dependence on steady delivery of blood-born nutrients and neuroactive substances makes it exceptionally vulnerable to age-related declines in vascular functions and to alterations of its own vascular properties. As blood-born oxygen is critically important for brain work, measures of tissue oxygenation may hold promise as predictors of brain atrophy. Transition of blood from an unstable oxygenated to a default deoxygenated state (i.e., from relatively high concentration of unstable oxyhemoglobin to increased concentration of deoxyhemoglobin) can be monitored with *in vivo* MRI by measuring T2* relaxation times.[19,20] Although T2* is sensitive to many factors that introduce local inhomogenenity of the magnetic field, in the cerebral cortex it provides an indirect index of metabolism via rate of clearance of oxygenated blood.

Recent findings in older humans and a rodent model by Small and his colleagues suggest that basal rate of tissue oxygenation at rest may be associated with regional deterioration of the specific hippocampal regions of the medial temporal system of older adults and related to declarative memory performance.[20,21] However, Small and his colleagues examined only hippocampal and entorhinal regions and did not compute true T2* values. Thus, it is unclear whether the observed effects are unique to the hippocampal–entorhinal system and whether they reflect true differences in relaxation rates. If such differences are observed in other regions, it is important to establish whether their regional pattern mirrors the pattern of age-related shrinkage.

To determine whether differential effects of age on basal brain oxygenation indices are restricted to the medial–temporal structures, we studied age differences in neocortical (superior frontal gyrus and primary visual cortex) and medial–temporal (hippocampus and entorhinal cortex) T2* values. The latter were computed from a multi-echo susceptibility weighted imaging sequence (SWI; axial plane, eight echoes, TE = 10 – 80 ms, voxel = $1 \times 1 \times 2$ mm$^3$, slice thickness = 2 mm) for each voxel. Regions of interest were identified on the true T1-weighted image (first echo, TE = 10 ms) and marked with a standard-size probe. The mean T2* within the probe was measured with test–retest reliability of regional measures for one (fixed) rater was ICC(3) $\geq$ 0.90 across the ROIs.

Inasmuch as shorter T2* reflects higher deoxyhemoglobin to oxyhemoglobin ratio, advanced age was associated with higher basal deoxyhemoglobin concentration (main effect of age: $F(1, 68) = 46.23$, $P < 0.001$). Some regions evidenced greater T2* values than others (main effect of ROI: $F(3, 204) = 11.39$, $P < 0.001$). Most notably, age-related differences in basal oxygenation rate varied across the examined ROIs: Age $\times$ ROI: $F(3, 204) = 10.22$, $P < 0.001$. Specifically, significantly lower T2* was observed in PFC and hippocampus of the older adults, whereas little or no age differences were evident in the entorhinal and primary visual cortices (see Fig. 2). Comparison of correlations with Steiger's Z*, which takes into account dependence between the correlated variables, revealed that HC and SFG correlations with age were significantly larger than EC–age correlation: $Z^* = 2.37$ and 1.88, $P < 0.01$ and $P < 0.05$ one-tailed, respectively. They were also significantly larger than the correlation between age and VC T2*: $Z^* = 3.51$ and 3.04, both $P < 0.001$, one-tailed. There were no differences in strength of association with age for SFG versus HC and EC versus VC. Thus, the pattern of age-related difference in resting T2* values seems to mirror the pattern of age-related shrinkage.

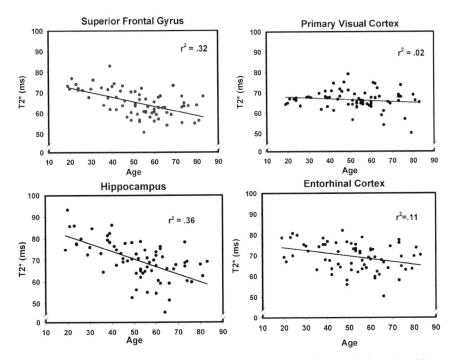

**FIGURE 2.** Regional T2* values as a function of age in four cortical regions. Note significant age-dependent shortening of T2* (corresponding to prolongation of relaxation rate) in prefrontal cortex (SFG) and hippocampus (HC). In contrast, susceptibility dependent relaxation rate in the primary visual cortex is unrelated to age. Correlations with age were significantly stronger for HC and SFG than for EC and VC.

In a longitudinal study currently under way in our laboratory, we will assess the possibility that local changes in tissue oxygenation may precede structural decline in the selected brain locales.

Multiple factors affect brain aging and among the most important are those that alter its vascular function.[9,22] Arterial hypertension accelerates age-related shrinkage of the PFC and the hippocampus and modifies the nonlinear trajectory of hippocampal aging.[15,17] Hypertension-related HC shrinkage is exacerbated by presence of lacunar infarcts, whereas no such influence on EC atrophy rates was found.[17] Persons with hypertension and other vascular disease factors show longitudinal declines in the regions that are usually stable in normal aging, such as the primary visual cortex.[23] In the resting T2* study (Fig. 3), we found reduced T2* values in 13 hypertensive participants compared to 13 normotensive controls matched on age, sex, and education. The difference, presumably reflecting reduced oxygenation, was observed across all examined ROIs: main effect of HBP: $F(1, 24) = 8.36$, $P < 0.008$; no HBP $\times$ ROI interaction ($F[3, 72] < 1$, ns).

## Regional T2* and Treated Hypertension

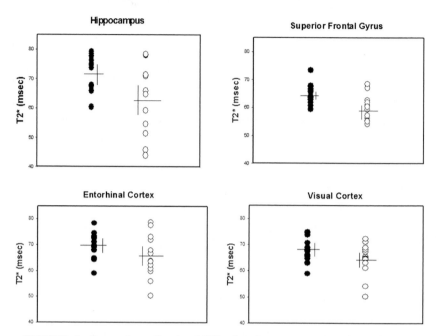

**FIGURE 3.** Comparison of regional T2* values between normotensive and hypertensive demographically adults. Vertical *bars* correspond to standard errors of the mean. Solid *circles* are normotensive and empty circles are hypertensive participants.

At this stage the interpretation of T2* findings is unclear. The major determinant of T2* signal in the brain tissue is local deposition of various iron-related compounds, that is, heme and nonheme iron.[24] As heme iron is blood born, its abundance is related to perfusion of the cortical tissue, mainly through a dense network of small vessels. On the other hand, the presence of nonheme iron in the brain is unrelated to blood flow, blood volume, or oxygen metabolism. In the absence of direct measures of brain oxygen metabolism, we can offer only circumstantial evidence in favor of the oxygenation interpretation of our T2* finding. Nonheme iron is especially plentiful in the basal ganglia and myelinated axons, not in the neocortical regions examined here, although, in degenerative disease, the hippocampus may also be prone to iron accumulation.[25,26] Nonheme iron may also accumulate in some (though not all) amyloid plaques and contribute to a reduction of T2* signal.[27] In the cerebral cortex, however, with notable exception of the primary motor regions, nonheme iron content is relatively low and relaxation rates do not show high correlation with iron concentrations assessed from postmortem studies.[28,29] Thus, it is likely that the observed T2* variations in the cortical regions reflect concentration of deoxyhemoglobin in the local vasculature more than that of nonheme iron. Disentangling those sources of age-related T2* shortening is a challenge we are currently addressing in a longitudinal study of healthy aging and its modifiers.

## CONCLUSIONS

The extant literature provides clear evidence that even "normal" ("successful") aging is associated with significant brain shrinkage. Such shrinkage is differential and affects polymodal association cortices, striatum, and cerebellum more than primary sensory cortices. Hippocampus and the white matter evidence nonlinear shrinkage that accelerates with age. The mechanisms of differential brain shrinkage are unclear, but vascular risk factors, even at moderate levels, may significantly accelerate its pace. Imaging modalities that interrogate local inhomogeneities of the magnetic field created by vascular phenomena, such as susceptibility weighted imaging,[24] are sensitive to metabolic and microvascular properties of brain tissue and may be well suited for evaluation of the effects of aging on the brain.

### ACKNOWLEDGMENT

This work was supported in part by a grant R37-AG-11230 from the National Institute on Aging. We thank Y-C.N. Chang for stimulating discussion of the topics covered in this article.

## REFERENCES

1. KEMPER, T. 1994. Neuroanatomical and neuropathological changes during aging and dementia. *In* Clinical Neurology of Aging. M.L. Albert & J. Knoefel, Eds.: 3–67. Oxford University Press. New York.
2. MORRISON, J.H. & P.R. HOF. 1997. Life and death of neurons in the aging brain. Science **278:** 412–419.
3. RIDDLE, D.R., W.E. SONNTAG & R.J. LICHTENWALNER. 2003. Microvascular plasticity in aging. Age. Res. Rev. **2:** 149–168.
4. ASHBURNER, J. & K.J. FRISTON. 2000. Voxel-based morphometry—The methods Neuroimage. **11:** 805–821.
5. DAVITZIKOS, C. 2004. Why voxel-based morphometric analysis should be used with great caution when characterizing group differences. Neuroimage. **23:** 17–20.
6. FISCHL, B., D.H. SALAT, E. BUSA, *et al.* 2002. Whole brain segmentation: automated labeling of neuroanatomical structures in the human brain. Neuron. **33:** 341–355.
7. THOMPSON, P.M., J.N. GIEDD, R.P. WOODS, *et al.* 2000. Growth patterns in the developing brain detected by using continuum mechanical tensor maps. Nature **404:** 190–193.

8. RAZ, N., F. GUNNING-DIXON, D. HEAD, *et al.* 2004. Aging, sexual dimorphism, and hemispheric asymmetry of the cerebral cortex: replicability of regional differences in volume. Neurobiol. Aging **25:** 377–396.
9. DE LEEUW, F.E., J.C. DE GROOT & M.M.B. BRETELER. 2001. White matter changes: frequency and risk factors. *In* The Matter of White Matter: Clinical and Pathophysiological Aspects of White Matter Disease Related to Cognitive Decline and Vascular Dementia. L.D. Pantoni & A. Inzitari Wallin, Eds.: 19–33. Academic Pharmaceutical Productions. Utrecht, the Netherlands.
10. PANTONI, L., J.H. GARCIA & J.A. GUTIERREZ. 1996. Cerebral white matter is highly vulnerable to ischemia. Stroke **27:** 1641–1646.
11. RAZ, N. 2004. The aging brain observed *in vivo*: Differential changes and their modifiers. *In* Cognitive Neuroscience of Aging: Linking Cognitive and Cerebral Aging. R. Cabeza, L. Nyberg & D.C. Park, Eds.: 17–55. Oxford University Press. New York.
12. JERNIGAN, T.L., S.L. ARCHIBALD, C. FENEMA-NOTESTINE, *et al.* 2001. Effects of age on tissues and regions of the cerebrum and cerebellum. Neurobiol. Aging **22:** 581–594.
13. FJELL, A.M., K.B. WALHOVD, I. REINVANG, *et al.* 2005. Age does not increase rate of forgetting over weeks—neuroanatomical volumes and visual memory across the adult life-span. J. Int. Neuropsychol. Soc. **11:** 2–15.
14. PFEFFERBAUM, A., E.V. SULLIVAN, M.J. ROSENBLOOM, *et al.* 1998. A controlled study of cortical gray matter and ventricular changes in alcoholic men over a 5-year interval. Arch. Gen. Psychiatry. **55:** 905–912.
15. RAZ, N., U. LINDENBERGER, K.M. RODRIGUE, *et al.* 2005. Regional brain changes in aging healthy adults: general trends, individual differences, and modifiers. Cereb. Cortex. **15:** 1676–1689.
16. RESNICK, S.M., D.L. PHAM, M.A. KRAUT, *et al.* 2003. Longitudinal magnetic resonance imaging studies of older adults: a shrinking brain. J. Neurosci. **23:** 3295–3301.
17. DU, A.T., N. SCHUFF, L.L. CHAO, *et al.* 2006. Age effects on atrophy rates of entorhinal cortex and hippocampus. Neurobiol. Aging **27:** 733–740.
18. RAZ, N., F.M. GUNNING, D. HEAD, *et al.* 1997. Selective aging of the human cerebral cortex observed *in vivo*: differential vulnerability of the prefrontal gray matter. Cereb. Cortex. **7:** 268–282.
19. OGAWA, S., T.M. LEE, A.S. NAYAK, *et al.* 1990. Oxygenation-sensitive contrast in magnetic resonance image of rodent brain at high magnetic fields. Magn. Reson. Med. **14:** 68–78.
20. SMALL, S.A., E.X. WU, D. BARTSCH, *et al.* 2000. Imaging physiologic dysfunction of individual hippocampal subregions in humans and genetically modified mice. Neuron. **28:** 653–664.
21. SMALL, S.A., W.Y. TSAI, R. DELAPAZ, *et al.* 2002. Imaging hippocampal function across the human life span: is memory decline normal or not? Ann. Neurol. **51:** 290–295.
22. RAZ, N., K.M. RODRIGUE & J.D. ACKER. 2003. Hypertension and the brain: vulnerability of the prefrontal regions and executive functions. Behav. Neurosci. **17:** 1169–1180.
23. RAZ, N., K.M. RODRIGUE, K.M. KENNEDY, *et al.* Effects of age and vascular health on changes in brain and cognition: a longitudinal study. Submitted.
24. HAACKE, E.M., Y. XU, Y-C.N. CHENG, *et al.* 2004. Susceptibility weighted imaging (SWI). Mag. Res. Med. **52:** 612–618.

25. BARTZOKIS, G., T.A. TISHLER, P.H. LU, *et al.* 2006. Brain ferritin iron may influence age- and gender-related risks of neurodegeneration. Neurobiol. Aging **22:** [Epub ahead of print].

26. QUINTANA, C., S. BELLEFQIH, J.Y. LAVAL, *et al.* 2006. Study of the localization of iron, ferritin, and hemosiderin in Alzheimer's disease hippocampus by analytical microscopy at the subcellular level. J. Struct. Biol. **153:** 42–54.

27. VANHOUTTE, G., I. DEWACHTER, P. BORGHGRAEF, *et al.* 2005. Noninvasive *in vivo* MRI detection of neuritic plaques associated with iron in APP[V717I] transgenic mice, a model for Alzheimer's disease. Magn. Reson. Med. **53:** 607–613.

28. OGG, R.J., J.W. LANGSTON, E.M. HAACKE, *et al.* 1999. The correlation between phase shifts in gradient-echo MR images and regional brain iron concentration. Magn. Reson. Imag. **17:** 1141–1148.

29. HARDY, P.A., D. GASH, R. YOKEL, *et al.* 2005. Correlation of R2 with total iron concentration in the brains of rhesus monkeys. J. Magn. Reson. Imag. **21:** 118–127.

# Linking Brain Imaging and Genomics in the Study of Alzheimer's Disease and Aging

ERIC M. REIMAN

*Banner Alzheimer's Institute, the Neurogenomics Division at the Translational Genomics Research Institute, the Department of Psychiatry at the University of Arizona, and the Arizona Alzheimer's Consortium, Phoenix, Arizona, USA*

ABSTRACT: My colleagues and I have been using positron emission tomography (PET) and magnetic resonance imaging (MRI) to detect and track the brain changes associated with Alzheimer's disease (AD) and normal brain aging in cognitively normal persons with two copies, one copy, and no copies of the apolipoprotein E (APOE) ε4 allele, a common AD susceptibility gene. In this review article, I consider how brain imaging techniques could be used to evaluate putative AD prevention therapies in cognitively normal APOE ε4 carriers and putative age-modifying therapies in cognitively normal APOE ε4 noncarriers, how they could help investigate the individual and aggregate effects of putative AD risk modifiers, and how they could help guide the investigation of a molecular mechanism associated with AD vulnerability and normal neurological aging. I suggest how high-resolution genome-wide genetic and transcriptomic studies could further help in the scientific understanding of AD, aging, and other common and genetically complex phenotypes, such as variation in normal human memory performance, and in the discovery and evaluation of promising treatments for these phenotypes. Finally, I illustrate the push–pull relationship between brain imaging, genomics research, and other neuroscientific research in the study of AD and aging.

KEYWORDS: positron emission tomography; magnetic resonance imaging; apolipoprotein E

## INTRODUCTION

Alzheimer's disease (AD) is the most common form of disabling cognitive impairment in older people. According to one community survey, the disorder afflicts about 10% of persons over 65 and almost half of those over 85 years of age.[1] By the time today's young adults become senior citizens the number of persons in these older age groups is projected to quadruple.[2] Given the

Address for correspondence: Eric M. Reiman, M.D., Banner Alzheimer's Institute, 901 East Willetta Street, Phoenix, Arizona 85006. Voice: 602-239-6999; fax: 602-239-6253.
Eric.Reiman@bannerhealth.com

Ann. N.Y. Acad. Sci. 1097: 94–113 (2007). © 2007 New York Academy of Sciences.
doi: 10.1196/annals.1379.011

physical, emotional, and financial toll AD currently takes on afflicted patients and their families, and the financially overwhelming toll AD and other age-related disorders are projected to take around the world, the identification of effective treatments to not only stop the progression but also prevent the onset of AD is an urgent public health priority. This prevention imperative is even more striking when one considers the growing number of molecular targets at which to aim promising new treatments, the growing range of suggested disease-slowing and -prevention therapies that are ready to be evaluated in clinical trials,[3] and the public health impact of an even modestly effective prevention therapy.

It is commonly agreed that an effective treatment for the prevention of AD would have an enormous public health benefit, that AD treatments are most likely to be effective when administered in the earliest stages of the disorder, before the disease takes its ravaging toll on the brain, and that many patients with mild cognitive impairment (MCI) already have significant neuropathology in this early clinical stage of AD.[4] Indeed, a prevention therapy that delayed the onset of AD by only 5 years has the potential to reduce the number of afflicted persons by half,[5] and it may be possible to identify prevention therapies significantly more effective than that. Despite the imperative to find an effective treatment for the primary prevention of AD, it would take thousands of healthy volunteers and many years—for example, longer than the life of a pharmaceutical company's patent—to evaluate the most promising treatments. With the discovery of a common susceptibility gene for late-onset AD, my colleagues and I were struck by the idea of using imaging techniques to detect and track brain changes associated with the predisposition to AD in carriers of this gene, and we became engrossed by the idea of developing a brain imaging strategy to identify an effective prevention therapy without having to lose a generation.

In this article, I briefly review how the original discovery of a common AD susceptibility gene led us to use brain imaging techniques in the unusually early detection and tracking of AD in cognitively normal persons at genetic risk for this disorder and to provide a foundation for the cost-effective evaluation of primary prevention therapies; how our brain imaging findings have subsequently led to the investigation of new genetic and nongenetic AD risk factors, molecular mechanisms, and therapeutic strategies; and how recently developed high-resolution whole-genome approaches to the analysis of inherited and expressed genes are contributing to these and other endeavors, including new approaches to the study of normal neurological aging and normal human memory.

## GENETIC RISK FACTORS: A FOUNDATION FOR THE STUDY OF AD

In my opinion, more scientific progress has been made in the scientific understanding of AD and the discovery of promising new AD therapies than that related to any other common neurological or psychiatric disorder—and the major springboard for this progress has been the discovery of genetic risk factors for this particular disease. Many AD cases with dementia onset before the age of 60 ("early-onset AD") have been attributed to more than 100 mutations of the presenilin 1 (PS1) gene on chromosome 14, the presenilin 2 gene on chromosome 1, and the amyloid precursor protein (APP) gene on chromosome 21.[6] These genes, which cause an autosomal dominant form of early-onset AD (and which also may account for a very small number of late-onset cases), have provided compelling support for the "amyloid-cascade" hypothesis of AD; have provided a target at which to aim new treatments; and have provided further encouragement for the discovery of amyloid-modifying medications and immunization therapies. Meantime, about 30% of far more common late-onset AD cases have been attributed to the apolipoprotein E (APOE) ε4 allele on chromosome 19, which increases a person's susceptibility to, but is not itself, a sufficient cause of AD.[7,8] While it is not yet established how the APOE protein (i.e., the product of different APOE alleles) contributes to the risk of AD, this protein is the major cholesterol transporter in the brain.[9] Variants of this protein have been suggested to differentially affect the aggregation of amyloid and development of neuritic plaques (a cardinal neuropathological feature of AD),[10] the phosphorylation of tau,[11] the development of neurofibrillary tangles (another cardinal neuropathological feature of AD), mitochondrial neurotoxicity,[12] and the vulnerability of neurons to these and other suggested pathogenic processes.[13] This discovery has provided further encouragement for the evaluation of cholesterol-lowering and insulin-sensitizing therapies in ongoing clinical trials of AD.[12]

The APOE gene has three common variants, ε2, ε3, and ε4, giving rise to six possible APE genotypes: ε2ε2, ε2ε3, ε3ε3 (the most common genotype), ε2ε4, ε3ε4, and ε4ε4. In comparison with the ε3ε3 genotype, each additional copy of the ε4 allele in a person's APOE genotype is associated with a higher risk of late-onset AD and a slightly younger median age at dementia onset.[7,8] Conversely, the presence of an ε2 allele in a person's APOE genotype is associated with a decreased risk of AD and an older median age at dementia onset.[7] Of relevance to the study of aging itself, the APOE ε4 allele is also associated with a higher risk of coronary artery disease and decreased longevity, whereas the APOE ε2 allele is generally associated with a lower risk of coronary artery disease, increased longevity and, indeed, a higher chance of becoming a centenarian.[14] While the frequency of the ε4 allele and its relationship to AD risk appears to vary in populations with different genetic backgrounds, one copy of the ε4 allele is found in almost one-fourth of Americans and about one-third of those with a reported history of dementia in a first-degree relative, and two copies of the ε4 allele is found in 2–3% of the American population and about 5% of those with a reported history of dementia in a first-degree relative.[9,14] The association between the APOE ε4 allele and AD risk has now been reported in hundreds of studies.

While the APOE ε4 allele may account for about 30% of late-onset AD cases, the search is on for a set of additional susceptibility genes, which altogether may account for another 50% of the risk for the disorder.[15] Why have these susceptibility genes been so elusive? Here are a few possible explanations: First, it is unlikely that another gene will account for such a high percentage of late-onset cases.[16] Second, there is some heterogeneity in the clinical assessment of AD cases and elderly controls (about one-third of whom may have AD neuropathology despite the absence of dementia or MCI.[17] Third, there is likely to be heterogeneity in the genetic and nongenetic causes of AD and in the genetic backgrounds of different samples. Fourth, sample sizes in most genetic association studies may be too small to have adequate statistical power. Fifth, there has been a need for whole genome single-nucleotide polymorphism (SNP) platforms with sufficiently high resolution to read "the genetic book of life" in genetic association studies of unrelated cases and controls.[18] Finally, there has been a need for more sophisticated whole genome data analysis techniques, which not only correct for heterogeneity in the subjects' genetic background,[19] but which permit the simultaneous analysis of multiple SNP (rather than separate analyses of each individual SNP), which are likely to contribute to common and genetically complex phenotypes like AD, and results in a single statistic.[20] The recent development of genetic platforms that permit the simultaneous assessment of more than 500,000 SNP throughout the human genome, the continued development of platforms of more than one million SNP, the development of algorithms to evaluate and control for individual differences in genetic backgrounds,[19,21] and the development of compound genetic association algorithms to simultaneously investigate the aggregate effects of several candidate genes[20,21] may have watershed effects of the discovery of susceptibility genes for AD and other common and genetically complex pathological and normal phenotypes.

We have been using an individualized genome-wide screen with more than 500,000 SNP to investigate genes involved in the susceptibility to AD in clinically and neuropathologically well-characterized cases and controls. Preliminary findings from our neurogenomics laboratory support the long-held suggestion that APOE locus is associated with the highest risk of AD and that genome-wide screens may begin to have the resolution to detect genes involved in the vulnerability to common phenotypes.[16] Illustrating the power of this new genotyping technology, Andreas Papassotiropoulos, Dietrich Stephan, and our colleagues used this high-resolution genome-wide platform to analyze pooled DNA from young adults who were stratified on the basis of the recall memory performance.[22] This analysis identified a genomic locus encoding the brain protein KIBRA, which permitted us to demonstrate that *KIBRA T* carriers performed recall memory tests better than noncarriers in three independent normal cohorts. Gene expression studies found that the *KIBRA* gene is expressed in the hippocampus and other brain regions. A functional magnetic resonance imaging (MRI) study suggested the hippocampus of *KIBRA*

*T* noncarriers had to work harder during a memory task to perform the task as well as the carriers. This study led us to consider the role of KIBRA and related molecular events in normal human memory and to begin to conduct preclinical studies of candidate memory-enhancing compounds suggested to affect these molecular events. While this gene does not appear to be involved in the risk of AD, it suggests the promise of new genetics technology in the study of common multigenic phenotypes, and the complementary roles that genetic and imaging studies may play in this line of investigation.

As discussed below, my colleagues and I have capitalized on the use of brain imaging techniques to detect and track brain changes associated with the predisposition to AD in cognitively normal persons at three levels of genetic risk for AD: APOE ε4 homozygotes, heterozygotes (all with the ε3ε4 genotype), and noncarriers.[14,23–27] We have used our imaging data to estimate the number of cognitively normal APOE ε4 heterozygotes needed to evaluate promising prevention therapies in a 2-year clinical trial.[25] We have also used our imaging data to propose the use of positron emission tomography (PET) as a quantitative presymptomatic endophenotype for the assessment of other putative genetic and nongenetic AD risk factors,[27] and we have begun to use it to evaluate a putative genetic risk score generated from a cluster of cholesterol-related genes.[28] In other studies, we are using our imaging findings to guide the selection of metabolically affected brain regions to evaluate in ongoing gene expression studies of laser-capture microdissected neurons and astroglia cells; and we are using brain imaging in putative transgenic mouse models of AD, which have some but not all of the histopathological features of the disorder in the effort to provide an indicator of disease progression that could help bridge the gap between studies of AD in persons and laboratory animals.[29–31] Finally, we hope that our high-resolution genome-wide SNP study of AD cases and controls will help us to further characterize persons at risk for this disorder and further enrich clinical trials of putative primary prevention therapies in our imaging studies.

## BRAIN IMAGING IN THE STUDY OF ALZHEIMER'S DEMENTIA AND MCI

To date, fluorodeoxyglucose positron emission tomography (FDG PET) and volumetric MRI have provided the best established markers of disease progression in patients with Alzheimer's dementia and MCI.[32–36] FDG PET studies find that patients with Alzheimer's dementia have abnormally low measurements of the cerebral metabolic rate for glucose (CMRgl) in the precuneus and posterior cingulate, parietal, and temporal cortex, abnormally low frontal and whole brain measurements in more severely affected patients—reductions that are correlated with dementia severity and progressively decline over time.[32–37] It has been suggested that the earliest CMRgl reductions are in adjacent regions of the posterior cingulate cortex and precuneus.[38] The CMRgl reductions could reflect the density or activity of terminal neuronal fields (some of which may originate in medial temporal regions), the density or activity of perisynaptic astroglial cells, metabolic abnormalities, the combined effects of atrophy and partial volume averaging (image blurring), or a combination of these factors. (However, they do not appear to be solely attributable to atrophy and partial volume averaging.[39] In patients with mild dementia, the pattern of CMRgl reductions has been suggested to predict subsequent clinical decline and the histopathological diagnosis of AD with about 93% sensitivity and about 75% specificity.[40] Using baseline and 1-year follow-up PET images acquired in patients with Alzheimer's dementia, we estimated the number of patients needed to evaluate the effectiveness of putative disease-slowing treatments to slow down the brain imaging declines.[32] In comparison with the use of traditional clinical endpoints, we suggested that FDG PET could be used to help evaluate putative disease-slowing treatments in proof-of-concept studies (e.g., early phase 2 clinical trials) with about one-tenth the number of patients. In phase 2 or phase 3 clinical studies, FDG PET could also help determine whether a treatment's clinical benefits are related to disease-slowing rather than compensatory effects.[41]

Volumetric MRI has been even more extensively studied than FDG PET as a marker of disease progression in patients with AD. Using MRI, patients with AD have accelerated rates of hippocampal, entorhinal cortex, regional gray matter and whole brain atrophy.[33,34,42] Smaller hippocampal and entorhinal cortex volumes are correlated with dementia severity, correlated with neuronal loss in post-mortem brain tissue, and predictive of subsequent clinical decline, but not specific for the neuropathological diagnosis of AD. Rates of hippocampal, entorhinal cortex, and whole brain atrophy have been used to estimate the number of Alzheimer's dementia patients needed to evaluate putative disease-slowing treatments.[33,34,36] Like FDG PET measurements, these MRI measurements could help evaluate putative disease-slowing treatments in proof-of-concept studies with about one-tenth the number of patients,[33] and they could help determine whether a treatment's clinical benefits are related to disease-slowing effects.

Researchers have recently developed promising PET and single photon emission computed tomography (SPECT) radioligand techniques for the assessment of fibrillary amyloid deposition in the living human brain.[43–45] To date, the most widely used radioligand is [11]C-labeled Pittsburgh Compound B (PIB), for which tracer-kinetic models and most but not all of their underlying assumptions have been most fully evaluated.[44–51] Using this radiotracer method, patients with Alzheimer's dementia have increased fibrillar amyloid deposition, including the same posterior cingulate, precuneus, parietal, temporal, and frontal regions associated with reduced CMRgl in FDG PET studies.[47,48] It remains to be determined how early fibrillar amyloid binding occurs, though it has been reported in some elderly normal persons using PET as it has in neuropathological studies; the extent to which this binding progresses or, instead, levels off as recently suggested;[50] how it compares to other bioimaging and clinical measurements in predicting subsequent clinical decline and the histopathological diagnosis of AD; and the extent to which it could provide an indirect measure of the concentration of soluble amyloid oligomers, which may be more toxic than plaques themselves in the pathogenesis of AD.

Since many patients with MCI (including but perhaps not limited to the amnestic subtype) have AD neuropathology[4] and increased rates of subsequent progression to Alzheimer's dementia,[52] there has been great interest in using imaging techniques in MCI patients to help in the early detection and tracking of AD and in the evaluation of putative disease slowing (i.e., secondary prevention therapies) in these patients. In patients with amnestic MCI, lower regional CMRgl, smaller hippocampal and entorhinal cortex volumes, and higher rates of CMRgl decline and hippocampal, entorhinal cortex, whole brain and regional gray matter atrophy are associated with increased rates of conversion to Alzheimer's dementia.[34,42,53] There is growing interest in the use of these imaging techniques in MCI clinical trials to reduce the number of patients needed to detect the effects of a disease-slowing treatment and to do so without having to wait several years to determine whether or when they convert to Alzheimer's dementia.[35,36,41]

In preliminary imaging studies, patients with MCI appear to have intermediate levels of fibrillar amyloid deposition.[46] It remains to be seen whether these intermediate levels are related to mild but progressive fibrillary amyloid deposition in this overall group or instead reflect two subgroups with and without high levels of fibrillar amyloid, and it remains to be determined whether fibrillar amyloid deposition in these patients is progressive. Since almost 30% of MCI patients who progress to dementia may have neuropathological diagnoses other than AD (but involving the hippocampus),[54] fibrillar amyloid imaging techniques may have particular promise in the diagnosis of AD and in selection of MCI subjects in clinical trials of putative amyloid-modifying treatments.

Because of the emerging role of volumetric MRI and FDG PET in the detection and tracking of AD and in the evaluation of putative disease-slowing treatments, the NIH and industry have been supporting a 5-year $60 million study known as the Alzheimer's disease neuroimaging initiative (ADNI) [www.adni-info.org]. In this study, about 200 patients with Alzheimer's dementia, 400 patients with amnestic MCI, and 200 elderly control subjects from more than 50 American sites are being followed approximately every 6 months (depending on the subject group) for 2–3 years using MRI, clinical ratings and neuropsychological tests, and blood and urine biomarkers (in all of the subjects) and FDG PET (in about half of the subjects). Well over 20% of these subjects are also providing cerebrospinal fluid samples at their baseline and 1-year visits, and PIB PET will also be included in almost 100 of these subjects. This study promises to further characterize and compare the statistical power of MRI and FDG PET, other biomarker measurements, and clinical ratings in multicenter clinical trials. It will further establish how baseline measurements and short-term bioimaging and other biomarker changes predict subsequent rates of clinical decline and conversion from MCI to Alzheimer's dementia. It has already led to standardized data acquisition and real-time quality assurance procedures that may be relevant to clinical trials. Finally, it will provide public access to a common database and (sufficiently well justified) biological specimens, making it possible to directly compare different methods and measurements, helping to determine which of these tests to incorporate in clinical trials, to develop and test new image analysis techniques, and to capitalize in the role of complementary data sets in the detection and tracking of AD.

Already, researchers have begun to embed brain imaging techniques in clinical trials of putative disease-modifying treatments. I personally believe that two (or three) imaging modalities are preferable to one in some of these studies.[41] Using both FDG PET and volumetric MRI, researchers could provide converging support for a putative treatment's disease-modifying effects, overcoming modality specific confounds. These potential confounds include a treatment's effects on brain swelling using MRI (as suggested in the aborted clinical trial of the first putative immunization therapy for the treatment of AD, which found accelerated rates of brain volume loss in the active treatment[55] and its effects on regional brain activity of CMRgl using PET independent of its effects on disease progression. Furthermore, embedded imaging studies could provide the data needed to suggest that these measurements are "reasonably likely therapeutic surrogates" to support the claim that a treatment has a disease-modifying effect, since researchers must be able to show that an effect on the therapeutic surrogate predicts a beneficial clinical effect. Fibrillar amyloid imaging has the potential to investigate a putative treatment's effects on fibrillar amyloid deposition, but may not be close enough to the clinical endpoint (i.e., it may be too early an event that is less able to predict a clinical effect than the other imaging endpoints that may be better indicators of neuronal and synaptic close and better predictors of clinical outcome).

## BRAIN IMAGING IN THE STUDY OF COGNITIVELY NORMAL PERSONS AT DIFFERENTIAL RISK FOR AD

We have been using FDG PET and MRI to study cognitively normal persons with two copies, one copy, and no copies of the APOE ε4 allele.[14,23-27] In these studies, newspaper ads were used to recruit healthy volunteers who understood that they would receive no information about their APOE genotype and consented to participate in our studies. Initially, we compared FDG PET measurements in 11 cognitively normal APOE ε4 homozygotes (who have a particularly high risk of AD) and 22 ε4 noncarriers, 50–65 years of age, who were individually matched for their gender, age, and educational level. Although the two subject groups did not have significant differences in any of their clinical ratings or neuropsychological tests, the ε4 homozygotes had significantly reduced CMRgl in each of the same posterior cingulate, precuneus, parietal, temporal, and prefrontal regions as previously studied patients with Alzheimer's dementia.[14] In this initial study, the APOE ε4 homozygotes also had significantly reduced CMRgl in frontal regions previously found in PET, MRI, and neuropathological studies to be preferentially affected by normal aging. At the time, we raised the possibility the APOE ε4 allele increases the risk and hastens the onset of AD by accelerating normal aging processes.[14] However, we have not been able to reproduce these additional prefrontal CMRgl reductions in our studies of other APOE ε4 carriers.[24,27] The two groups did not have significant differences in their hippocampal volumes, and PET continued to distinguish the groups even after controlling for their hippocampus volumes.[23] Based on these and other findings, we suggested that PET was more sensitive than MRI hippocampal volume measurements in detecting the earliest brain changes associated with the predisposition to AD and that hippocampal volume tended to decline later, in conjunction with subtle memory declines. Even so, our preliminary voxel-based morphometry studies suggest that cognitively normal APOE ε4 carriers have abnormal reductions in regional gray matter density.[56] We subsequently extended our PET findings to 11 cognitively normal ε4 heterozygotes (all of whom had perfect scores on their mini-mental state examinations)—a group that accounts for almost one-fourth of the population and could be readily enrolled in primary prevention studies.[24] Finally, we showed the APOE ε4 carriers had greater 2-year rates of CMRgl decline than ε4 noncarriers in these and other brain regions implicated in PET or histopathological studies of AD.[25] Based on these findings, we estimated the number of cognitively normal APOE ε4 heterozygotes needed to evaluate a putative primary prevention therapy in a 2-year clinical trial (TABLE 1).[26,57] We are now developing a research program that is designed to test promising primary prevention therapies in just this way.

TABLE 1. Number of cognitively normal APOE-3/4's per treatment group needed to detect an effect with 80% power in 2 years

|                | Treatment effect | | | |
|----------------|------|------|------|------|
|                | 20%  | 30%  | 40%  | 50%  |
| Thalamus       | 78   | 35   | 21   | 14   |
| Parahippocampal| 129  | 58   | 33   | 22   |
| Cingulate      | 130  | 58   | 33   | 22   |
| Temporal       | 155  | 70   | 40   | 27   |
| Basal forebrain| 167  | 75   | 43   | 29   |
| Prefrontal     | 179  | 80   | 46   | 29   |
| Combined       | 39   | 19   | 12   | 8    |

$P = 0.01$ (two-tailed), uncorrected for multiple comparisons.
Adapted from Reiman et al., 2004[26] with permission.

In the same study, we also characterized rates of 2-year CMRgl decline in APOE ε4 noncarriers.[25] We suggested these declines, which include but are not limited to prefrontal and anterior cingulate brain regions previously found to be preferentially affected by normal aging, provide an indicator of normal aging processes relatively free of the risk for AD. Indeed, we estimated the number of ε4 noncarriers that could be used to evaluate promising age-modifying treatments (e.g., antioxidants, aerobic exercise, etc.) in a 2-year clinical trial.[25]

To investigate whether the CMRgl abnormalities could be detected even earlier, we compared FDG PET images from 12 APOE ε4 heterozygotes and 15 ε4 noncarriers 20–39 years of age (mean age 30 years). The young adult APOE ε4 heterozygotes had significantly reduced CMRgl in the same brain regions as patients with AD, almost 50 years before the estimated median age of dementia onset in ε4 heterozygotes and prior to the known histopathological features of AD.[26] A cross-sectional comparison with our older subjects suggests that these very early (perhaps even developmental) CMRgl reductions do not progress between young adulthood and late middle age, yet predict regions that are going to reflect subsequent CMRgl declines and fibrillar amyloid deposition. This study raises the possibility of unusually early, perhaps even developmental brain changes in persons at risk for late-onset AD, which eventually conspire with normal aging processes to elicit the biological and clinical features of AD. Further, it suggests a window of many years for the introduction of a safe, well tolerated, and effective primary prevention therapy.

We are now studying a large number of cognitively normal APOE ε4 homozygotes, heterozygotes, and noncarriers 47–68 years of age every 2 years using FDG PET, MRI, and a 4-h battery of clinical ratings and neuropsychological tests. We are interested in demonstrating the extent to which baseline CMRgl reductions and 2-year rates of CMRgl decline predict subsequent rates of cognitive decline and conversion to MCI and AD. FDG PET studies of patients with MCI[58,59] and older cognitively normal APOE ε4 heterozygotes who presented to a clinic with memory concerns[60] suggest that baseline CMRgl abnormalities and 2-year CMRgl declines in our implicated regions will predict subsequent decline, which would provide further support for the use of PET as a reasonable likely therapeutic surrogate in primary prevention trials.

We recently compared the FDG PET images of 160 cognitively normal persons 47–68 years of age, including 36 APOE ε4 homozgyotes, 46 ε4 heterozygotes, and 78 noncarriers. APOE ε4 gene dose (i.e., the number of ε4 alleles in a person's APOE genotype, reflecting three levels of genetic risk for late-onset AD) was significantly correlated with lower CMRgl in and only in each of the brain regions previously shown to be affected in patients with Alzheimer's dementia (FIG. 1).[27] (The reductions were not solely attributable to the combined effects of atrophy and partial-volume averaging). Based on this finding, we suggested that PET (and eventually MRI,

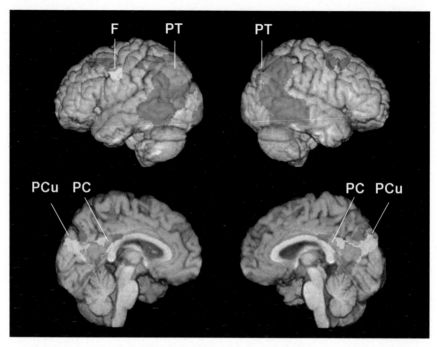

**FIGURE 1.** Correlations between APOE ε4 gene dose and lower CMRgl (shown in *blue*, $P < 0.005$, uncorrected for multiple comparisons) in cognitively normal, late middle-aged persons are projected onto the lateral and medial surfaces of the left and right cerebral hemispheres and shown in relationship to brain regions preferentially affected in an earlier PET study of patients with probable AD[2] (shown in *purple*). Significant correlations were observed bilaterally in the posterior cingulate (PC), precuneus (PCu), and parietotemporal (PT) cortex bilaterally and in the left frontal (F) cortex. Reproduced from Reiman *et al.*, 2005[27] with permission.

as suggested in the Alexander *et al.* abstract[61] could be used as a quantitative presymptomatic endophenotype (a measurement more closely related to disease susceptibility than the clinical syndrome itself) to help assess the individual and aggregate effects of putative genetic and nongenetic modifiers of AD risk.[27] As a complement to retrospective observational studies of older Alzheimer's dementia cases and controls, which typically require retrospective assessment of antecedent risk modifiers, this endophenotype could permit the concurrent and prospective evaluation of these putative risk modifiers prior to the onset of symptoms, minimizing the potentially confounding effects of differential survival or inaccurate or biased recall of the antecedent risk modifier and providing easier access to accurate presymptomatic measurements of a putative biological risk modifier. As a complement to prospective longitudinal cohort studies, this endophenotype could provide information about the putative risk factor without having to study many subjects or wait many years to determine whether or when they develop symptoms. Finally, this endophenotype could help overcome the confounding effects of individual differences in cognitive reserve capacity, which may compensate for AD neuropathology and mask its clinical expression.

## THE PUSH–PULL RELATIONSHIP BETWEEN BRAIN IMAGING AND GENOMIC STUDIES

Just as the discovery of the APOE ε4 allele has galvanized our use of brain imaging in the unusually early detection and tracking of AD and the development of a cost-effective way to assess putative treatments for the primary prevention of AD, our imaging studies have inspired subsequent genomic studies to further characterize AD risk factors and consider the molecular contributions to the metabolic brain abnormalities found even before the onset of plaques and tangles in persons at risk for AD. Here, I briefly consider several examples.

### *Example: Endophenotypic Assessment of a Putative AD Genetic Risk Factor*

Recently, Papassotiropoulos and his colleagues used a set association analysis to implicate a cluster of nine cholesterol-related genes in the risk of AD in 545 European cases and controls.[21] Based on these findings, the researchers proposed the calculation of a cholesterol-related genetic risk score (CREGS) to estimate a person's risk for AD, and they found that CREGS was correlated with cerebrospinal fluid levels of the final cholesterol catabolite 24S-hydroxycholesterol in a small number of normal volunteers. We recently used our proposed endophenotype to further investigate the relationship between CREGS and the genetic risk for AD. Using PET images and DNA from our ongoing American studies and with the help of our European colleagues, we found a significant correlation between CREGS and CMRgl reductions in and only in AD-affected brain regions, even after the individuals' APOE ε4 gene dose is included in the CREGS score.[28]

### *Example: Informing Transcriptomic Studies and Drug Discovery*

We have begun to use information about the distribution of histopathological abnormalities in patients with AD and the distribution of metabolic alterations associated with the predisposition to AD to investigate the genes that are differentially affected by AD. Using high-quality brain tissue from the entorhinal cortex, laser-capture microdissected neurons, and genome-wide microarray platforms, we compared the expression of genes from tangle-bearing and non-tangle-bearing neurons from the same AD patients and non-tangle-bearing neurons from nondemented, histopathologically normal controls to identify genes that are differentially expressed in relationship to neurofibrillary pathology.[62] Using a genome-wide small interfering RNA platform, we are investigating which of the genes, when silenced, interferes with the expression and phosphorylation of tau, molecular events that have been implicated in neurofibrillary pathology. Together, these studies may provide information about molecular events in neurofibrillary pathology and provide targets at which to aim new treatments. In a similar fashion, we have begun to compare the genes that are differentially expressed in laser-capture microdissected neurons from several of the brain regions that are preferentially affected by, or relatively spared in patients affected by, and cognitively normal persons at risk for AD (e.g., regions of posterior cingulate and visual cortex, respectively) to provide new information about the molecular events involved in early pathogenesis of AD. At the same time, we have begun to compare the genes that are differentially expressed in brain regions that are preferentially affected by or relatively spared in the normal aged brain (e.g., regions of frontal and visual cortex, respectively) to provide information about the molecular substrates of normal brain aging.

Based in part on our finding of CMRgl abnormalities in persons affected by and at risk for AD, on transcriptomic studies in APOE knockout mice, and observational and interventional studies, a pharmaceutical company was encouraged to launch a set of clinical trials of rosiglitazone, an insulin-sensitizing medication, in the treatment of AD in patients who are stratified for the presence or absence of the APOE ε4 allele.[12] (A separate clinical trial raised the possibility that rosiglitazone was beneficial in the APOE ε4 non-carriers, but not in the carriers—based on a finding that must be considered exploratory at this time but which has potentially interesting pharmacogenetic implications.[63] One of these clinical trials is using FDG PET as its primary therapeutic endpoint, (and MRI as a secondary endpoint), supporting the use of imaging in proof-of-concept clinical trials of putative AD disease-slowing treatments.

### Example: Developing Analytical Tools That Leverage Complementary Complex Data Sets from the Same Individuals

As different brain imaging, genetic, transcriptomic, and proteomic technologies continue to advance, there is an increasing need for data analysis tools that extract meaningful information from these complex and potentially complementary data sets in a more powerful way and with fewer statistical type 1 errors (i.e., chance findings) due to the problem of multiple comparisons. As a complement to traditional univariate statistical analyses, which separately analyze each regional brain, inherited or expressed gene, or protein measurement, we and others have begun using multivariate statistical algorithms to extract information about the patterns within complex data sets. Led by Gene Alexander, we have been using the Scaled Subprofile Model (SSM) network analysis to characterize the MRI patterns of regional gray matter atrophy associated with aging,[64] AD,[65] and APOE ε4 gene dose.[61] We have suggested how this strategy may aid in the detection and tracking of AD, AD risk, and normal brain aging, and we have suggested how it could be used in the evaluation of putative AD disease-modifying, AD prevention, and antiaging therapies.[64] As previously noted, researchers have begun to develop, test, and apply algorithms to simultaneously analyze the contributions of multiple SNP to common and genetically complex phenotypes like AD.[20,21] Led by Kewei Chen, we have been developing an application of partial least squares (PLS) to characterize in a single measurement the relationship between two or more complementary, complex data sets from the same individual. In preliminary studies, we have used this approach to characterize the relationship between a person's PET pattern of CMRgl and MRI pattern of regional gray matter density, to distinguish older from younger adults without any overlap between groups, and to characterize an extremely strong correlation between PLS-generated PET/MRI scores and APOE ε4 gene dose.[66,67] We continue to refine, test, and apply this method in the hope of characterizing the relationships among any combination of a person's PET, MRI, genetic, transcriptomic, proteomic, clinical, and neuropsychological data sets, to track the progression of AD, AD risk, and aging, and evaluate putative disease-modifying, prevention, and antiaging therapies with even greater power.

### *Example: Developing an Indicator of AD Progression in Laboratory Animals*

Capitalizing on the discovery of genes that cause early-onset autosomal-dominant AD, researchers have developed several promising transgenic mouse lines that are being used to help clarify disease mechanisms and screen promising new treatments.[68–71] Unfortunately, these and other animal models have some but not all of the features of AD, and there are limitations to the use of behavioral tests to assess disease progression in these animals. We have been using functional and structural imaging techniques to provide a biological indicator of AD progression that could be used to help bridge the gap between the study of persons and laboratory animals, to help in the study of disease mechanisms, and to help in the screening of promising new treatments. Using FDG autoradiography, we found that aged PDAPP mice had CMRgl reductions in posterior cingulate CMRgl that were more pronounced in the aged animal than in the younger animals.[29] Unfortunately, we found the PDAPP mice also had a truncated corpus callosum,[73,73] which could limit our ability to compare the same brain region, and transgenic and wild-type animals, and which would confound the interpretation of small animal PET studies due to the limited spatial resolution of PET and potentially confounding partial-volume averaging effects.[74] More recently, we have sought to extend this finding to other transgenic mouse lines with less extensive white matter pathology.[75] We have also developed an automated algorithm to compute whole brain atrophy rates from sequential MRI in mice, which could be used to help characterize changes in whole brain atrophy in the appropriate transgenic or nontransgenic animal model of AD,[76] as it can in humans.[77] This method could also be used to help characterize the time-course of potentially confounding effects of amyloid-modifying treatments on brain swelling,[55] which could influence the design of clinical trials using MRI as a therapeutic endpoint.

## CONCLUSION

Brain imaging techniques have a demonstrated role in the early detection and tracking of AD, an emerging role in the evaluation of putative disease-slowing and -prevention therapies, and promising roles in the tracking of normal brain aging and the evaluation of age-modifying treatments. Imaging techniques can also be used to evaluate the individual and aggregate effects of putative AD risk modifiers, and they can help guide the investigation of molecular mechanisms associated with AD vulnerability and normal neurological aging. In a complementary fashion, high-resolution genome wide genetic association studies promise to identify some of the remaining susceptibility genes that account for up to 70% of the risk for AD and also identify some of the genes associated with normal aging. New methodological developments promise to enhance the push–pull relationship between brain imaging, genomics research, and other neuroscientific research in the study of AD and aging. Given the prevention imperative, we are excited about the chance to use PET in cognitively normal APOE ε4 carriers to help identify promising treatments for the primary prevention of AD in the most cost-effective way.

### ACKNOWLEDGMENTS

The author thanks his colleagues and collaborators at the Banner Alzheimer's Institute, the Translational Genomics Research Institute, Mayo Clinic Arizona, other institutions in the Arizona Alzheimer's Consortium, and the University of Zurich for their contributions to the brain imaging and genomics studies described here. These studies were supported by the National Institute of Mental Health (RO1 MH057899), the National Institute on Aging (RO1 MH057899, P30 AG19610, RO1 AG023193, and UO1 AG024904), the Alzheimer's Association, Kronos Life Sciences, the Banner Alzheimer's Foundation, and the state of Arizona.

# REFERENCES

1. EVANS, D.A., H.H. FUNKENSTEIN, M.S. ALBERT, et al. 1989. Prevalence of Alzheimer's disease in a community population of older persons: higher than previously reported. JAMA **262:** 2551–2556.
2. BROOKMEYER, R., S. GRAY & C. KAWAS. 1998. Projections of Alzheimer's disease in the United States and the public health impact of delaying disease onset. Am. J. Public Health **88:** 1337–1342.
3. CASELLI, R.J., T.G. BEACH, R. YAARI & E.M. REIMAN. 2006. Alzheimer's disease: a century later. J. Clin. Psychiatry **67:** 1784–1800.
4. MARKESBERRY, W.R., F.A. SCHMITT, R.J. KRYSCIO, et al. 2006. Neuropathologic substrate of mild cognitive impairment. Arch. Neurol. **63:** 38–46.
5. KHACHATURIAN, Z.S. 1992. The five-five, ten-ten plan for Alzheimer's disease (editorial). Neurobiol. Aging **13:** 197–198.
6. PAPASSOTIROPOULOS, A., M. FOUNTOULAKIS, T. DUNCKLEY, et al. 2006. Genetics, transcriptomics, and proteomics of Alzheimer's disease. J. Clin. Psychiatry **67:** 652–670.
7. CORDER, E.H., A.M. SAUNDERS, W.J. SRITTMATTER, et al. 1993. Gene dose of apolipoprotein E type 4 allele and the risk of Alzheimer's disease in late onset families. Science **261:** 921–924.
8. FARRER, L.A., L.A. CUPPLES, J.L. HAIANES, et al. 1997. Effects of age, sex, and ethnicity on the association between apolipoprotein E genotype and Alzheimer disease. A meta-analysis. APOE and Alzheimer Disease Meta Analysis Consortium. JAMA **278:** 1349–1356.
9. MAHLEY, R.W. 1988. Apolipoprotein E: cholesterol transport protein with expanding role in cell biology. Science **240:** 622–630.
10. WISNIEWSKI, T., E.M. CASTANO, A. GOLABEK, et al. 1994. Acceleration of Alzheimer's fibril formation by apolipoprotein E in vitro. Am. J. Pathol. **145:** 1030–1035.
11. STRITTMATTER, W.J., K.H. WEISGRABER, M. GOEDERT, et al. 1994. Hypothesis: microtubule instability and paired helical filament formation in the Alzheimer disease brain are related to apolipoprotein E genotype. Exp. Nerol. **25:** 163–171.
12. ROSES, A.D., A.M. SAUNDERS, Y. HUANG, et al. 2006. Complex disease-associated pharmacogenetics: drug efficacy, drug safety, and confirmation of a pathogenetic hypothesis (Alzheimer's disease). Pharmacogenomics J. **13:** [Epub ahead of print].
13. MIYATA, M. & J.D. SMITH. 1996. Apolipoprotein E allele-specific antioxidant activity and effects on cytotoxicity by oxidative insults and amyloid peptides. Nat. Genet. **14:** 55–61.
14. REIMAN, E.M., R.J. CASELLI, L.S. YUN, et al. 1996. Preclinical evidence of Alzheimer's disease in persons homozygous for the ε4 allele for apolipoprotein E. N. Engl. J. Med. **334:** 752–758.
15. GATZ, M., C.A. REYNOLDS, L. FRATIGLIONI, et al. 2006. Role of genes and environments for explaining Alzheimer disease. Arch. Gen. Psychiatry **63:** 168–174.
16. PEARSON, J.V., M.J. HUENTELMAN, R.F. HALPERIN, et al. 2007. Identification of the genetic basis for complex disorders by use of pooling-based genomewide single-nucleotide-polymorphism association studies. Am. J. Hum. Genet. **80:** 126–139.

17. BENNETT, D.A., J.A. SCHNEIDER, Z. ARVANITAKIS, et al. 2006. Neuropathology of older persons without cognitive impairment from two community-based studies. Neurology **66:** 1837–1844.

18. CRAIG, D.W. & D.A. STEPHAN. 2005. Applications of whole-genome high-density SNP genotyping. Expert Rev. Mol. Diagn. **5:** 159–170.

19. PRITCHARD, J.K. & N.A. ROSENBERG. 1999. Use of unlinked genetic markers to detect population stratification in association studies. Am. J. Hum. Genet. **65:** 220–228.

20. HOH, J., A. WILLE & J. OTT. 2001. Trimming, weighting, and grouping SNPs in human case-control association studies. Genome Res. **11:** 2115–2119.

21. PAPASSOTIROPOULOS, A., A. WOLLMEER, M. TSOLAKI, et al. 2005. A cluster of cholesterol-related genes confers susceptibility for Alzheimer's disease. J. Clin. Psychiatry **66:** 940–947.

22. PAPASSOTIROPOULOS, A., D.A. STEPHAN, M. HUENTELMAN, et al. 2006. Common KIBRA alleles are associated with human memory performance. Science **314:** 475–478.

23. REIMAN, E.M., A. UECKER, R.J. CASELLI, et al. 1998. Hippocampal volumes in cognitively normal persons at genetic risk for Alzheimer's disease. Ann. Neurol. **44:** 288–291.

24. REIMAN, E.M., R.J. CASELLI, K. CHEN, et al. 2001a. Declining brain activity in cognitively normal apolipoprotein E ε4 heterozygotes: a foundation for using positron emission tomography to efficiently test treatments to prevent Alzheimer's disease. Proc. Nat. Acad. Sci. USA **98:** 3334–3339.

25. REIMAN, E.M., R.J. CASELLI, G.E. ALEXANDER & K. CHEN. 2001b. Tracking the decline in cerebral glucose metabolism in persons and laboratory animals at genetic risk for Alzheimer's disease. Clin. Neurosci. Res. **1:** 194–206.

26. REIMAN, E.M., K. CHEN, G.E. ALEXANDER, et al. 2004. Functional brain abnormalities in young adults at genetic risk for late-onset Alzheimer's dementia. Proc. Nat. Acad. Sci. USA **101:** 284–289.

27. REIMAN, E.M., K. CHEN, G.E. ALEXANDER, et al. 2005. Correlations between apolipoprotein ε4 gene dose and brain-imaging measurements of regional hypometabolism. Proc. Natl. Acad. Sci. USA **102:** 8299–8302.

28. REIMAN, E.M., K. CHEN, R.J. CASELLI, et al. 2005. Correlations between cholesterol-related genetic risk scores and lower brain-imaging measurements of regional glucose metabolism. Soc. Neurosci. Abstr. Washington, DC.

29. REIMAN, E.M., A. UECKER, F. GONZALEZ-LIMA, et al. 2000. Tracking Alzheimer's disease in transgenic mice using fluorodeoxyglucose autoradiography. Neuroreport **11:** 987–991.

30. VALLA, J., K. CHEN, J.D. BERNDT, et al. 2002. Effects of image resolution on autoradiographic measurements of posterior cingulate activity in PDAPP mice: implications for functional brain imaging studies of transgenic mouse models of Alzheimer's disease. Neuroimage **16:** 1–6.

31. VAALLA, J., L. SCHNEIDER & E.M. REIMAN. 2006. Age- and transgene-related changes in regional cerebral metabolism in PSAPP mice. Brain Res. **1116:** 194–200.

32. ALEXANDER, G.E., K. CHEN, P. PIETRINI, et al. 2002. Longitudinal PET evaluation of cerebral metabolic decline in dementia: a potential outcome measure in Alzheimer's disease treatment studies. Am. J. Psychiatry **159:** 738–745.

33. Fox, N.C., S. Cousens, R. Scahill, *et al.* 2000. Using serial registered brain magnetic resonance imaging to measure disease progression in Alzheimer disease: power calculations and estimates of sample size to detect treatment effects. Arch. Neurol. **57:** 333–335.

34. Jack, C.R. Jr, M.M. Shiung, J.L. Gunter, *et al.* 2004. Comparison of different MRI brain atrophy rate measures with clinical disease progression in AD. Neurology **62:** 591–600.

35. Morris, J.C., K.A. Quaid, D.M. Holtzman, *et al.* 2005. Role of biomarkers in studies of presymptomatic Alzheimer's disease. J. Alz. Dementia **1:** 145–151.

36. Thal, L.J., K. Kantarci, E.M. Reiman, *et al.* 2006. The role of biomarkers in clinical trials for Alzheimer disease. Alz. Dis. Assoc. Disord. **20:** 6–15.

37. Minoshima, S., B. Giordani, S. Berent, *et al.* 1997. Metabolic reduction in the posterior cingulate cortex in very early Alzheimer's disease. Ann. Neurol. **42:** 85–94.

38. Minoshima, S., N.L. Foster, D.E. Kuhl. 1994. Posterior cingulate cortex in Alzheimer's disease. Lancet **344:** 895.

39. Ibanez, V., P. Pietrini, G.E. Alexander, *et al.* 1998. Regional glucose metabolic abnormalities are not the result of atrophy in Alzheimer's disease. Neurology **50:** 1585–1593.

40. Silverman, D.H., G.W. Small, C.Y. Chang, *et al.* 2001. Positron emission tomography in evaluation of dementia: Regional brain metabolism and long-term outcome. JAMA **286:** 2120–2127.

41. Reiman, E.M., R.J. Caselli, K. Chen & G.E. Alexander. 2004b. Positron emission tomography and magnetic resonance imaging in the study of cognitively normal persons at differential genetic risk of Alzheimer's dementia. *In* The Living Brain and Alzheimer's. B.T. Hyman, J.F. Demonet, Y. Christen. Eds.: pp. 152–77. J.F. Demonet & Y. Christen Springer-Verlag. Berlin Heidelberg.

42. Chetelat, G., B. Landeau, F. Eustache, *et al.* 2005. Using voxel-based morphometry to map the structural changes associated with rapid conversion in MCI: a longitudinal MRI study. Neuroimage **27:** 934–946.

43. Shoghi-Jadid, K., G.W. Small, E.D. Agdeppa, *et al.* 2002. Localization of neurofibrillary tangles (NFTs) and beta-amyloid plaques (APs) in the brains of living patients with Alzheimer's disease. Am. J. Geriatr. Psychiatry **10:** 24–35.

44. Klunk, W.E., H. Engler, A. Nordbert, *et al.* 2004. Imaging brain amyloid in Alzheimer's disease with Pittsburgh Compound-B. Ann. Neurol. **55:** 306–319.

45. Verhoeff, N.P., A.A. Wilson, S. Takeshita, *et al.* 2004. *In-vivo* imaging of Alzheimer disease beta-amyloid with [11C]SB-13 PET. Am. J. Geriatr. Psychiatry **12:** 584–595.

46. Lopresti, B.J., W.E. Klunk, C.A. Mathis, *et al.* 2005. Simplified quantification of Pittsburgh Compound B amyloid imaging PET studies: a comparative analysis. J. Nucl. Med. **46:** 1959–1972.

47. Kemppainen, N.M., S. Aalto, I.A. Wilson, *et al.* 2006. Voxel-based analysis of PET amyloid ligand [$^{11}$C]PIB uptake in Alzheimer disease. Neurology **67:** 1–6.

48. Ziolko, S.K., L.A. Weissfeld, W.E. Klunk, *et al.* 2006. Evaluation of voxel-based methods for the statistical analysis of PIB PET amyloid imaging studies in Alzheimer's disease. Neuroimage **33:** 94–102.

49. Mintun, M.A., G.N. Larossa, Y.I. Sheline, *et al.* 2006. [11C]PIB in a nondemented population: potential antecedent marker of Alzheimer disease. Neurology **67:** 446–452.

50. ENGLER, H., A. FORSBERG, O. ALMKVIST, *et al.* 2006. Two-year follow-up of amyloid deposition in patients with Alzheimer's disease. Brain **129**: 2856–2866.
51. FAGAN, A.M., M.A. MINTUN, R.H. MACH, *et al.* 2006. Inverse relation between *in vivo* amyloid imaging load and cerebrospinal fluid $A\beta_{42}$ in humans. Ann. Neurol. **59**: 512–519.
52. PETERSEN, R.C., G.E. SMITH, S.C. WARING, *et al.* 1999. Mild cognitive impairment: clinical characterization and outcome. Arch. Neurol. **56**: 303–308.
53. JACK, C.R., R.C. PETERSEN, Y.C. XU, *et al.* 1999. Prediction of AD with MRI-based hippocampal volume in mild cognitive impairment. Neurology **52**: 1397–1403.
54. JICHA, G.A., J.E. PARISI, D.W. DICKSON, *et al.* 2006. Neuropathologic outcome of mild cognitive impairment following progression to clinical dementia. Arch. Neurol. **63**: 647–648.
55. FOX, N.C., R.S. BLACK, S. GILMAN, *et al.* 2005. Effects of Abeta immunization (AN1792) on MRI measures of cerebral volume in Alzheimer disease. Neurology **64**: 1563–1572.
56. ALEXANDER, G.E., K. CHEN, E.M. REIMAN, *et al.* 2003. APOE ε4 dose effect on gray matter atrophy in cognitively normal adults. Soc. Neurosci. Abstr. New Orleans.
57. REIMAN, E.M., R.J. CASELLI, K. CHEN, *et al.* 2001. Declining brain activity in cognitively normal apolipoprotein E ε4 heterozygotes: a foundation for testing Alzheimer's prevention therapies. Proc. Natl. Acad. Sci. USA **98**: 3334–3339.
58. DRZEZGA, A., N. LAUTENSCHLAGER, H. SIEBNER, *et al.* 2003. Cerebral metabolic changes accompanying conversion of mild cognitive impairment into Alzheimer's disease: a PET follow-up study. Eur. J. Nucl. Med. **30**: 1104–1113.
59. DRZEZGA, A., T. GRIMMER, M. RIEMENSCHNEIDER, *et al.* 2005. Prediction of individual clinical outcome in MCI by means of genetic assessment and [18]F-FDG PET. J. Nucl. Med. **46**: 1625–1632.
60. SMALL, G.W., L.M. ERCOLI, D.H.S. SILVERMAN, *et al.* 2000. Cerebral metabolic and cognitive decline in persons at genetic risk for Alzheimer's disease. Proc. Natl. Acad. Sci. USA **97**: 6037–6042.
61. ALEXANDER, G.E., J.L. ETNIER, E.M. REIMAN, *et al.* 2004. Interactive effects of APOE ε4 and physical fitness on gray matter in cognitively normal adults. Soc. Neurosci. Abstr. San Diego.
62. DUNCKLEY, T., T.G. BEACH, K.E. RAMSEY, *et al.* 2006. Gene expression correlates of neurofibrillary tangles in Alzheimer's disease. Neurobiol Aging **27**: 1359–1371.
63. RISNER, M.E., A.M. SAUNDERS, J.F. ALTMAN, *et al.* 2006. Efficacy of rosiglitazone in a genetically defined population with mild-to-moderate Alzheimer's disease. Pharmacogenomics J. **6**: 222–224.
64. ALEXANDER, G.E., K. CHEN, T.L. MERKLEY, *et al.* 2006. Regional network of magnetic resonance imaging gray matter volume in healthy aging. Neuroreport **17**: 951–958.
65. ALEXANDER, G.E., K. CHEN, M. ASCHENBRENNER, *et al.* 2006. Regional network pattern of MRI gray matter volume in Alzheimer's dementia. J. Alz. Dementia **2**(Suppl 1):S66.
66. CHEN, K., E.M. REIMAN, R. CASELLI, *et al.* 2004. Linking functional and structural brain images with multivariate network analyses: description and application using the partial least square method. Soc. Nucl. Med. 51st Ann. Meeting Abstr. Philadelphia.

67. CHEN, K., E.M. REIMAN, G.E. ALEXANDER, *et al*. 2006. Using partial least squares to demonstrate a correlation between combined PET/MRI scores and apolipoprotein E ε4 gene dose. ICAD. Madrid.

68. GAMES, D., D. ADAMS, R. ALESSANDRINI, *et al*. 1995. Alzheimer-type neuropathology in transgenic mice overexpressing V717F β-amyloid precursor protein. Nature **373:** 523–527.

69. HSIAO, K., P. CHAPMAN, S. NILSEN, *et al*. 1996. Correlative memory deficits, Aβ elevation, and amyloid plaques in transgenic mice. Science **274:** 99–102.

70. HOLCOMB, L., M.N. GORDON, E. MCGOWAN, *et al*. 1998. Accelerated Alzheimer-type phenotype in transgenic mice carrying both mutant amyloid precursor protein and presenilin 1 transgenes. Nat. Med. **4:** 97–100.

71. ODDO, S., A. CACCAMO, J.D. SHEPHERD, *et al*. 2003. Triple-transgenic model of Alzheimer's disease with plaques and tangles: intracellular Abeta and synaptic dysfunction. Neuron **39:** 409–421.

72. GONZALEZ-LIMA, F., J.D. BERNDT, J.E. VALLA, *et al*. 2001. Reduced corpus callosum, fornix and hippocampus in PDAPP transgenic mouse model of Alzheimer's disease. Neuroreport **12:** 2375–2379.

73. VALLA, J., L.E. SCHNEIDER, F. GONZALEZ-LIMA & E.M. REIMAN. 2006a. Nonprogressive transgene-related callosal and hippocampal changes in PDAAP mice. Neuroreport **17:** 829–832.

74. VALLA, J., K. CHEN, J.D. BERNDT, *et al*. 2002. Effects of image resolution on autoradiographic measurements of posterior cingulate activity in PDAPP mice: implications for functional brain imaging studies of transgenic mouse model of Alzheimer's disease. Neuroimage **16:** 1–6.

75. VALLA, J., L.E. SCHNEIDER & E.M. REIMAN. 2006b. Age and transgene-related changes in regional cerebral metabolism in PSAPP mice. Brain Res. **1116:** 194–200.

76. CHEN, K., E.M. REIMAN, T. HE, *et al*. 2002. Evaluation of an iterative principal component analysis for detecting whole brain volume change in small animal magnetic resonance imaging. Neurobiol. Aging **23:** S353 abstr.

77. CHEN, K., E.M. REIMAN, G.E. ALEXANDER, *et al*. 2004. An automated algorithm for the computation of brain volume change from sequential MRIs using an iterative principal component analysis and its evaluation for the assessment of whole-brain atrophy rates in patients with probable Alzheimer's disease. Neuroimage **22:** 134–143.

# Imaging and CSF Studies in the Preclinical Diagnosis of Alzheimer's Disease

M. J. DE LEON,[a,b] L. MOSCONI,[a] K. BLENNOW,[c] S. DESANTI,[a]
R. ZINKOWSKI,[d] P. D. MEHTA,[e] D. PRATICO,[f] W. TSUI,[a,b]
L. A. SAINT LOUIS,[g] L. SOBANSKA,[a] M. BRYS,[a] Y. LI,[a] K. RICH,[a]
J. RINNE,[h] AND H. RUSINEK[a]

[a] Center for Brain Health, New York University School of Medicine, New York, New York, USA

[b] Nathan Kline Institute, Orangeburg, New York, New York, USA

[c] Department of Clinical Chemistry, Sahlgren's University Hospital, Mölndal, Sweden

[d] Applied NeuroSolutions, Vernon Hills, Illinois, USA

[e] Department of Immunology, Institute for Basic Research, Staten Island, New York, USA

[f] Department of Pharmacology, University of Pennsylvania, Philadelphia, Pennslyvania, USA

[g] CDR Radiology, New York, New York, USA

[h] Turku PET Centre and Turku Imanet, Turku, Finland

ABSTRACT: It is widely believed that the path to early and effective treatment for Alzheimer's disease (AD) requires the development of early diagnostic markers that are both sensitive and specific. To this aim, using longitudinal study designs, we and others have examined magnetic resonance imaging (MRI), 2-fluoro-2-deoxy-D-glucose-positron emission tomography (FDG/PET), and cerebrospinal fluid (CSF) biomarkers in cognitively normal elderly (NL) subjects and in patients with mild cognitive impairment (MCI). Such investigations have led to the often replicated findings that structural evidence of hippocampal atrophy as determined by MRI, as well as metabolic evidence from FDG-PET scan of hippocampal damage, predicts the conversion from MCI to AD. In this article we present a growing body of evidence of even earlier diagnosis. Brain pathology can be detected in NL subjects and used to predict future transition to MCI. This prediction is enabled by examinations revealing reduced glucose metabolism in the hippocampal

Address for correspondence: Dr. Mony de Leon, Center for Brain Health, NYU School of Medicine, Department of Psychiatry, 560 First Ave., New York, N.Y. 10016. Voice: 212-263-5805; fax: 212-263-3270.

mony.deleon@med.nyu.edu

Ann. N.Y. Acad. Sci. 1097: 114–145 (2007). © 2007 New York Academy of Sciences.
doi: 10.1196/annals.1379.012

formation (hippocampus and entorhinal cortex [EC]) as well as by the rate of medial temporal lobe atrophy as determined by MRI. However, neither regional atrophy nor glucose metabolism reductions are specific for AD. These measures provide secondary not primary evidence for AD. Consequently, we will also summarize recent efforts to improve the diagnostic specificity by combining imaging with CSF biomarkers and most recently by evaluating amyloid imaging using PET. We conclude that the combined use of conventional imaging, that is MRI or FDG-PET, with selected CSF biomarkers incrementally contributes to the early and specific diagnosis of AD. Moreover, selected combinations of imaging and CSF biomarkers measures are of importance in monitoring the course of AD and thus relevant to evaluating clinical trials.

KEYWORDS: MCI; Alzheimer's disease; longitudinal imaging; CSF biomarkers; early diagnosis

## INTRODUCTION

The prevalence of Alzheimer's disease (AD) is expected to double every 20 years.[1] Worldwide in 2000, more than 25 million persons had dementia, 50–60% of which were AD. These numbers are estimated to rise to 63 million in 2030 and 114 million in 2050.[2] Feeding this trend is an estimated annual incidence of mild cognitive impairment (MCI) of about 1–2% in population studies[3,4] and about 5–9% in clinical samples.[5-9] Prevalence rates for MCI in those over 65 years range between 3% for a neuropsychologically defined isolated amnestic subtype[4,10] and as high as 25% when all cognitive subtypes of MCI are considered.[10] The annual rates of transition between MCI and AD have been estimated between 10% and 15% for the amnestic subtype,[11] but remain unknown for the other MCI subtypes. Little is known about predictors of future MCI for normal elderly (NL) subjects.[12] Part of the uncertainty is due to the reliance on unreliable and nonstandard cognitive evaluation techniques[10] and undeveloped biological markers. Recent reports show that a substantial number of MCI patients are reclassified as NL on follow-up,[3] and many MCI do not progress to dementia. In other words, clinical diagnostic evaluations, including neuropsychological tests, in the NL stages of function have not been shown to be useful for the prediction of future MCI, nor are they specific for the prediction of AD at the MCI stage. As reported by the biomarkers in AD working group of the Reagan Research Institute,[13] with improved understandings of the pathophysiology of AD and the promise of mechanism-based and preventative therapeutic approaches, there is an urgent need to develop biomarkers for early diagnosis.

The goal of this article is to highlight both the pathological context and the recent work in imaging and cerebrospinal fluid (CSF) biological markers that have set the stage for developing promising antecedent markers for AD. However, it should be noted that the summaries are not complete as they tend to emphasize our recent studies. The imaging sections of this review will focus on 2-fluoro-2-deoxy-D-glucose-positron emission tomography (FDG/PET) and magnetic resonance imaging (MRI) procedures that have been shown to predict and track the course of AD from NL to MCI[5,14,15] and from NL to AD.[14] In spite of this success, imaging modalities are not widely accepted because neither MRI tissue volume reductions nor FDG-PET glucose metabolism reductions are specific for AD, are costly, and they require intensive high-precision processing. CSF measures of total tau (T-tau) and Aβ42 levels are individually sensitive though not highly specific for AD and not sensitive to disease progression. Moreover, CSF Aβ42 levels are not easily interpreted because CSF Aβ is not exclusively brain derived and production and clearance are not well characterized. Therefore, the interpretation of abnormal concentrations of either T-tau or CSF Aβ42 is problematic and of limited use. However, recent studies have shown that the combined use of these analytes is of diagnostic value for AD.[16] Moreover, two other CSF analytes with valuable and complementary properties were individually validated: P-tau231, which has demonstrated AD specificity[17–19] and is predictive of decline from MCI to AD, and Isoprostane (IsoP), a sensitive marker of oxidative damage (diagnostic specificity unknown) that is similarly predictive of AD and uniquely sensitive to disease progression.[20–22] In addition, experimental amyloid imaging protocols were recently developed[23–27] and one PET tracer for brain fibrillar Aβ, Pittsburgh compound B (PIB),[28] became available as a research tool. Overall, we offer that these modalities, when combined, offer the potential for an early and specific diagnosis of AD.

## THE NEUROPATHOLOGY OF EARLY AD

The principal hallmarks of AD include: Aβ deposition in extracellular plaques and vascular walls, the accumulation of intracellular neurofibrillary tangles (NFT), synaptic damage, and neuronal and brain volume losses (atrophy).[29–32] The hippocampal formation, which includes the entorhinal cortex (EC), hippocampus, and subiculum, comprises the regions most vulnerable to the early deposition of NFT with synaptic damage[32–37] and neuronal and volume losses.[36,38–42] Specifically, a pattern of early hippocampal formation NFT deposition,[43–51] with relative sparing of the neocortex,[44,45,47,52,53] is often found in studies of nondemented elderly (this term includes both normal and MCI patients). Braak's neuropathology studies show NFT and neuropil thread pathology in the EC and hippocampus in the most mildly affected individuals.[54] On the other hand, Thal[55] showed that for Aβ, plaque deposition occurs first in the neocortex and EC regions before hippocampal involvement. However, which lesions occur first is unclear as both plaque-only and tangle-only nondemented cases have been observed.

Studies with transgenic (Tg) mice suggest that human Aβ oligomers induce tau pathology,[56] disrupt neuronal function,[57] and cause memory dysfunction.[58]

Several reports indicate that the Aβ oligomers may be in equilibrium with the fibrillar Aβ[59,60] suggesting that the fibrillar Aβ load (estimated using PIB-PET), may be a potentially useful surrogate marker. In this regard, the fibrillar Aβ burden shows limited association with either cognitive impairment[61,62] or brain damage[63] and may only provide an indirect measure of the active pathophysiology. Nevertheless, plaque pathology remains of intrinsic diagnostic importance. Currently there is no CSF assay available for the soluble Aβ oligomers.

In a prospective study of normal aging, Morris *et al.*[64] followed a group of NL subjects to autopsy that transitioned to and died at the MCI stage. The control group of NL subjects who remained NL did not show appreciable Aβ depositions at postmortem, whereas Aβ plaques were restricted to those NL subjects who developed MCI. On the other hand, tangle pathology was found in 20% of the normal controls and in all the MCI. Two interpretations of these results are possible—tangle deposition may precede Aβ lesion depositions in future AD patients or there may be greater diagnostic specificity associated with Aβ lesions. In either case, both lesions are needed for the pathological diagnosis of AD. Since cross-sectional preclinical data cannot separate aging from disease effects, these Aβ and tauopathy data set the stage for developing longitudinal biomarker studies. Of value in estimating the sequence of events to be expected *in vivo*, other studies show that both tau and Aβ pathology precede EC and hippocampus neuronal losses in nondemented and preclinical AD patients.[65] However, once the AD process is under way, the extent of hippocampal neuronal loss exceeds the number of NFT lesions.[66] This underlies our working hypothesis that the CSF biomarkers of tau and Aβ will contribute to imaging measures of progressive atrophy and glucose metabolism reductions in the prediction of cognitive decline.

## CSF STUDIES IN AD

### CSF Tau Studies

Two types of CSF measures for tau pathology are in use for AD: total tau (T-tau) and markers for several of the known isoforms (X) of hyperphosphorylated tau (P-TauX). T-tau, the first biomarker to be available, is the most widely used. The evidence consistently demonstrates elevated CSF concentrations of T-tau in AD and in MCI compared to NL controls.[16,67] Moreover, 11 studies show that CSF T-tau in combination with Aβ42 predicts the conversion from MCI to AD.[67] Equivalent prediction accuracies between CSF T-tau and P-tau231-235 were reported by Arai *et al.*,[68] and by Hansson *et al.* using CSF T-tau and P-tau181,[69] and by our group in collaboration with Kaj Blennow using CSF T-tau and P-tau231 (see below). However, very little is known about CSF T-tau or P-tau X levels in normal aging. Some cross-sectional studies show age-related elevations in T-tau[70] and some not.[71,72] P-tauX are not yet studied.

The T-tau level is not specific for AD as it is also elevated in other neurodegenerative diseases,[73,74] and in acute stroke,[75] where the T-tau but not the P-tau181 levels are increased and later return to normal.[75] Immunohistochemistry studies of several P-tau epitopes (phosphorylation sites) support the early diagnostic potential for P-tau231. Hyman's group observed that the P-tau231 antibodies intensely stained all stages of tangle pathology in the EC and hippocampus of AD patients.[76] P-tau231 was particularly effective at the early Braak stage III of NFT involvement. Others have shown in Braak stage ll (EC) that brain P-tau immunoreactivity is present prior to histological NFT accumulation.[77] Moreover, in nondemented elderly, the number of P-tau231-stained EC tangles was inversely associated with declarative memory function.[78]

P-tau231 offers diagnostic specificity for AD. The levels of P-tau231, but not T-tau, were consistently elevated in AD as compared with frontotemporal dementia (FTD), Lewy body dementia (LBD), vascular dementia, and NL elderly controls.[17] Recent work extended the specificity of P-tau231 for AD in studies with major depression[18] and CJD.[19] In addition, our preliminary studies show that P-tau231 shows promising specificity at the MCI stage (prior to a diagnosis of probable AD) against FTD cases (specificity and sensitivity both 75%). Similarly, others demonstrated the advantage of P-tau181 over T-tau in comparisons between AD with FTD[79,80] and with non-AD dementias.[81,82] Only one study found that P-tau181 did not differentiate AD from LBD.[74] While less is known about CSF P-tau 396–404, Iqbal reported that this P-tau assay, but not T-tau differentiated AD from vascular dementia and NL.[83]

Overall, the CSF T-tau likely reflects both the normal metabolism of tau and the nonspecific release of tau following neuronal damage, whereas CSF P-tau231 reflects abnormal tau metabolism that is both sensitive and specific for early brain AD.[84]

### CSF Aβ Studies

The genetic mutations causing early-onset familial AD (FAD) elevate the production of Aβ, particularly Aβ42,[85] and this results in increased brain Aβ deposition with a consequent reduction of the CSF levels.[86,87] A recent FAD study of patients with presenilin-1 gene mutations demonstrated CSF Aβ42 reductions in advance of clinical symptoms.[88] We recently observed widespread MRglc reductions in asymptomatic carriers of the PS1 mutation (see below) but both FDG-PET and CSF modalities have not been examined in the same subjects. CSF Aβ studies by Mehta, Blennow, and many others consistently show that relative to normal control, Aβ42 levels are also reduced in late onset AD (see reviews)[16,67] and in MCI.[69,89] A few longitudinal studies report preliminary evidence for Aβ42 levels to decrease in AD over time, however, the magnitude of change has limited diagnostic value.[74,90] There are no replicated reports of elevated CSF Aβ42 levels in either FAD or late-onset AD. Overall these CSF Aβ data are difficult to interpret because samples were derived from multiple collaborating sites with potentially different thresholds for recognizing "early" AD. Longitudinal NL data are limited, and the effects of normal aging on CSF turnover and Aβ production and clearance are poorly understood.[91–93] It has been experimentally demonstrated that with increasing age, amyloid plaques start to accumulate in the brain and may act as a sink for soluble Aβ.[94] Based on this view, assuming constant Aβ production, one would predict that age-related plaque deposition would be associated with decreased CSF Aβ levels. However, reduced Aβ clearance due to age may have confounded the longitudinal studies that failed to show differential changes in CSF Aβ42. Moreover, recent observations of reduced CSF Aβ levels in other dementias without plaque formation, alternatively suggest that reduced neuronal production of Aβ is yet another consideration in the interpretation of low CSF levels. The diagnostic utility of CSF Aβ40 as an AD biomarker is less well understood than Aβ42. A limited number of reports have shown elevated CSF Aβ40 levels with increasing age.[95,96] However, several studies failed to observe diagnostic differences between AD and NL.[97,98]

### CSF Isoprostane Studies

IsoPs are biochemically stable, prostaglandin-like compounds formed by free radical peroxidation of fatty acids. Because of increasing evidence demonstrating that oxidative stress and subtle inflammatory processes play an important role in AD pathology, detection of oxidized products from lipid peroxidation such IsoP may be helpful in the early diagnosis of AD.[99,100]

Postmortem AD studies by both the Montine and Pratico groups show elevated brain[101] and CSF IsoP levels.[102] These studies show a correlation between neuronal oxidation[101] and Braak staging of neurofibrillary pathology.[100] *In vivo*, there is consensus that CSF IsoP levels are elevated in AD[103,104] and MCI.[20,21] Our MCI data show elevated CSF IsoP levels that increase longitudinally,[20] are associated with progressive brain damage, and predict future decline to AD (see below). There is no biological basis to expect that IsoP levels are specific for AD and there are no data on normal human aging. However, Pratico *et al.* showed that elevated CSF IsoP levels distinguished AD from FTD patients[105] and Montine *et al.* showed that elevated IsoP distinguished AD from other dementias.[106]

### Correction for the CSF Dilution of X-Tau and IsoP Concentrations

Given the progressive brain damage in AD, it is surprising that CSF concentrations of T-tau and P-tauX are not consistently found to be progressive. Only a few longitudinal AD studies report increases in T-tau levels,[107–109] while many others do not show changes.[74,110–114] With similar uncertainty for P-tau231, one small study showed that in AD longitudinal levels decrease,[114] while we and others[22,68] did not find longitudinal P-tau231effects. While potential explanations for the negative longitudinal X-tau findings include short follow-up intervals and variability in the pathologic course of AD (production and clearance), our recent findings suggest that brain atrophy and an increased volume of CSF causes dilution of these proteins that, if uncorrected, confound detection of their longitudinal changes. We observed that only after controlling for the progressive ventricular enlargement in MCI and the consequent dilution of the P-tau231 concentration, were significant longitudinal increases in total loads detected[115] (see below). This finding has been replicated and extended to T-tau and IsoP.[22]

Our rationale for the ventricular volume correction is based on observations, that brain-derived proteins, such as tau, have higher levels in the ventricular than in lumbar CSF. Reiber[116] has shown that the ventricular to lumbar concentration ratio is 1.5:1 for tau and 18:1 for S-100B. Similarly, Quinn *et al.* reported that in postmortem AD, ventricular IsoP levels were twofold higher than lumbar cistern samples.[22] For systemically derived proteins,[117] ventricular to lumbar ratios <1 are found (e.g., albumin 1:205, and Aβ 1:2 [Blennow unpublished communication]).

Curiously, the recently discontinued Elan immunotherapy trial demonstrated among antibody responders, decreased brain volume, increased ventricular volume, and decreased T-tau levels.[118] The reduced tau finding was interpreted as a possible therapeutic effect but the dilution of tau was not considered. In summary, it is generally accepted that lumbar CSF X-tau and Aβ4X concentrations are potentially useful surrogate markers of brain AD. However, the poor understanding of the physiological mechanisms governing protein production and clearance from brain[119] and accumulations in CSF and plasma may limit the clinical utility of the CSF protein levels. We propose that volume-corrected measures of total loads of specific CSF analytes are important in interpreting the results of CSF biomarker studies.

## NEUROIMAGING STUDIES OF AD

### *Neuroimaging Markers for MCI and AD*

In 1989 the first study was published showing that qualitative estimates of hippocampal atrophy in MCI predicted decline to AD (see FIG. 1).[120] This finding has been replicated[121,122] and more recently, predictions of future AD were demonstrated with hippocampal volume,[123–124] and with hippocampal perfusion.[125] These early studies also demonstrated that the prevalence of hippocampal atrophy increased with age and was very common in MCI and AD (see FIG. 2).[126]

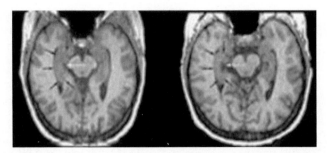

**FIGURE 1.** *Arrows* highlight the body of the hippocampus on an axial MRI image. Image on right is from an elderly patient with atrophy (increased CSF and decreased hippocampal size) and image on left from an NL volunteer.

## HIPPOCAMPAL ATROPHY AND AGE
### (N=405)

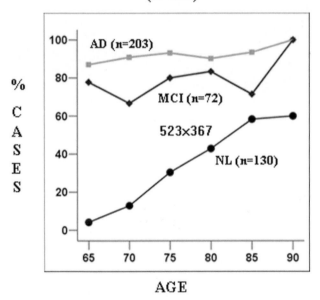

**FIGURE 2.** Frequency of hippocampal atrophy as a function of age and the diagnosis of MCI or AD.

Recent findings additionally show that reduced EC size can discriminate between MCI and NL)[127–132] and accurately predict future conversion of MCI subjects to AD.[5,128,132,133] There is also evidence to show that size or glucose metabolism (MRglc) in temporal neocortex,[134–137] and posterior cingulate gyrus,[125] can predict the MCI conversion to AD. In 2001, using FDG-PET, we published the first imaging study predicting the decline of NL to MCI. This finding was based on EC MRglc reductions. This study also showed that EC

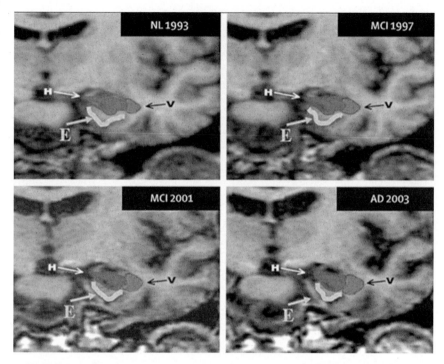

**FIGURE 3.** Ten-year time series demonstrating hippocampal, entorhinal cortex, and ventricular changes on MRI in association with clinical decline from normal to MCI to AD. Images were coregistered and displayed at a single slice at the level of the Pes hippocampus.

reductions predicted future hippocampal glucose metabolism reductions.[5] We recently showed using serial MRI that the medial temporal lobe atrophy rate during the normal stage, estimated with an automated regional boundary shift protocol, predicts the future conversion of NL to MCI.[15] Previously, Jack *et al.* demonstrated that NL patients that converted to MCI showed a greater rate of hippocampal volume loss than nondeclining subjects. However, baseline prediction of future decline to MCI was not observed.[9] Overall, these MRI-PET studies indicate the potential of hippocampal formation imaging measures to predict transitions related to AD as well as to describe disease progression from NL to MCI and to AD[138] levels of impairment (see FIG. 3).

However, the regional MRI brain volume or metabolism reductions determined by FDG-PET are not disease specific. Apart from the value in detecting stroke, normal pressure hydrocephalus, and Cruetzfeldt-Jakob disease (CJD),[139] reliable MRI markers to separate FTD and LBD from AD do not exist.[140–142] For example, both the EC and hippocampal volumes are reduced in AD and FTD as compared to controls, and, these anatomical changes do not distinguish between the two disorders.[140] Also, longitudinal whole brain atrophy changes estimated from the boundary shift integral method fail to distinguish the abnormal rates of atrophic change characteristic of both AD and FTD.[141,142]

On the other hand, FDG-PET studies have demonstrated that patterns of MRglc reduction have some differential diagnostic value. A reduced frontal MRglc with preserved posterior association area MRglc appears to be useful for recognition of FTD, but only in the earlier stages.[143] Also, reduced occipital MRglc, not found with AD, is useful for the diagnosis of LBD.[144] While there is clinical evidence validating the FDG-PET differential diagnosis, only limited numbers of FDG-PET diagnoses have been confirmed at autopsy.[145] There are virtually no studies showing that MRglc changes can be used to differentiate among these neurodegenerative disorders prior to overt symptom onset.

Only recently have PET Aβ imaging studies appeared in the literature. The pioneering reports of PIB by Klunk and Mathis and FDDNP by the UCLA group demonstrated that the compounds were valid markers of AD pathology. Specifically, PIB was reported as a marker for fibrillar Aβ[146] and FDDNP for both fibrillar Aβ and tangle pathology.[27] The widespread availability of the PIB compound has contributed to its rapid development and demonstration of its utility in AD.[146] One cross-sectional PIB study demonstrated the inverse relationship between brain fibrillar Aβ depositions and CSF Aβ42 levels.[86]

There is also a recent study of the brain regional distribution of PIB and MRglc in very mild AD patients, showing little regional relationship.[146] This is likely due to well-known differing distributions of fibrillar Aβ and NFT pathology in the early stages of disease.[55] As reviewed above, tangle pathology is more closely associated with neuronal damage than is plaque pathology. The diffuse amyloid and Aβ oligomers, potentially affecting neuronal function, are not imaged with PIB-PET. Moreover, several recent American Academy of Neurology (AAN) 2006 abstracts report elevated PIB binding in about 50% of MCI patients and in a (lesser) number of NL elderly. The prognostic significance of these PIB findings in MCI and NL remains unknown.

## NYU STUDIES IN THE EARLY DIAGNOSIS OF AD

### *MRI Studies*

*Hippocampal Size, a Marker in MCI for Future AD*

Using qualitative image analysis techniques, our early CT and subsequent MRI studies showed that the hippocampal size reduction found in MCI is a predictor of future AD.[120,121] In more recent cross-sectional and prediction studies using regional brain volumes, we observed that the hippocampal volume was the superior anatomical measurement to significantly classify MCI and elderly NL controls.[147,148] When contrasting MCI and AD patients, inclusion of the fusiform gyrus volume in the model significantly improved the ability of the hippocampal volume to separate the groups.[134] These data provide strong evidence that AD-related volume losses are most sensitively detected in the hippocampus in MCI, and indicate that in predicting the transition to dementia, it is important to consider both hippocampal and temporal lobe neocortical volume reductions.

*Hippocampal Size and Declarative Memory Performance*

In cross-sectional studies of NL and MCI, as compared with a temporal lobe neocortical reference volume, the hippocampal volume showed an anatomically unique correlation to delayed verbal recall.[147,149] In a 4-year follow-up study of 44 NL subjects, we observed that reduced delayed recall performance was predicted by a smaller baseline hippocampus[150] ($R^2 = 0.65$, $P < 0.001$).

*Neuropathological Validation Studies of the MRI Hippocampal Volume*

We completed a neuropathology study validating the MRI hippocampal volume.[151] Specifically, the hippocampal volumes from 16 AD and 4 NL were determined from hemispheric tissue sections and from comparably sliced postmortem T1-weighted MRI scans. Unbiased estimates were made of the number of hippocampal neurons. The results showed a strong correlation between the MRI and the tissue-derived hippocampal volumes, $r = 0.97$, $P < 0.001$. Restricting the analysis to the AD group left the correlation unchanged, $r = 0.97$, $P < 0.001$. The difference in the hippocampal volumes between normal and AD groups was 42% for the MRI data, and after adjusting for tissue shrinkage during specimen processing, 40% for the tissue data. Moreover, both the tissue-based and the MRI-based hippocampal volume measurements were significantly associated with the number of hippocampal neurons, ($r = 0.91$, $P < 0.001$ and $r = 0.90$, $P < 0.01$, respectively, see FIG. 4).

*Neuropathological Validation Studies of the MRI Entorhinal Cortex Surface Area*

We validated the MRI measurement of the surface area of the EC.[131] The gray and white matter boundaries of the entorhinal and perirhinal cortices (EC) are poorly demarcated on MRI making total cortical ribbon volume studies unreliable with standard MRI imaging protocols. Several recent studies have used partial estimates of the EC ribbon to avoid this problem and applied this to AD and to MCI.[129,152,153] Using postmortem materials we validated an MRI image analysis method that avoided this problem by estimating the surface area

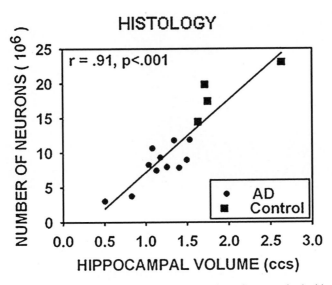

**FIGURE 4.** The relationship between the total number of neurons in the hippocampus and the hippocampal volume.

of the EC (the sum across slices of the ribbon lengths multiplied by the slice thickness). We used serial 3 mm sections stained with cresyl violet to define three measurements: a histology-based EC volume, a histology-determined EC surface area, and EC surface area based on sulcal and gyral landmarks visible on MRI (EC-MRI). We studied 16 AD patients and 4 NL controls. The histology surface area was measured between the most medial boundary (pyriform cortex, or amygdala, or presubiculum, or parasubiculum) and the most lateral aspect (alternatively referred to as perirhinal or transentorhinal cortex). Using the MRI landmark method, the surface area was bounded medially (superiorly) by the sulcus semianularis on anterior sections and the medial parahippocampal gyrus on posterior sections. The lateral (inferior) boundary, in the anterior sections was the depth of the rhinal sulcus and in the posterior sections, the depth of the collateral sulcus. The results showed that the histology-based volume of the EC was significantly related to both surface area measurements: histological $r = 0.94$, $P < 0.001$; and landmark $r = 0.91$, $P < 0.001$. Between the two groups, the following measures were significantly ($P < 0.01$) reduced in AD: volume 61%, histological surface area 49%, and landmark surface area 45%. An *in vivo* study of 8 NL and 8 mildly impaired AD patients included in the same publication, found significant between group differences of 27% for the landmark EC method and 12% differences for the hippocampal volume.[131] Individually, the EC correctly classified 100% of the controls and 87% of the AD group. By comparison, the hippocampus classified 88% of the controls and 75% of the AD patients. Multivariate logistic regression models

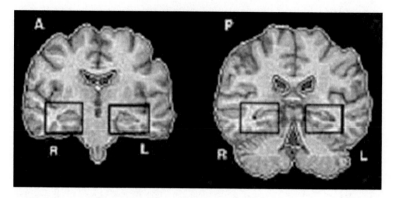

**FIGURE 5.** Anterior and posterior limits of the medial temporal lobe regions (box shaped) sampled using the regional boundary shift method. Since the focus of this study was the annual rate of tissue loss, this study sacrificed anatomical accuracy for the ability to detect atrophy rate with the highest possible precision and in an automated manner.

showed that the EC measure was superior to the hippocampus in the diagnostic classification of the groups ($X^2$ (1) = 22.2, $P < 0.001$).

*Semiautomated Medial Temporal Lobe Atrophy Predicts the Conversion from NL to MCI*

Brain atrophy rate was assessed using an automated procedure entailing a modification of the Boundary-Shift Algorithm (BSA) of Fox.[154,155] Analyses were restricted to sampling the MTL and whole brain (see FIG. 5). Forty-five NL elderly subjects were given a comprehensive battery of clinical and neuropsychological tests at baseline and every 2 years for three follow-ups (2, 4, and 6 years).[15] The same 1.5T MRI machine and T1-weighted high-resolution sequence were acquired at baseline and the 2-year follow-up. By the 6-year time point, a total of 13 subjects had declined. The results show that the annualized rates of MTL change between the baseline and 2-year exams best separated ($P < 0.05$) the declining and nondeclining NL groups. At baseline, and at follow-up, whole brain atrophy was also increased in the decliners, but this measure did not show good predictive ability. Of particular interest, the NL group that declined to MCI after the second scan ($n = 6$) also showed a significantly elevated MTL atrophy rate (0.7% per year) as compared with the 32 nondeclining NL group (0.3% per year), $t$ (36) = $-3.1$, $P < 0.01$. After controlling for age, gender, education, and the rate of whole brain atrophy, the MTL rate incremented the prediction and the overall accuracy was 89% (40/45), with 94% specificity (30/32) and 77% sensitivity (10/13). This image analysis involves a minimal user intervention (selection of the first and last coronal hippocampal slice), but it does require high-resolution serial MRI and stringent quality control of the MRI system.

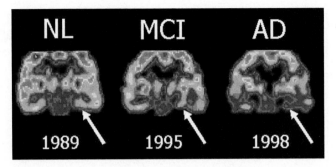

**FIGURE 6.** Longitudinal metabolic reductions on FDG-PET. FDG-PET scans in a 71-year-old cognitively normal woman at baseline (1989) and over 9 years. During this observation period the patient declined to MCI and later was diagnosed with Alzheimer's disease, which was confirmed at autopsy. For each observation a coronal PET scan is depicted at the level of the entorhinal cortex and anterior hippocampus. Arrows point to the progressively darker image of the inferior surface of the entorhinal cortex, which indicates progressive reductions in glucose metabolism.

## *FDG-PET Studies*

### *EC Glucose Metabolism Predicts Conversion from NL to MCI*

In a longitudinal FDG-PET study of NL, mean age $= 72$ years, range 60–80 years), the EC was sampled on MRI based on the above described postmortem-validated anatomical criteria.[131] These and other regions-of-interest (ROI) were used to sample coregistered PET scans (see FIG. 6). We reported[5] that baseline EC MRglc reductions accurately predicted decline to MCI with a sensitivity of 83%, $n = 12$, and a specificity of 85%, $n = 13$, $(X^2 (1) = 20.8, P < 0.001$, odds ratio $= 1.42$, confidence interval (95%) $= 1.08–1.88$). Those NL subjects that progressed to MCI showed, at follow-up, significant MRglc reductions in the hippocampus and temporal neocortex as compared with nondeclining NL. These results advanced our appreciation of the EC pathology that occurs early in the course of AD.

### *The Automated and Anatomy-Validated FDG-PET HIPMask Sampling Procedure*

We developed an automated and anatomically precise sampling technique (HIPMask) to study the hippocampus on PET.[156] This technique combines automated nonlinear size normalization procedures[157] with the anatomical precision of the "gold-standard" ROI approach. The HIPMask is derived from and was validated on MRI in elderly NL, MCI, and AD brains after

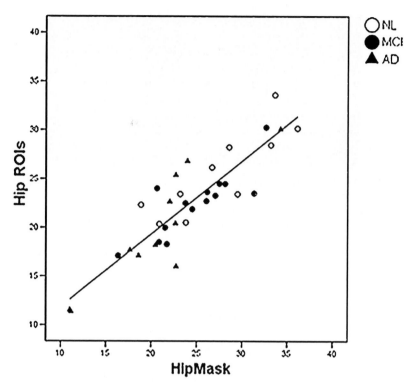

**FIGURE 7.** Scatterplot showing the strong relationship between the individually determined hippocampal MRglc and automated sampling of the hippocampus using the HIP-Mask. The data are shown for normal, MCI, and AD patients.

nonlinear spatial normalization to a common reference space. The HIP-Mask is the result of a "training" procedure that maximizes the overlap across subjects while minimizing the volume of false-positive (non-HIP) voxels. Validation using an independent sample demonstrated that on average 96% (range 82–100%) of the content of the HipMask is true hippocampus tissue, as determined with respect to the individual MRI-ROI. The HIPMask was also tested for agreement with the hippocampus ROI sampling method (see FIG. 7). A high correlation was found between the ROI and the HIPMask MRglc measures separately for NL ($r = 0.91$), MCI ($r = 0.88$), and AD ($r = 0.87$) groups ($Ps < 0.001$).[156] Moreover, the ROI and the HIPMask showed relative to NL, equivalent hippocampus MRglc reductions in MCI (ROI:14%, HIPMask:10%) and AD (ROI:31%, HIPMask:33%) ($Ps < 0.05$). Overall, these results demonstrate that the HIPMask method precisely samples the hippocampus on PET and that automated procedures are suitable for sampling the hippocampus.

## Hippocampal MRglc Predicts Decline from NL Aging to AD

We completed the longitudinal study of 78 NL elderly subjects that were followed over a period averaging 9 years (range 7 to 14 years).[14] At study end, 19 declined to MCI (NL-MCI), 6 were diagnosed AD (NL-AD) with 2 confirmed at autopsy, and 5 to other diagnostic outcomes. At baseline and longitudinally, using the HIPMask[156] to examine the hippocampus and Statistical Parametric Mapping (SPM)[158] for all voxels from the entire brain, our results show that hippocampus MRglc was the only predictor of future cognitive decline from NL. The time between the baseline PET and the onset of MCI/AD was 9 ± 2 years. Neocortical regional voxel clusters were not found for significant prediction effects. At baseline (when all the subjects were NL), as compared to NL-NL, the hippocampus MRglc was reduced 26% in NL-AD, $P = 0.002$, and 15% in NL-MCI ($P = 0.01$) [$F(3,75) = 5.23$, $P = 0.002$].

Significant ($Ps < 0.05$) longitudinal effects were found for the hippocampus MRglc. The annual rate of hippocampus MRglc reduction was greater for NL-AD ($4.4 \pm 0.7\%$, $P < 0.001$) and NL-MCI ($2.4 \pm 0.2\%$, $P > 0.01$) relative to NL-NL ($0.8 \pm 0.3\%$). We conclude that reduced hippocampal metabolism, in the normal stages of cognition, is a sensitive marker of future AD.

## FDG-PET MRglc Is Superior to MRI Volume in the Diagnosis of MCI

Cross-sectional data were used to test three hypotheses: (1) EC and hippocampus measures from either modality are superior to temporal neocortical measures in the discrimination of NL ($n = 11$) and MCI ($n = 15$); (2) neocortical measures are most useful in the separation of AD ($n = 12$) from MCI; (3) measures of PET MRglc provide greater diagnostic accuracy than MRI volume.[148] The three groups were matched on age (75 years), education (15 years), and gender (40–50% female). FDG-PET and MRI scans were coregistered to enable volume sampling and atrophy correction. Logistic regression analyses showed two significant regional PET classifiers of NL and MCI: the EC (85%) and hippocampus (73%) MRglc. For MRI-based discrimination only the hippocampus (73%) was significant. For separation of MCI and AD, high significance was found in middle/inferior temporal gyri on both PET and MRI (both with 81% accuracy) while PET contributed additional regions. Hippocampus and temporal cortex MRglc and volume measures significantly classified AD and NL (78–100%). With a frequency of significant findings of nearly 2:1, regional MRglc measures were superior to volume measures in classifying the three groups. These cross-sectional effects, observed after atrophy correction, suggest that in MCI, hippocampus changes precede neocortical changes and that metabolism reductions can be detected prior to volume losses.

*Qualitative Rating of MTL Hypometabolism in MCI and AD*

Visual inspection is the preferred technique for clinical evaluation of FDG-PET images. Traditionally, the evaluation of AD has focused on the presence of posterior cortical (predominantly parietal and posterior cingulate cortex [PCC]) hypometabolism. However, the usefulness of cortical hypometabolism in classifying patients with MCI is inconsistent, a finding we also observed in quantitative studies.[14,148] Conversely, studies using precise MRglc sampling, show consistent evidence for MTL MRglc reductions in MCI.[5,148,156,159] In the absence of prior FDG-PET studies of MCI or AD using an MTL visual rating, we developed and tested a visual rating scale for MTL hypometabolism.[160] We examined 75 subjects in three age- and gender-balanced groups (27 NL, 26 MCI, and 22 AD). Four-point visual rating scales were developed to separately evaluate hypometabolism in MTL and in the cortex. For validation purposes, the visual MTL ratings were compared with quantitative hippocampus MRglc data extracted using MRI coregistered ROI.[5]

High intra- and interrater reliabilities were found for both the MTL and cortical ratings, (ICC $= 0.98$, $Ps < 0.001$). The validation results show that the MTL rating and the hippocampus ROI MRglc measures are highly correlated ($r = -0.76$, $P < 0.001$) and yield comparable diagnostic accuracies for AD versus NL (rating:81% and ROI: 77%), and MCI versus NL (rating:74% and ROI: 67%) ($Ps < 0.001$). In differentiating MCI from NL, the addition of MTL to the cortical ratings significantly improves the diagnostic accuracy from 62% ($P > 0.05$) to 78% ($P < 0.05$). These results show that a visual MTL rating procedure is reliable, yields a diagnostic accuracy equal to the quantitative ROI measures, and like quantitative data is clinically more sensitive than cortical ratings for patients with MCI.[160]

*Hypometabolism Exceeds Atrophy in Presymptomatic*
*Early-Onset Familial AD*

In collaboration with Dr. Sandro Sorbi from the University of Florence (Italy), we found that FDG-PET MRglc reductions precede MRI atrophy in presymptomatic carriers from families with early-onset AD (FAD) due to mutations in the presenilin-1 gene (PS-1).[161] FAD is characterized by autosomal dominant inheritance with nearly 50% penetrance and a specific age of onset for a given pedigree.[162] Therefore, study of presymptomatic mutation carriers close to the expected age of onset provides unique information about preclinical AD-related brain changes. Seven asymptomatic individuals at genetic risk, from three Italian families with PS-1 FAD (Clinical Dementia Rating (CDR) = 0, age 35–49 years, 4/7 women, education $\geq 12$ years) and 7 age- and gender-matched NL controls received complete clinical, neuropsychological, MRI, and FDG-PET examinations. Patients were examined on average $13 \pm 9$ years (range 1–27 years) prior to estimated onset of the disease. Volumes of interest for the whole brain, hippocampus, EC, PCC, inferior parietal lobule (IPL), and superior temporal gyrus (STG) were drawn bilaterally on the MRI scans of all subjects and also used to sample the MRglc from the coregistered PET scans. For MRI, as compared to NL, after correcting for head size, volume reductions in FAD subjects were found only in the IPL (18%, $P \leq 0.01$). For PET, after atrophy correction and adjusting for pons MRglc, MRglc reductions ($Ps < 0.05$) were found in the whole brain (13%), hippocampus (12%), the left EC (21%), PCC (20%), IPL (17%), and the STG (12%) ($Ps < 0.05$). Overall, presymptomatic FAD patients show widespread MRglc reductions consistent with the typical AD PET pattern in the relative absence of structural brain atrophy. These data further suggest that PET MRglc measures contribute to the presymptomatic diagnosis of AD.

## CSF Biomarker Studies

### The Incremental Diagnostic Value of CSF and MRI Hippocampus Markers in MCI

In a 2-year longitudinal study of MCI patients and normal controls, we examined the hypothesis that CSF markers for these pathological features improve the diagnostic accuracy over memory and MRI–hippocampal volume evaluations.[20] Relative to control, MCI patients showed decreased memory and hippocampal volumes and elevated CSF concentrations of P-tau231 and IsoP. These two CSF measures consistently improved the diagnostic accuracy over the memory measures and the IsoP measure incremented the accuracy of the hippocampal volume achieving overall diagnostic accuracies of about 90%. These results demonstrate that CSF biomarkers for AD contribute to the characterization of MCI.

### MRI Correction for the Ventricular Volume Dilution of Tau

In a 1-year follow-up study of NL elderly ($n = 10$, GDS = $1.6 + 0.5$, MMSE = $29.4 + 0.7$, age = $62.5 + 9.2$) and MCI ($n = 8$, GDS = $3.0 + 0.4$, MMSE = $28.5 \pm 1.2$, age = $69.8 \pm 9.2$) we examined lumbar CSF levels (pg/mL) of P-tau231 and ventricular volume. The ventricular volume corrected for head-size (ratio) was greater in MCI at both baseline ($t$ (16) $=-2.1$, $P < 0.05$) and at follow-up ($t$ (16) $= -2.2$, $P < 0.05$). P-tau231 levels were elevated in the MCI group at baseline (Mann–Whitney $U = 14.0$, $P < 0.05$, $n = 18$) and at follow-up ($U = 6.0$, $P < 0.01$, $n = 18$). No longitudinal changes were observed in either P-tau231 or ventricular volume ($P > 0.05$). To control for possible dilution effects (see FIG. 8), we estimated ventricular CSF P-tau231 load (ng) by multiplying the P-tau231 level (pg/mL) by the ventricular volume (mL)

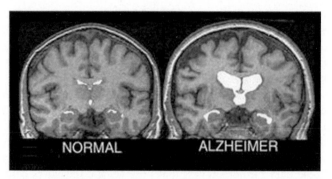

**FIGURE 8.** Ventricular anatomy highlighted in a control and in an AD patient. The lateral ventricle volumes range between 2 and 10 × and are progressive.

and dividing by 1,000.[115] P-tau231 loads were elevated in the MCI group at baseline (Mann–Whitney $U = 11$, $P < 0.01$, $n = 18$) and at follow-up ($U = 6$, $P = 0.001$, $n = 18$). In the longitudinal design, we observed a significant group by time interaction for the annualized P-tau231 load ($U = 12.0$, $P < 0.05$, $n = 18$). Post hoc examination showed a significant P-tau231 load increase restricted to the MCI group (Wilcoxon Signed Ranks Test $Z = -2.1$, $P < 0.05$, $n = 8$). We directly compared annualized longitudinal P-tau231 load and P-tau231 level changes, using two hierarchical linear regression models with reversed orders of entry, in the prediction of diagnostic group. At the first entry steps, only the delta P-tau231 load was related to group membership ($R^2 = 0.38$, ($F$ [1,16] $= 9.6$, $P < 0.01$). Comparing the second entry steps, the delta P-tau231 load uniquely increased the variance explained by the delta P-tau231 level ($R^2$ change $= 0.23$, $F$ [1,15] $= 5.8$, $P < 0.05$). This dilution correction was recently applied to T-tau and IsoP following a postmortem CSF validation study by the Seattle group.[22] The results confirm the earlier observation of longitudinal Tau load effects and extend this to include longitudinal IsoP load effects when concentration differences were not observed.

*CSF X-Tau Biomarkers Prediction Transition from MCI to AD*[163]

In collaboration with Kaj Blennow (University of Goteborg, Sweden) we studied a group of 41 MCI subjects, and examined the 2-year prediction of decline to AD (20 decliners and 21 nondecliners). The results show that both P-tau231 and T-tau gave overall correct predictions of 85% $Ps < 0.001$ ($X^2 = 16.6$ and $X^2 = 14.0$, respectively). IsoP yielded 81% ($X^2 = 15.3$, $P < 0.001$) and Aβ42, 71% ($X^2 = 7.8$, $P < 0.01$). The 2-year longitudinal data showed that IsoP changes correctly classified

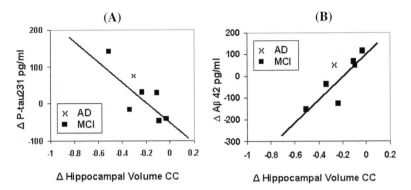

**FIGURE 9.** The longitudinal relationship in MCI between: (**A**) the changes in P-tau231 and changes in hippocampal volume, and in (**B**) between Aβ42 and hippocampal volume. The **x** shows the data for the MCI patient that transitioned to AD.[20]

81% of decliners ($X^2 = 9.6$, $P < 0.01$) and Aβ42, 71% ($X^2 = 5.6$, $P < 0.05$). However, neither P-tau231 nor T-tau showed significant longitudinal effects. Ventricular volume dilution correction studies are in progress.

*Longitudinal Correlation in MCI of AD-Related CSF Proteins with Hippocampal Volume*

Because of the known inverse relationships at postmortem between the hippocampus volume and tau pathology and, albeit to a lesser extent, between brain Aβ42 depositions and hippocampus volume reductions, we examined the hypothesis that these relationships could be observed *in vivo* using MRI and CSF measures.[20] Over a 1.5-year interval, in a preliminary analysis of 7 MCI subjects, we observed a strong relationship between hippocampus volume reductions and both elevations in P-tau231 concentrations ($r = -0.79$, $P < 0.05$) and reductions in Aβ42 concentrations ($r = 0.82$, $P < 0.05$). These observations show that the uncorrected longitudinal changes in three biomarkers for AD (hippocampus volume, Ptau231, and Aβ42) are correlated in MCI (see Fig. 9).

*11C-PIB Binding Is Increased in MCI and AD*

In collaboration with Juha Rinne at the Turku PET Center in Finland we used FDG-PET, PIB-PET, and MRI to examine 7 NL, 9 MCI, and 17 AD patients. PIB-PET data was dynamically collected and the "noninvasive Logan" analysis performed with the cerebellum as the reference using

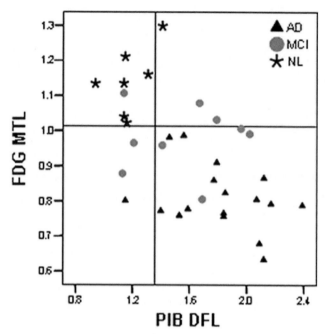

**FIGURE 10.** Scatterplot showing the relationship between FDG-PET (*y axis*) and PIB-PET (*x axis*) in the diagnosis of NL (*stars*), MCI (*circles*), and AD patients (*triangles*).

the 60–90 min scans. Voxel-based morphometry (VBM), as performed with SPM, was used for image registration, spatial normalization, and smoothing to standardize all brains to a common space.[164] Spatially normalized MRI templates were used to sample regional brain PIB uptake. Standard arterialized venous input functions were used to derive the FDG-PET regional MRglc. For FDG, the maximum regional omnibus diagnostic differences were found in the Medial Temporal Lobe (MTL) ($F$ (2,30) = 33.9, $P <$ 0.001) and for PIB, in the dorsolateral frontal (DFL) region ($F$ (2,30) =10.6, $P < 0.001$). Post-hoc tests show significant group differences between all three groups for FDG-MTL ($P$'s < 0.01), and for PIB-DFL, differences were found between the controls and both the MCI and the AD groups ($P$'s ≤ 0.05). In a logistic regression classifying AD and control, both FDG-MTL and PIB-DFL, individually, had high diagnostic accuracy, that is, 100% ($X^2$ (1) = 29, $P < 0.001$) and 92% ($X^2$ (1) = 18, $P < 0.001$), respectively. Logistic regression showed that the overall accuracy for distinguishing NL from MCI was 75% ($P < 0.05$) for both FDG and PIB. Combining the two measures by adding PIB-DFL to FDG-MTL improved the classification of NL and MCI to 94% ($X^2$ (1) = 4, $P < 0.05$, see FIG. 10). These data suggest that the use of these two PET techniques offers a potential for the sensitive and more specific diagnosis of AD.

# CONCLUSIONS

Drugs that modify the pathology of AD are now entering clinical trials. For treatment to be most effective, it is believed that the regimen must be started before significant downstream damage—that is, before clinical diagnosis of AD, at the stage of MCI, or even earlier. Patients with MCI are at high risk for dementia, but not all patients with MCI develop AD. Two complementary modalities, imaging and CSF biomarker studies, are making the early diagnosis of AD possible. Considerable data show that MRI and FDG-PET modalities are sensitive to early changes of AD. In fact there is evidence that during the normal stages of cognition, AD-related changes can be detected with imaging that offers meaningful diagnostic prediction. However, these imaging studies are not diagnostically specific as other degenerative diseases are known to affect brain structure and function. High concentrations of either CSF T-tau (an indicator of neuronal damage) or hyperphosphorylated P-tau (indicative of tau fibrillization and tangle formation), in combination with reduced concentrations of amyloid-$\beta$1–42 (a major component of senile plaques), can accurately identify patients with MCI who are at risk of developing AD.[67] A recent large study clearly showed that these CSF measures are predictive of future AD.[69] The 95% sensitivity and 83% specificity for the detection of preclinical AD in this MCI cohort is impressive, especially because further follow-up could improve the specificity if some patients with currently stable MCI or controls develop the disease. CSF and imaging modalities have complementary advantages. Our studies show that diagnostic separation between healthy people and those with MCI was raised to 94% when hippocampal volume measures were combined with either CSF measures of P-tau (87%) or IsoP (88%)[20] (a measure of lipid peroxidation[165]). Thus it appears that specific CSF analytes can contribute to MRI imaging and as estimated from other studies[17] can also provide diagnostic specificity for AD.

Recently, it has been shown that PET also enables imaging of amyloid accumulations, which in AD are inversely related to CSF A$\beta$42 concentrations. However, because the early amyloid burden spares the hippocampus, amyloid imaging is unlikely to replace the need for imaging the hippocampal formation with either PET or MRI, or for assessing CSF for P-tau, known to originate in the hippocampal formation in early AD. In conclusion, advances in the early diagnosis of AD, made possible by the combined use of CSF assays for A$\beta$ and tau pathology and imaging modalities, will encourage a revision of the current clinical standards for the diagnosis of the disease and provide the rationale for early treatment. As in many other diseases, early diagnosis when combined with preclinical treatment, could be the most effective strategy.

## ACKNOWLEDGMENTS

These projects were supported by NIH AG12101, AG08051, AG03051, and AG13616.

# REFERENCES

1. BROOKMEYER, R., S. GRAY & C. KAWAS. 1998. Projections of Alzheimer's disease in the United States and the public health impact of delaying disease onset. Am. J. Pub. Health **88:** 1337–1342.
2. WIMO, A., L. JONSSON & B. WINBLAD. 2006. An estimate of the worldwide prevalence and direct costs of dementia in 2003. Dement. Ger. Cogn. Dis. **21:** 175–181.
3. LARRIEU, S., L. LETENNEUR & J.M. ORGOGOZO. 2002. Incidence and outcome of mild cognitive impairment: a population-based prospective cohort. Neurology **59:** 1594-1599.
4. GANGULI, M., H.H. DODGE, C. SHEN & S.T. DEKOSKY. 2004. Mild cognitive impairment, amnestic type: an epidemiologic study. Neurology **63:** 115–121.
5. DE LEON, M.J., A. CONVIT, O.T. WOLF, *et al.* 2001. Prediction of cognitive decline in normal elderly subjects with 2-[18F]fluoro-2-deoxy-D-glucose/positron-emission tomography (FDG/PET). Proc. Natl. Acad. Sci. USA **98:** 10966–10971.
6. ADAK, S., K. ILLOUZ, W. GORMAN, *et al.* 2004. Predicting the rate of cognitive decline in aging and early Alzheimer disease. Neurology **63:** 108–114.
7. MARQUIS, S., M.M. MOORE, D.B. HOWIESON, *et al.* 2002. Independent predictors of cognitive decline in healthy elderly persons. Arch. Neurol. **59:** 601–606.
8. CSERNANSKY, J.G., L. WANG, J. SWANK, *et al.* 2005. Preclinical detection of Alzheimer's disease: hippocampal shape and volume predict dementia onset in the elderly. Neuroimage **25:** 783–792.
9. JACK, C.R., R.C. PETERSEN, Y. XU, *et al.* 2000. Rates of hippocampal atrophy correlate with change in clinical status in aging and AD. Neurology **55:** 484–489.
10. MANLY, J.J., S. BELL-MCGINTY, M.X. TANG, *et al.* 2005. Implementing diagnostic criteria and estimating frequency of mild cognitive impairment in an urban community. Arch. Neurol. **62:** 1739–1746.
11. PETERSEN, R.C., G.E. SMITH, S.C. WARING, *et al.* 1999. Mild cognitive impairment: clinical characterization and outcome. Arch. Neurol. **56:** 303–308.
12. FELDMAN, H.H. & C. JACOVA. 2005. Mild cognitive impairment. Am. J. Geriatr. Psychiatry **13:** 645–655.
13. CONSENSUS WORKING GROUP, CONSENSUS REPORT OF THE WORKING GROUP ON: "MOLECULAR AND BIOCHEMICAL MARKERS OF ALZHEIMER'S DISEASE." 1998. The Ronald and Nancy Reagan Research Institute of the Alzheimer's Association and the National Institute on Aging. Neurobiol. Aging **19:** 109–116.
14. MOSCONI, L., S. DE SANTI, J. LI, *et al.* 2006. Hippocampal hypometabolism predicts decline from normal aging to Alzheimer's disease. Neurobiol. Aging. In press.
15. RUSINEK, H., S. DE SANTI, D. FRID, *et al.* 2003. Regional brain atrophy rate predicts future cognitive decline: 6-year longitudinal MR imaging study of normal aging. Radiology **229:** 691–696.
16. BRYS, M., L. MOSCONI, S. DE SANTI, *et al.* 2006. CSF biomarkers for mild cognitive impairment. Aging Health **2:** 111–121.
17. BUERGER, K., R. ZINKOWSKI, S.J. TEIPEL, *et al.* 2002. Differential diagnosis of Alzheimer disease with cerebrospinal fluid levels of tau protein phosphorylated at threonine 231. Arch. Neurol. **59:** 1267–1272.

18. BUERGER, K., R. ZINKOWSKI, S.J. TEIPEL, *et al.* 2003. Differentiation of geriatric major depression from Alzheimer's disease with CSF tau protein phosphorylated at threonine 231. Am. J. Psychiatry **160:** 376–379.

19. BUERGER, K., M. OTTO, S.J. TEIPEL, *et al.* 2006. Dissociation between CSF total tau and tau protein phosphorylated at threonine 231 in Creutzfeldt-Jakob disease. Neurobiol. Aging **27:** 10–15.

20. DE LEON, M.J., S. DE SANTI, R. ZINKOWSKI, *et al.* 2006. Longitudinal CSF and MRI biomarkers improve the diagnosis of mild cognitive impairment. Neurobiol. Aging **27:** 394–401.

21. PRATICO, D., C.M. CLARK, F. LIUN, *et al.* 2002. Increase of brain oxidative stress in mild cognitive impairment: a possible predictor of Alzheimer disease. Arch. Neurol. **59:** 972–976.

22. QUINN, J.F., K.S. MONTINE, M. MOORE, *et al.* 2004. Suppression of longitudinal increase in CSF $F_2$-isoprostanes in Alzheimer's disease. J. Alzheimer's Dis. **6:** 93–97.

23. BENVENISTE, H., G. EINSTEIN, K.R. KIM, *et al.* 1999. Detection of neuritic plaques in Alzheimer's disease by magnetic resonance microscopy. Proc. Natl. Acad. Sci. USA **96:** 14079–14084.

24. ZHEN, W., H. HAN, M. ANGUIANO, *et al.* 1999. Synthesis and amyloid binding properties of rhenium complexes: preliminary progress toward a reagent for SPECT imaging of Alzheimer's disease brain. J. Med. Chem. **42:** 2805–2815.

25. SKOVRONSKY, D.M., B. ZHANG, M.P. KUNG, *et al.* 2000. In vivo detection of amyloid plaques in a mouse model of Alzheimer's disease. Proc. Natl. Acad. Sci. USA **97:** 7609–7614.

26. WENGENACK, T.M., G.L. CURRAN & J.F. PODUSLO. 2000. Targeting Alzheimer amyloid plaques *in vivo*. Nat. Biotechnol. **18:** 868–872.

27. AGDEPPA, E.D., V. KEPE, J. LIU, *et al.* 2001. Binding characteristics of radiofluorinated 6-dialkylamino-2-naphthylethylidene derivatives as positron emission tomography imaging probes for beta-amyloid plaques in Alzheimer's disease. J. Neurosci. **21:** 1–5.

28. MATHIS, C.A., B.J. BACSKAI, S.T. KAJDASZ, *et al.* 2002. A lipophilic thioflavin-T derivative for positron emission tomography (PET) imaging of amyloid in brain. Bioorg. Med. Chem. Lett. **12:** 295–298.

29. BALL, M.J. 1978. Topographic distribution of neurofibrillary tangles and granulovascular degeneration in hippocampal cortex of aging and demented patients. A quantitative study. Acta Neuropathologica (Berlin) **42:** 73–80.

30. BALL, M.J., V. HACHINSKI, A. FOX, *et al.* 1985. A new definition of Alzheimer's disease: a hippocampal dementia. Lancet **1:** 14–16.

31. BRAAK, H. 1985. On areas of transition between entorhinal allocortex and temporal isocortex in the human brain. Normal morphology and lamina-specific pathology in Alzheimer's disease. Acta Neuropathol (Berl) **68:** 325–332.

32. BRAAK, H. & E. BRAAK. 1991. Neuropathological staging of Alzheimer-related changes. Acta Neuropathologica **82:** 239–259.

33. AMARAL, D.G. & R. INSAUSTI. 1990. Hippocampal formation. *In*: G. Paxinos, Ed.: 711–755. The Human Nervous System. Academic Press. San Diego.

34. LORENTE DE NO, R. 1934. Studies on the structure of the cerebral cortex. II. Continuation of the study of the ammonic system. J. Psychologie Neurologie **46:** 113–177.

35. ARNOLD, S.E., B.T. HYMAN, J. FLORY, *et al.* 1991. The topographical and neuroanatomical distribution of neurofibrillary tangles and neuritic plaques in the cerebral cortex of patients with Alzheimer's disease. Cereb. Cortex **1**: 103–116.
36. HYMAN, B.T., G.W. VAN HOESEN, A.R. DAMASIO & C.L. BARNES. 1984. Alzheimer's disease: cell-specific pathology isolates the hippocampal formation. Science **225**: 1168–1170.
37. HYMAN, B.T., G.W. VAN HOESEN & A.R. DAMASIO. 1990. Memory-related neural systems in Alzheimer's disease: an anatomic study. Neurology **40**: 1721–1730.
38. BALL, M.J. 1977. Neuronal loss, neurofibrillary tangles and granulovacuolar degeneration in the hippocampus with ageing and dementia. Acta Neuropathologica (Berlin) **37**: 111–118.
39. BOBINSKI, M.J., J. WEGIEL, H.M. WISNIEWSKI, *et al.* 1996. Neurofibrillary pathology—correlation with hippocampal formation atrophy in Alzheimer disease. Neurobiol. Aging **17**: 909–919.
40. BOBINSKI, M., J. WEGIEL, M. TARNAWSKI, *et al.* 1997. Relationships between regional neuronal loss and neurofibrillary changes in the hippocampal formation and duration and severity of Alzheimer disease. J. Neuropath. Exp. Neurol. **56**: 414–420.
41. DE LA MONTE, S.M. 1989. Quantitation of cerebral atrophy in preclinical and end-stage Alzheimer's disease. Ann. Neurol. **25**: 450–459.
42. GOMEZ-ISLA, T., J.L. PRICE, D.W. MCKEEL, JR., *et al.* 1996. Profound loss of layer II entorhinal cortex neurons occurs in very mild Alzheimer's disease. J. Neurosci. **16**: 4491–4500.
43. HUBBARD, B.M., G.W. FENTON & J.M. ANDERSON. 1990. A quantitative histological study of early clinical and preclinical Alzheimer's disease. Neuropathol. App. Neurobiol. **16**: 111–121.
44. PRICE, J.L., P.B. DAVIS, J.C. MORRIS & D.L. WHITE. 1991. The distribution of tangles, plaques and related immunohistochemical markers in healthy aging and Alzheimer's disease. Neurobiol. Aging **12**: 295–312.
45. ARRIAGADA, P.V., K. MARZLOFF & B.T. HYMAN. 1992. Distribution of Alzheimer-type pathologic changes in nondemented elderly individuals matches the pattern in Alzheimer's disease. Neurology **42**: 1681–1688.
46. GIANNAKOPOULOS, P., P.R. HOF, S. MOTTIER, *et al.* 1994. Neuropathological changes in the cerebral cortex of 1258 cases from a geriatric hospital: retrospective clinicopathological evaluation of a 10-year autopsy population. Acta Neuropathologica **87**: 456–468.
47. ULRICH, J. 1985. Alzheimer changes in nondemented patients younger than sixty-five: Possible early stages of Alzheimer's disease and senile dementia of Alzheimer type. Ann. Neurol. **17**: 273–277.
48. VERMERSCH, P., B. FRIGARD, J.-P. DAVID, *et al.* 1992. Presence of abnormally phosphorylated Tau proteins in the entorhinal cortex of aged non-demented subjects. Neurosci. Lett. **144**: 143–146.
49. JELLINGER, K.A. 1995. Alzheimer's changes in non-demented and demented patients. Acta Neuropathologica **89**: 112–113.
50. GUILLOZET, A.L., S. WEINTRAUB, D.C. MASH & M.M. MESULAM. 2003. Neurofibrillary tangles, amyloid, and memory in aging and mild cognitive impairment. Arch. Neurol. **60**: 729–736.
51. GIANNAKOPOULOS, P., F.R. HERRMANN, T. BUSSIERE, *et al.* 2003. Tangle and neuron numbers, but not amyloid load, predict cognitive status in Alzheimer's disease. Neurology **60**: 1495–1500.

52. LANGUI, D., A. PROBST & J. ULRICH. 1995. Alzheimer's changes in non-demented and demented patients: A statistical approach to their relationships. Acta Neuropathol. **89:** 57–62.

53. MORRIS, J.C., D.W. MCKEEL, M. STORANDT, *et al.* 1991. Very mild Alzheimer's disease: Informant-based clinical, psychometric, and pathological distinction from normal aging. Neurology **41:** 469–478.

54. BRAAK, H. & E. BRAAK. 1997. Aspects of cortical destruction in Alzheimer's disease. *In* Connections, Cognition and Alzheimer's Disease. B.T. Hyman, C. Duyckaerts & Y. Christen, Eds.: 1-16. Springer-Verlag. Berlin.

55. THAL, D.R., U. RUB, M. ORANTES & H. BRAAK. 2002. Phases of A beta-deposition in the human brain and its relevance for the development of AD. Neurology **58:** 1791–1800.

56. ODDO, S., A. CACCAMO, L. TRAN, *et al.* 2006. Temporal profile of amyloid-beta (abeta) oligomerization in an *in vivo* model of Alzheimer disease: a link between abeta and tau pathology. J. Biol. Chem. **281:** 1599–1604.

57. TOWNSEND, M., G. SHANKAR, T. MEHTA, *et al.* 2006. Effects of secreted oligomers of amyloid {beta}-protein on hippocampal synaptic plasticity: a potent role for trimers. J. Physiol. (Lond). **572**(Pt 2)**:** 477–492.

58. LESNE, S., M.T. KOH, L. KOTILINEK, *et al.* 2006. A specific amyloid-[beta] protein assembly in the brain impairs memory. Nature **440:** 352–357.

59. TANZI, R.E. 2005. The synaptic A[beta] hypothesis of Alzheimer disease. Nat. Neurosci. **8:** 977–979.

60. GANDY, S. 2005. The role of cerebral amyloid beta accumulation in common forms of Alzheimer disease. Rev. J. Clin. Invest. **115:** 1121–1129.

61. HULETTE, C.M., K.A. WELSH-BOHMER, A.M. SAUNDERS, *et al.* 1998. Neuropathological and neuropsychological changes in "normal" aging: evidence for preclinical Alzheimer disease in cognitively normal individuals. J. Neuropath. Exp. Neurol. **57:** 1168–1174.

62. HAROUTUNIAN, V., D.P. PERL, D.P. PUROHIT, *et al.* 1998. Regional distribution of neuritic plaques in the nondemented elderly and subjects with very mild Alzheimer disease. Arch. Neurol. **55:** 1185–1191.

63. ADLARD, P.A. & J.C. VICKERS. 2002. Morphologically distinct plaque types differentially affect dendritic structure and organisation in the early and late stages of Alzheimer's disease. Acta Neuropathologica **103:** 377–383.

64. MORRIS, J.C., M. STORANDT, D.W. MCKEEL, *et al.* 1996. Cerebral amyloid deposition and diffuse plaques in "normal" aging: Evidence for presymptomatic and very mild Alzheimer's disease. Neurology **46:** 707–719.

65. PRICE, J.L., A.I. KO, M.J. WADE, *et al.* 2001. Neuron number in the entorhinal cortex and CA1 in preclinical Alzheimer disease. Arch. Neurol. **58:** 1395–1402.

66. KRIL, J.J., S. PATEL, A.J. HARDING & G.M. HALLIDAY. 2002. Neuron loss from the hippocampus of Alzheimer's disease exceeds extracellular neurofibrillary tangle formation. Acta Neuropathologica **103:** 370–376.

67. BLENNOW, K. & H. HAMPEL. 2003. CSF markers for incipient Alzheimer's disease. Lancet Neurol. **2:** 605–613.

68. ARAI, H., K. ISHIGURO, H. OHNA, *et al.* 2000. CSF phosphorylated tau protein and mild cognitive impairment: A prospective study. Exp. Neurol. **166:** 201–203.

69. HANSSON, O., H. ZETTERBERG, P. BUCHHAVE, *et al.* 2006. Association between CSF biomarkers and incipient Alzheimer's disease in patients with mild cognitive impairment: a follow-up study. Lancet Neurol. **5:** 228–234.

70. BUERGER NEE, B.K., F. PADBERG, T. NOLDE, *et al.* 1999. Cerebrospinal fluid tau protein shows a better discrimination in young old (<70 years) than in old patients with Alzheimer's disease compared with controls. Neurosci Lett. **277:** 21–24.

71. HULSTAERT, F., K. BLENNOW, A. IVANOIU, *et al.* 1999. Improved discrimination of AD patients using β-amyloid (1–42) and tau levels in CSF. Neurology **52:** 1555–1562.

72. ANDREASEN, N., L. MINTHON, P. DAVIDSSON, *et al.* 2001. Evaluation of CSF-tau and CSF-Abeta42 as diagnostic markers for Alzheimer disease in clinical practice. Arch. Neurol. **58:** 373–379.

73. ARAI, H., Y. MORIKAWA, M. HIGUCHI, *et al.* 1997. Cerebrospinal fluid tau levels in neurodegenerative diseases with distinct tau-related pathology. Biochem. Biophys. Res. Commun. **236:** 262–264.

74. MOLLENHAUER, B., M. BIBL, C. TRENKWALDER, *et al.* 2005. Follow-up investigations in cerebrospinal fluid of patients with dementia with Lewy bodies and Alzheimer's disease. J. Neural Transm. **112:** 933–948.

75. HESSE, C., L. ROSENGREN, N. ANDREASEN, *et al.* 2001. Transient increase in total tau but not phospho-tau in human cerebrospinal fluid after acute stroke. Neurosci. Lett. **297:** 187–190.

76. AUGUSTINACK, J.C., A. SCHNEIDER, E.M. MANDELKOW & B.T. HYMAN. 2002. Specific tau phosphorylation sites correlate with severity of neuronal cytopathology in Alzheimer's disease. Acta Neuropathologica **103:** 26–35.

77. MUKAETOVA-LADINSKA, E.B., F. GARCIA-SIERA, J. HURT, *et al.* 2000. Staging of cytoskeletal and beta-amyloid changes in human isocortex reveals biphasic synaptic protein response during progression of Alzheimer's disease. Am. J. Pathol. **157:** 623–636.

78. MITCHELL, T.W., E.J. MUFSON, J.A. SCHNEIDER, *et al.* 2002. Parahippocampal tau pathology in healthy aging, mild cognitive impairment, and early Alzheimer's disease. Ann. Neurol. **51:** 182–189.

79. VANMECHELEN, E., H. VANDERSTICHELE, P. DAVIDSSON, *et al.* 2000. Quantification of tau phosphorylated at threonine 181 in human cerebrospinal fluid: a sandwich ELISA with a synthetic phosphopeptide for standardization. Neurosci. Lett. **285:** 49–52.

80. SJOGREN, M., P. DAVIDSSON, M. TULLBERG, *et al.* 2001. Both total and phosphorylated tau are increased in Alzheimer's disease. J. Neurol. Neurosurg. Psychiatry **70:** 624–630.

81. ISHIGURO, K., H. OHNO, H. ARAI, *et al.* 1999. Phosphorylated tau in human cerebrospinal fluid is a diagnostic marker for Alzheimer's disease. Neurosci. Lett. **270:** 91–94.

82. PARNETTI, L., A. LANARI, S. AMICI, *et al.* 2001. Phospho-Tau International Study, G., CSF phosphorylated tau is a possible marker for discriminating Alzheimer's disease from dementia with Lewy bodies. Phospho-Tau International Study Group. Neurol. Sci. **22:** 77–78.

83. HU, Y.Y., S.S. HE, X. WANG, *et al.* 2002. Levels of nonphosphorylated and phosphorylated tau in cerebrospinal fluid of Alzheimer's disease patients: an ultrasensitive bienzyme-substrate-recycle enzyme-linked immunosorbent assay. Am. J. Pathol. **160:** 1269–1278.

84. MITCHELL, A. & N. BRINDLE. 2003. CSF phosphorylated tau–does it constitute an accurate biological test for Alzheimer's disease? Int. J. Geriat. Psychiat. **18:** 407–411.

85. HARDY, J. & D.J. SELKOE. 2002. The amyloid hypothesis of Alzheimer's disease: progress and problems on the road to therapeutics. Science **297:** 353–356.

86. FAGAN, A.M., M.A. MINTUN, R.H. MACH, *et al.* 2006. Inverse relation between *in vivo* amyloid imaging load and cerebrospinal fluid. Ann. Neurol. **3:** 512–519.

87. DEMATTOS, R.B., K.R. BALES, M. PARSADANIAN, *et al.* 2002. Plaque-associated disruption of CSF and plasma amyloid-beta (Abeta) equilibrium in a mouse model of Alzheimer's disease. J. Neurochem. **81:** 229–236.

88. MOONIS, M.M., J.M. SWEARER, M.P. DAYAW, *et al.* 2005. Familial Alzheimer disease: decreases in CSF A[beta]42 levels precede cognitive decline. Neurology **65:** 323–325.

89. ANDREASEN, N. & K. BLENNOW. 2005. CSF biomarkers for mild cognitive impairment and early Alzheimer's disease. Clin. Neurol. Neurosurg. **107:** 165–173.

90. TAPIOLA, T., T. PIRTTILA, M. MIKKONEN, *et al.* 2000. Three-year follow-up of cerebrospinal fluid tau, B-amyloid 42 and 40 concentrations in Alzheimer's disease. Neurosci. Lett. **280:** 119–122.

91. BADING, J.R., S. YAMADA, J.B. MACKIC, *et al.* 2002. Brain clearance of Alzheimer's amyloid-beta40 in the squirrel monkey: a SPECT study in a primate model of cerebral amyloid angiopathy. J. Drug Target. **10:** 359–368.

92. SILVERBERG, G.D., E. LEVINTHAL, E.V. SULLIVAN, *et al.* 2002. Assessment of low-flow CSF drainage as a treatment for AD: results of a randomized pilot study. Neurology **59:** 1139–1145.

93. SILVERBERG, G.D.H. 2001. The cerebrospinal fluid production rate is reduced in dementia of the Alzheimer's type. Neurology **57:** 1763–1766.

94. DEMATTOS, R.B., K.R. BALES, D.J. CUMMINS, *et al.* 2001. Peripheral anti-Abeta antibody alters CNS and plasma Abeta clearance and decreases brain Abeta burden in a mouse model of Alzheimer's disease. Proc. Natl. Acad. Sci. USA **98:** 8850–8855.

95. FUKUYAMA, R., T. MIZUNO, S. MORI, *et al.* 2000. Age-dependent change in the levels of Abeta40 and Abeta42 in cerebrospinal fluid from control subjects, and a decrease in the ratio of Abeta42 to Abeta40 level in cerebrospinal fluid from Alzheimer's disease patients. Eur. Neurol. **43:** 155–160.

96. SHOJI, M., M. KANAI, E. MATSUBARA, *et al.* 2001. The levels of cerebrospinal fluid Abeta40 and Abeta42(43) are regulated age-dependently. Neurobiol. Aging **22:** 209–215.

97. KANAI, M., E. MATSUBARA, K. ISOE, *et al.* 1998. Longitudinal study of cerebrospinal fluid levels of tau, A beta1-40, and A beta1-42(43) in Alzheimer's disease: a study in Japan. Ann. Neurol. **44:** 17–26.

98. MEHTA, P.D., T. PIRTTILA, S.P. MEHTA, *et al.* 2000. Plasma and cerebrospinal fluid levels of amyloid beta proteins 1-40 and 1-42 in Alzheimer disease. Arch. Neurol. **57:** 100–105.

99. MARKESBERY, W.R. & J.M. CARNEY. 1999. Oxidative alterations in Alzheimer's disease. Brain Pathol. (Zurich, Switzerland) **9:** 133–146.

100. MONTINE, T.J., W.R. MARKESBERY, J.D. MORROW & L.J. ROBERTS. 1998. Cerebrospinal fluid F2-isoprostane levels are increased in Alzheimer's disease. Ann. Neurol. **44:** 410–413.

101. MONTINE, T.J., W.R. MARKESBERY, W. ZACKERT, *et al.* 1999. The magnitude of brain lipid peroxidation correlates with the extent of degeneration but not with density of neuritic plaques or neurofibrillary tangles or with APOE genotype in Alzheimer's disease patients. Am. J. Pathol. **155:** 863–868.

102. PRATICO, D., V. MY LEE, J.Q. TROJANOWSKI, *et al.* 1998. Increased F2-isoprostanes in Alzheimer's disease: evidence for enhanced lipid peroxidation *in vivo*. FASEB J **12:** 1777–1783.

103. MONTINE, T.J., M.F. BEAL, M.E. CUDKOWICZ, *et al.* 1999. Increased CSF F2-isoprostane concentration in probable AD. Neurology **52:** 562–565.

104. PRATICO, D., C.M. CLARK, V.M. LEE, *et al.* 2000. Increased 8,12-iso-iPF2alpha-VI in Alzheimer's disease: correlation of a noninvasive index of lipid peroxidation with disease severity. Ann. Neurol. **48:** 809–812.

105. YAO, Y., V. ZHUKAREVA, S. SUNG, *et al.* 2003. Enhanced brain levels of 8,12-iso-iPF2{alpha}-VI differentiate AD from frontotemporal dementia. Neurology **61:** 475–478.

106. MONTINE, T.J., J.A. KAYE, K.S. MONTINE, *et al.* 2001. Cerebrospinal fluid abeta42, tau, and F$_2$-isoprostane concentrations in patients with Alzheimer disease, other dementias, and in age-matched controls. Arch. Pathol. Lab. Med. **125:** 510–512.

107. BLOMBERG, M., M. JENSEN, H. BASUN, *et al.* 1996. Increasing cerebrospinal fluid tau levels in a subgroup of Alzheimer patients with apolipoprotien E allele ε4 during 14 months follow-up. Neurosci. Lett. **214:** 163–166.

108. ARAI, H., M. TERAJIMA, M. MIURA, *et al.* 1997. Effect of genetic risk factors and disease progression on the cerebrospinal fluid tau levels in Alzheimer's disease. JAGS **45:** 1228–1231.

109. KANAI, M., M. SHIZUKA, K. URAKAMI, *et al.* 1999. Apolipoprotein E4 accelerates dementia and increases cerebrospinal fluid tau levels in Alzheimer's disease. Neurosci. Lett. **267:** 65–68.

110. SUNDERLAND, T., B. WOLOZIN, D. GALASKO, *et al.* 1999. Longitudinal stability of CSF tau levels in Alzheimer patients. Biol. Psychiatry **46:** 750–755.

111. NISHIMURA, T., M. TAKEDA, Y. NAKAMURA, *et al.* 1998. Basic and clinical studies on the measurement of tau protein in cerebrospinal fluid as a biological marker for Alzheimer's disease and related disorders: multicenter study in Japan. Methods Findings Exp. Clin. Pharmacol. **20:** 227–235.

112. ANDREASEN, N., L. MINTHON, A. CLARBERG, *et al.* 1999. Sensitivity, specificity, and stability of CSF-tau in AD in a community-based patient sample. Neurology **53:** 1488–1494.

113. ANDREASEN, N., L. MINTHON & E. VANMECHELEN. 1999. Cerebrospinal fluid tau and Abeta42 as predictors of development of Alzheimer's disease in patients with mild cognitive impairment. Neurosci. Lett. **273:** 5–8.

114. HAMPEL, H., K. BUERGER, R. KOHNKEN, *et al.* 2001. Tracking of Alzheimer's disease progression with cerebrospinal fluid tau protein phosphorylated at threonine 231. Ann. Neurol. **49:** 545–546.

115. DE LEON, M.J., C.Y. SEGAL, C.Y. TARSHISH, *et al.* 2002. Longitudinal CSF tau load increases in mild cognitive impairment. Neurosci. Lett. **333:** 183–186.

116. REIBER, H. 2001. Dynamics of brain-derived proteins in cerebrospinal fluid. Clinica Chimica Acta **310:** 173–186.

117. KUO, Y.M., T.A. KOKJOHN, M.D. WATSON, *et al.* 2000. Elevated abeta42 in skeletal muscle of Alzheimer disease patients suggests peripheral alterations of abetaPP metabolism. Am. J. Pathol. **156:** 797–805.

118. FOX, N.C., R.S. BLACK, S.F. GILMAN, *et al.* 2005. for the AN1792(QS-21)-201 Study Team, Effects of A[beta] immunization (AN1792) on MRI measures of cerebral volume in Alzheimer disease. Neurology **64:** 1563–1572.

119. PRESTON, S.D., P.V. STEART, A. WILKINSON, *et al.* 2003. Capillary and arterial cerebral amyloid angiopathy in Alzheimer's disease: defining the perivascular route for the elimination of amyloid beta from the human brain. Neuropathol. App. Neurobiol. **29:** 106–117.

120. DE LEON, M.J., A.E. GEORGE, L.A. STYLOPOULOS, *et al.* 1989. Early marker for Alzheimer's disease: the atrophic hippocampus. Lancet **2:** 672–673.

121. DE LEON, M.J., J. GOLOMB, A.E. GEORGE, *et al.* 1993. The radiologic prediction of Alzheimer's disease: the atrophic hippocampal formation. Am. J. Neuroradiol. **14:** 897–906.

122. VISSER, P.J., P. SCHELTENS, F.R.J. VERBY, *et al.* 1999. Medial temporal lobe atrophy and memory dysfunction as predictors for dementia in subjects with mild cognitive impairment. J. Neurol. **246:** 477–485.

123. JACK, C.R., JR., R.C. PETERSEN, Y.C. XU, *et al.* 1999. Prediction of AD with MRI-based hippocampal volume in mild cognitive impairment. Neurology **52:** 1397–1403.

124. WOLF, H., V. JELIC, H.J. GERTZ, *et al.* 2003. A critical discussion of the role of neuroimaging in mild cognitive impairment. Acta Neurologica Scandinavica. Supplementum **179:** 52–76.

125. JOHNSON, K.A., K. JONES, B.L. HOLMAN, *et al.* 1998. Preclinical prediction of Alzheimer's disease using SPECT. Neurology **50:** 1563–1571.

126. DE LEON, M.J., A.E. GEORGE, J. GOLOMB, *et al.* 1997. Frequency of hippocampal formation atrophy in normal aging and Alzheimer's disease. Neurobiol. Aging **18:** 1–11.

127. DU, A.T., N. SCHUFF, D. AMEND, *et al.* 2001. Magnetic resonance imaging of the entorhinal cortex and hippocampus in mild cognitive impairment and Alzheimer's disease. J. Neurol. Neurosurg. Psychiatry **71:** 441–447.

128. DICKERSON, B.C., I. GONCHAROVA, M.P. SULLIVAN, *et al.* 2001. MRI-derived entorhinal and hippocampal atrophy in incipient and very mild Alzheimer's disease. Neurobiol. Aging **22:** 747–754.

129. XU, Y., C.R.J. JACK, P.C. O'BRIEN, *et al.* 2000. Usefulness of MRI measures of entorhinal cortex versus hippocampus in AD. Neurology **54:** 1760–1767.

130. JUOTTONEN, K., M.P. LAAKSO, R. INSAUSTI, *et al.* 1998. Volumes of the entorhinal and perirhinal cortices in Alzheimer's disease. Neurobiol. Aging **19:** 15–22.

131. BOBINSKI, M., M.J. DE LEON, A. CONVIT, *et al.* 1999. MRI of entorhinal cortex in mild Alzheimer's disease. Lancet **353:** 38–40.

132. DE TOLEDO-MORRELL, L., I. GONCHAROVA, B. DICKERSON, *et al.* 2000. From healthy aging to early Alzheimer's disease: *in vivo* detection of entorhinal cortex atrophy. Ann. N.Y. Acad. Sci. **911:** 240–253.

133. KILLIANY, R.J., T. GOMEZ-ISLA, M. MOSS, *et al.* 2000. Use of structural magnetic resonance imaging to predict who will get Alzheimer's disease. Ann. Neurol. **47:** 430–439.

134. CONVIT, A., J. DE ASIS, M.J. DE LEON, *et al.* 2000. Atrophy of the medial occipitotemporal, inferior, and middle temporal gyri in non-demented elderly predict decline to Alzheimer's disease. Neurobiol. Aging **21:** 19–26.

135. PIETRINI, P., N.P. AZARI, C.L. GRADY, *et al.* 1993. Pattern of cerebral metabolic interactions in a subject with isolated amnesia at risk for Alzheimer's disease: a longitudinal evaluation. Dementia **4:** 94–101.

136. BERENT, S., B. GIORDANI, N. FOSTER, *et al.* 1999. Neuropsychological function and cerebral glucose utilization in isolated memory impairment and Alzheimer's disease. J. Psychiat. Res. **33:** 7–16.

137. ARNAIZ, E., V. JELIC, O. ALMKVIST, et al. 2001. Impaired cerebral glucose metabolism and cognitive functioning predict deterioration in mild cognitive impairment. Neuroreport 12: 851–855.
138. RUSINEK, H., Y. ENDO, S. DE SANTI, et al. 2004. Atrophy rate in medial temporal lobe during progression of Alzheimer disease. Neurology 63: 2354–2359.
139. COLLIE, D.A., R.J. SELLAR, M. ZEIDLER, et al. 2001. MRI of Creutzfeldt-Jakob disease: imaging features and recommended MRI protocol. Clin. Radiol. 56: 726–739.
140. FRISONI, G.B., M.P. LAAKSO, A. BELTRAMELLO, et al. 1999. Hippocampal and entorhinal cortex atrophy in frontotemporal dementia and Alzheimer's disease. Neurology 52: 91–100.
141. O'BRIEN, J.T., S. PALING, R. BARBER, et al. 2001. Progressive brain atrophy on serial MRI in dementia with Lewy bodies, AD, and vascular dementia. Neurology 56: 1386–1388.
142. CHAN, D., N.C. FOX, R. JENKINS, et al. 2001. Rates of global and regional cerebral atrophy in AD and frontotemporal dementia. Neurology 57: 1756–1763.
143. DIEHL-SCHMID, J., T. GRIMMER, A. DRZEZGA, et al. 2007. Decline of cerebral glucose metabolism in frontotemporal dementia: a longitudinal 18F-FDG-PET-study. Neurobiol. Aging 28: 1060–1063.
144. MCKEITH, I.G., D.W. DICKSON, J. LOWE, et al. 2005. For the Consortium on DLB, diagnosis and management of dementia with Lewy bodies: third report of the DLB consortium. Neurology 65: 1863–1872.
145. SILVERMAN, D.H.S., G.W. SMALL, C.Y. CHANG, et al. 2001. Positron emission tomography in evaluation of dementia: regional brain metabolism and long-term outcome. JAMA 286: 2120–2127.
146. KLUNK, W.E., H. ENGLER, A. NORDBERG, et al. 2004. Imaging brain amyloid in Alzheimer's disease with Pittsburgh Compound-B.[see comment]. Ann. Neurol. 55: 306–319.
147. CONVIT, A., M.J. DE LEON, C. TARSHISH, et al. 1997. Specific hippocampal volume reductions in individuals at risk for Alzheimer's disease. Neurobiol. Aging 18: 131–138.
148. DE SANTI, S., M.J. DE LEON, H. RUSINEK, et al. 2001. Hippocampal formation glucose metabolism and volume losses in MCI and AD. Neurobiol. Aging 22: 529–539.
149. GOLOMB, J., A. KLUGER, M.J. DE LEON, et al. 1994. Hippocampal formation size in normal human aging: a correlate of delayed secondary memory performance. Learn. Mem. 1: 45–54.
150. GOLOMB, J., A. KLUGER, M.J. DE LEON, et al. 1996. Hippocampal formation size predicts declining memory performance in normal aging. Neurology 47: 810–813.
151. BOBINSKI, M., M.J. DE LEON, J. WEGIEL, et al. 2000. The histological validation of postmortem magnetic resonance imaging-determined hippocampal volume in Alzheimer's disease. Neuroscience 95: 721–725.
152. KILLIANY, R.J., B.T. HYMAN, T. GOMEZ-ISLA, et al. 2002. MRI measures of entorhinal cortex vs. hippocampus in preclinical AD. Neurology 58: 1188–1196.
153. DE TOLEDO-MORRELL, L., T.R. STOUB, M. BULGAKOVA, et al. 2004. MRI-derived entorhinal volume is a good predictor of conversion from MCI to AD. Neurobiol. Aging 25: 1197–1203.

154. FREEBOROUGH, P.A., R.P. WOODS & N.C. FOX. 1996. Accurate registration of serial 3D MR brain images and its application to visualizing change in neurodegenerative disorders. J. Comp. Assist. Tom. **20:** 1012–1022.

155. FOX, N.C. & P.A. FREEBOROUGH. 1997. Brain atrophy progression measured from registered serial MRI: validation and application to Alzheimer's disease. J. Mag. Res. Imag. **7:** 1069–1075.

156. MOSCONI, L., W.H. TSUI, S. DE SANTI, *et al.* 2005. Reduced hippocampal metabolism in mild cognitive impairment and Alzheimer's disease: automated FDG-PET image analysis. Neurology **64:** 1860–1867.

157. FRISTON, K., J. ASHBURNER, C. FRITH, *et al.* 1995. Spatial registration and normalization of images. Hum. Brain Map. **3:** 165–189.

158. FRISTON, K.J., C.D. FRITH, P.F. LIDDLE & R.S.J. FRACKOWIAK. 1991. Comparing functional (PET) images: the assessment of significant change. J. Cereb. Blood Flow Metab. **11:** 690–699.

159. NESTOR, P.J., T.D. FRYER, P. SMIELEWSKI & J.R. HODGES. 2003. Limbic hypometabolism in Alzheimer's disease and mild cognitive impairment. Ann. Neurol. **54:** 343–351.

160. MOSCONI, L., S. DE SANTI, Y. LI, *et al.* 2006. Visual rating of medial temporal lobe metabolism in mild cognitive impairment and Alzheimer's disease using FDG-PET. Eur. J. Nucl. Med. **33:** 210–221.

161. MOSCONI, L., S. SORBI, M.J. DE LEON, *et al.* 2006. Hypometabolism exceeds atrophy in presymptomatic early-onset familial Alzheimer's disease. J. Nucl. Med. **47:** 1778–1786.

162. TANZI, R.E. & L. BERTRAM. 2001. New frontiers in Alzheimer's disease genetics. Neuron. **32:** 181–184.

163. BUERGER, K., S.J. TEIPEL, R. ZINKOWSKI, *et al.* 2002. CSF tau protein phosphorylated at threonine 231 correlates with cognitive decline in MCI subjects. Neurology **59:** 627–629.

164. GOOD, C.D., R.I. SCAHILL, N.C. FOX, *et al.* 2002. Automatic differentiation of anatomical patterns in the human brain: validation with studies of degenerative dementias. Neuroimage **17:** 29–46.

165. PRATICO, D., J.A. LAWSON, J. ROKACH & G.A. FITZGERALD. 2001. The isoprostanes in biology and medicine. Trends Endocrinol. Metab. **12:** 243–247.

# Functional MRI Studies of Associative Encoding in Normal Aging, Mild Cognitive Impairment, and Alzheimer's Disease

REISA SPERLING

*Department of Neurology, Memory Disorders Unit, Brigham and Women's Hospital, Alzheimer's Disease Research Center and Gerontology Research Unit, Massachusetts General Hospital, Massachusetts, USA*

*Department of Neurology, Harvard Medical School, Massachusetts, USA*

ABSTRACT: Functional magnetic resonance imaging (fMRI) is a non-invasive neuroimaging technique that can be used to study the neural correlates of complex cognitive processes, and the alterations in these processes that occur in the course of normal aging or superimposed neurodegenerative disease. Our studies have focused on the neural substrates of successful associative encoding, particularly of face–name associations. We have found that the specific regions of the hippocampus and prefrontal cortices are critical for successful memory in both young and healthy older subjects. Our fMRI studies, as well as those of several other groups, have consistently demonstrated that, compared to cognitively intact older subjects, patients with clinical Alzheimer's disease (AD) have decreased fMRI activation in the hippocampus and related structures within the medial temporal lobe during the encoding of new memories. More recently, fMRI studies of subjects at risk for AD, by virtue of their genetics or evidence of mild cognitive impairment (MCI), have yielded variable results. Some of these studies, including our own, suggest that there may be a phase of paradoxically increased activation early in the course of prodromal AD. Further studies to validate fMRI in these populations are needed, particularly longitudinal studies to investigate the pattern of alterations in functional activity over the course of prodromal AD and the relationship to AD pathology.

KEYWORDS: fMRI; aging; Alzheimer's disease; hippocampus; memory

## INTRODUCTION

Alzheimer's disease (AD) affects 1 of every 10 individuals over the age of 65 years, and remains one of the most feared consequences associated with

Address for correspondence: Reisa Sperling, M.D., Memory Disorders Unit, 221 Longwood Avenue, Boston, MA 02215. Voice: 617-732-8085; fax: 617-264-5212.
reisa@rics.bwh.harvard.edu

Ann. N.Y. Acad. Sci. 1097: 146–155 (2007). © 2007 New York Academy of Sciences.
doi: 10.1196/annals.1379.009

aging. The past decade has seen remarkable advances in our understanding of the pathophysiological process of AD, yet we lack a detailed understanding of how the pathology of AD results in the emergent clinical syndrome of memory impairment. Furthermore, it remains quite difficult to reliably differentiate the earliest symptoms of AD from the memory changes that may occur in the course of normal aging. Functional neuroimaging techniques hold tremendous promise in elucidating the neural underpinnings of memory impairment in AD, and the neural alterations that occur in the process of aging.

Functional magnetic resonance imaging (fMRI) is a noninvasive imaging technique that enables the assessment of brain function during complex cognitive processes, such as memory and learning. Although fMRI is an indirect measure of neural activity, it provides a "window" into the functional alterations that occur in aging and age-associated neurodegenerative diseases.

Our own fMRI work has focused primarily on associative memory processes, in particular face–name associations. Converging evidence suggests that one primary role of the hippocampal formation in episodic encoding is to form new associations between previously unrelated items of information.[1,2] Learning the names of new individuals we encounter can be thought of as a particularly difficult cross-modal, noncontextual, paired-associate memory task. Difficulty remembering proper names is the most common memory complaint of older individuals visiting memory clinics.[3,4] Several neuropsychological studies have also suggested that difficult paired-associate memory tasks may be particularly useful in detecting the earliest memory impairment in AD.[5–7] Multiple fMRI studies have recently reported that associative memory paradigms produce robust activation of the anterior hippocampal formation,[8–10] and our own fMRI studies in young subjects using a face–name associative encoding task confirm these findings.[11–13]

## fMRI ALTERATIONS IN NORMAL AGING

Our initial studies in aging utilized a "block design" fMRI paradigm, which compared the fMRI activation during the encoding of Novel face–name pairs to the viewing of Repeated face–name pairs (see FIG. 1). All of the face–name pairs are unfamiliar to the subjects, are taken from a library of 700 faces ranging

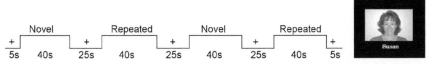

**FIGURE 1.** The block design fMRI paradigm (shown on left) alternates epochs of Novel face–name pairs (shown only once during the experiment) with Repeated face–name pairs (a male and female face–name pair, each shown 42 times over the course of the experiment), as well as periods of visual fixation on a cross-hair. The face–name stimuli (example shown on the right) are unfamiliar faces paired with fictional first names.

from age 18 years through 87 years, and are varied in gender and ethnicity.[12] Each face is paired with a fictional name, taken from Internet lists of the most popular names from each decade.

Our first fMRI study of normal aging compared 10 young controls and 10 older controls.[14] We found that young and older subjects showed an overall similar pattern of fMRI activation for the Novel versus Repeated contrast. Both young and older subjects activated the anterior hippocampal formation during novel encoding ($P < 0.001$), although older subjects' hippocampal activation was more limited in extent. Using a random-effects, between-group comparison of the Novel versus Repeated contrast, young and older controls differed primarily in the pattern of prefrontal and parietal activation. Older subjects showed less prefrontal and greater parietal activation than young for the Novel versus Repeated contrast. Interestingly, this difference was driven by continued prefrontal activation to Repeated stimuli in the older controls.

To follow up on this finding, and also to try to enhance encoding success in older subjects, our next experiment utilized an event-related fMRI paradigm to examine the response to repeated stimulus exposure.[15] In this study, we examined 12 older controls during encoding of face–name pairs that were each shown three times. We were particularly interested in the pattern of activation for face–name pairs that were subsequently remembered correctly with high confidence (i.e., successful encoding). We found that during the initial encoding trial for successfully encoding face–name pairs, the older controls showed robust anterior hippocampal activation, similar to the pattern we had observed in young subjects with single encoding trials.[13] During the second and third encoding trials, however, there was no significant hippocampal activation, and in fact there was evidence of the MR signal in the hippocampus being suppressed to below baseline levels (see FIG. 2). Interestingly, the prefrontal cortex showed a different response to repeated stimulus exposure, with continued activation above baseline even on the third encoding trial. We concluded that the memory benefits of repeated stimulus exposure in normal aging are likely due to neocortical mechanisms rather than any additional encoding activity in the medial temporal lobe.

In a recent event-related fMRI study, we compared 17 young and 17 older subjects during associative encoding with a large number of face–name pairs, each shown only once for 3.75 sec.[16] In this study, subjects were tested immediately after scanning on each of the 230 face–name pairs shown during the fMRI. We used a forced-choice recognition test, with each face paired with two names: the correct name and a name that was paired with a different face during scanning. Subjects were also asked to indicate high or low confidence in their choice. Older subjects performed significantly worse than younger subjects on this task, so we confined our analyses to those face–name pairs that were successfully remembered compared to those that were forgotten. Our study demonstrated that both young and older subjects showed significantly greater hippocampal activation during the encoding of face–name pairs

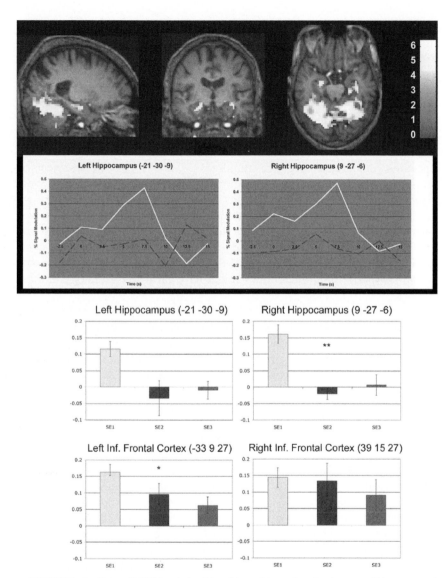

**FIGURE 2.** Group fMRI data in healthy older subjects showing increased hippocampal activation for the first successful encoding trial compared to second and third encoding trials. Statistical maps for activation in the first encoding trial greater than the second (shown on *top left*) with extracted time courses of MRI signal (shown on *bottom left*) demonstrate significant differences in the hippocampus. Region of interest analyses of fMRI signal change (shown on *right*) revealed that the hippocampal signal returns to baseline or below on the second and third encoding trial (*top right*) whereas prefrontal cortices show continued activation for all three trials (*bottom right*).

that were successfully remembered compared to forgotten pairs ($P < 0.005$). We found a similar extent and magnitude of activation in the hippocampus comparing young and older controls.

In this experiment, we also examined areas of the brain that showed memory-related "deactivations," that is, a decrease in MR signal associated with task. Other researchers had reported that young subjects demonstrated deactivation in medial parietal regions during successful encoding,[17] but this had not been examined in older individuals. We found that young subjects showed very significant deactivation in the precuneus and posterior cingulate during successful encoding compared to forgotten stimuli ($P < 0.00001$), but older subjects as a group did not show evidence of differential deactivation responses in these regions. We then subdivided the older group on the basis of their postscan test performance, and found that the high-performing older subjects showed greater deactivation in the precuneus than the low-performing older subjects ($P < 0.01$). The precuneus and posterior cingulate are regions of great interest in MCI and AD (see below), and thus we speculated that perhaps some of the low-performing older adults might have early AD pathology in these regions.

Our experiments in cognitively intact older control subjects have consistently demonstrated that older subjects are able to activate their hippocampus during successful associative encoding. Furthermore, our findings suggest that age-related changes in memory performance may be due primarily to alterations in cortical regions or in the connections between the medial temporal lobe and neocortical regions.

### fMRI Alterations in Mild AD

Although fMRI is a relative newcomer to the field of AD, studies of novel encoding in mild AD patients have consistently found decreased fMRI activation in hippocampal and parahippocampal regions compared to older controls.[18–24] Our own work, using the block-design face–name paradigm, has found that AD patients demonstrate significantly less hippocampal activation in the Novel versus Repeated comparison than Normal older controls.[14,25] Several groups, including our own, have also found evidence of increased activation in some neocortical regions in AD patients, which may represent a compensatory process in the setting of hippocampal failure.[14,24,26]

More recently, several groups have also reported alterations in the pattern of deactivation in AD patients.[27–31] These alterations in deactivation occur in a specific set of regions that has been characterized as the "default mode network."[32] Interestingly, the regions involved in the "default mode network" are strikingly similar to those regions that typically demonstrate evidence of fibrillar amyloid deposition binding with Pittsburgh Compound B (PIB) in positron emission tomography (PET) studies in AD,[30,33] as well as to the pattern of hypometabolism found on fluorodeoxyglucose (FDG) PET studies of AD patients[30,34–36] and subjects at-risk for AD;[37–39] and of hypoperfusion on resting MR perfusion studies in AD.[40,41]

Our own recent fMRI work suggest that the alterations in hippocampal activation and parietal deactivation over the course of MCI and AD are strongly correlated.[42] We have hypothesized that there is a distributed memory network, which is disrupted by the pathophysiological process of AD, which includes both medial temporal lobe systems and medial and lateral parietal regions involved in default mode activity. Our future studies will combine amyloid imaging with PIB and fMRI to determine whether amyloid deposition in parietal regions is associated with alterations in hippocampal activation.

## fMRI ALTERATIONS IN MILD COGNITIVE IMPAIRMENT

Relatively few studies have been published to date in subjects at-risk for AD, either MCI or genetically at-risk, and the results have been quite variable, ranging from hyperactivation[25,43–45] to hypoactivation.[18,22,46,47] MCI subjects with significantly impaired memory have shown consistently *decreased* medial temporal lobe (MTL) activation compared with controls.[22] At the other end of the spectrum, cognitively intact ApoE 4 carriers showed *increased* MTL activation compared to noncarriers,[43] with similar findings reported in asymptomatic offspring of autopsy-confirmed AD patients.[48] We believe that the variability in these results relates to the ability of the subjects to perform the fMRI task, and to the severity of the cognitive impairment along the continuum between normal aging and dementia.

Our own work has also suggested that older subjects with *very mild* cognitive impairment (MCI) also show evidence of increased MTL activation, and that the extent and location of hyperactivation is related to memory task demands and memory performance.[25,45] We hypothesize that MTL hyperactivation in very early stages of MCI may be a compensatory response to maintain memory performance in the setting of early AD pathology. Our recent work with more impaired MCI subjects suggests that the hippocampus fails in later stages of MCI.[42] In a recent study, utilizing independent component analyses (ICA), we found that MCI subjects with low Clinical Dementia Rating Scale Sum of Box scores (CDR-SB)[49] showed greater hippocampal activation compared to older controls, while MCI subjects with high CDR-SB showed very little hippocampal activation, similar to AD patients (see FIG. 3). Thus, we have hypothesized that there is a nonlinear trajectory of memory-related fMRI activity over the course of MCI and AD, such that there is an initial phase of hyperactivation in presymptomatic and very mildly impaired subjects, followed by decreased activation with progression of pathology and memory impairment. We are currently beginning a longitudinal fMRI study to track the evolution of memory-related fMRI activation over the course of MCI.

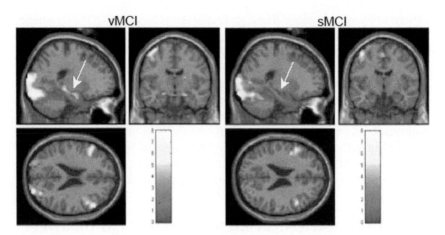

**FIGURE 3.** Group fMRI data in two groups of MCI subjects, based on the CDR Sum of Box score, was analyzed with ICA. Very mild impaired MCI (vMCI) subjects show significant hippocampal activation that is strongly linked to the timing of the fMRI paradigm ($P < 0.001$). More significantly impaired MCI (sMCI) subjects demonstrated very little hippocampal activation, despite similar or increased neocortical activation.

In summary, fMRI has shown evidence of specific alterations in memory networks that may be able to differentiate the process of normal aging from early AD. Further work is clearly needed to understand the relationship of these alterations to amyloid pathology, as well as tau pathology and neuronal loss. Future studies that combine fMRI with amyloid PET imaging, as well as volumetric MRI should prove particularly valuable in detecting the earliest pathological alterations.

## ACKNOWLEDGEMENT

This manuscript represents the work of many individuals who have contributed to these studies, in particular: Saul Miller, Kim Celone, Kristina Depeau, Elizabeth Chua, Eli Diamond, Andrew Cocchiarella, Erin Rand-Giovannetti, Brad Dickerson, Julie Bates, Vince Calhoun, Bruce Rosen, Douglas Greve, Ali Atri, Dorene Rentz, Deborah Blacker, Dennis Selkoe, and Marilyn Albert. Research funded by NIA (ROI-AG027435; DO1-AG04953; P50-AG005134) and the Harvard Center for Neurodegeneration and Repair.

## REFERENCES

1. Squire, L.R. & S. Zola-Morgan. 1991. The medial temporal lobe memory system. Science **253:** 1380–1386.

2. EICHENBAUM, H., G. SCHOENBAUM, B. YOUNG & M. BUNSEY. 1996. Functional organization of the hippocampal memory system. Proc. Natl. Acad. Sci. USA **93:** 13500–13507.

3. ZELINSKI, E.M. & M.J. GILEWSKI. 1988. Assessment of memory complaints by rating scales and questionnaires. Psychopharmacol. Bull. **24:** 523–529.

4. LEIRER, V.O., D.G. MORROW, J.I. SHEIKH & G.M. PARIANTE. 1990. Memory skills elders want to improve. Exp. Aging Res. **16:** 155–158.

5. MORRIS, J.C., D.W. MCKEEL JR., M. STORANDT, et al. 1991. Very mild Alzheimer's disease: informant-based clinical, psychometric, and pathologic distinction from normal aging [see comments]. Neurology **41:** 469–478.

6. FOWLER, K.S., M.M. SALING, E.L. CONWAY, et al. 2002. Paired associate performance in the early detection of DAT. J. Int. Neuropsychol. Soc. **8:** 58–71.

7. GALLO, D.A., A.L. SULLIVAN, K.R. DAFFNER, et al. 2004. Associative recognition in Alzheimer's disease: evidence for impaired recall-to-reject. Neuropsychology **18:** 556–563.

8. SMALL, S.A., A.S. NAVA, G.M. PERERA, et al. 2001. Circuit mechanisms underlying memory encoding and retrieval in the long axis of the hippocampal formation. Nat. Neurosci. **4:** 442–449.

9. ZEINEH, M.M., S.A. ENGEL, P.M. THOMPSON & S.Y. BOOKHEIMER. 2003. Dynamics of the hippocampus during encoding and retrieval of face–name pairs. Science **299:** 577–580.

10. KIRWAN, C.B. & C.E. STARK. 2004. Medial temporal lobe activation during encoding and retrieval of novel face–name pairs. Hippocampus **14:** 919–930.

11. SPERLING, R.A., J. BATES, A. COCCHIARELLA, et al. 2001. Encoding novel face–name associations: a functional MRI study. Hum. Brain Mapp. **14:** 129–139.

12. SPERLING, R.A., D. GREVE, A. DALE, et al. 2002. fMRI detection of pharmacologically induced memory impairment. Proc. Nat. Acad. Sci. **99:** 455–460.

13. SPERLING, R., E. CHUA, A. COCCHIARELLA, et al. 2003. Putting names to faces: successful encoding of associative memories activates the anterior hippocampal formation. Neuroimage **20:** 1400–1410.

14. SPERLING, R., J. BATES, E. CHUA, et al. 2003. fMRI studies of associative encoding in young and elderly controls and mild AD patients. J. Neurol. Neurosurg. Psychiatry **74:** 44–50.

15. RAND-GIOVANNETTI, E., E.F. CHUA, A.E. DRISCOLL, et al. 2006. Hippocampal and neocortical activation during repetitive encoding in older persons. Neurobiol. Aging **27:** 173–182.

16. MILLER, S., K. DEPEAU, E. DIAMOND, et al. 2006. fMRI activations and deactivations during successful associative encoding in normal aging. Ann. N. Y. Acad. Sci. This volume.

17. DASELAAR, S.M., S.E. PRINCE & R. CABEZA. 2004. When less means more: deactivations during encoding that predict subsequent memory. Neuroimage **23:** 921–927.

18. SMALL, S.A., G.M. PERERA, R. DELAPAZ, et al. 1999. Differential regional dysfunction of the hippocampal formation among elderly with memory decline and Alzheimer's disease. Ann. Neurol. **45:** 466–472.

19. ROMBOUTS, S.A., F. BARKHOF, D.J. VELTMAN, et al. 2000. Functional MR imaging in Alzheimer's disease during memory encoding. AJNR Am. J. Neuroradiol. **21:** 1869–1875.

20. KATO, T., D. KNOPMAN & H. LIU. 2001. Dissociation of regional activation in mild AD during visual encoding: a functional MRI study. Neurology **57:** 812–816.

21. GRON, G., D. BITTNER, B. SCHMITZ, *et al.* 2002. Subjective memory complaints: objective neural markers in patients with Alzheimer's disease and major depressive disorder. Ann. Neurol. **51:** 491–498.
22. MACHULDA, M.M., H.A. WARD, B. BOROWSKI, *et al.* 2003. Comparison of memory fMRI response among normal, MCI, and Alzheimer's patients. Neurology **61:** 500–506.
23. GOLBY, A., G. SILVERBERG, E. RACE, *et al.* 2005. Memory encoding in Alzheimer's disease: an fMRI study of explicit and implicit memory. Brain **128:** 773–787.
24. PARIENTE, J., S. COLE, R. HENSON, *et al.* 2005. Alzheimer's patients engage an alternative network during a memory task. Ann. Neurol. **58:** 870–879.
25. DICKERSON, B.C., D. SALAT, D. GREVE, *et al.* 2005. Increased hippocampal activation in mild cognitive impairment compared to normal aging and AD. Neurology **65:** 404–411.
26. GRADY, C.L., A.R. MCINTOSH, S. BEIG, *et al.* 2003. Evidence from functional neuroimaging of a compensatory prefrontal network in Alzheimer's disease. J. Neurosci. **23:** 986–993.
27. LUSTIG, C., A.Z. SNYDER, M. BHAKTA, *et al.* 2003. Functional deactivations: change with age and dementia of the Alzheimer type. Proc. Natl. Acad. Sci. USA **100:** 14504–14509.
28. GREICIUS, M.D., G. SRIVASTAVA, A.L. REISS & V. MENON. 2004. Default-mode network activity distinguishes Alzheimer's disease from healthy aging: evidence from functional MRI. Proc. Natl. Acad. Sci. USA **101:** 4637–4642.
29. ROMBOUTS, S.A., R. GOEKOOP, C.J. STAM, *et al.* 2005. Delayed rather than decreased BOLD response as a marker for early Alzheimer's disease. Neuroimage **26:** 1078–1085.
30. BUCKNER, R.L., A.Z. SNYDER, B.J. SHANNON, *et al.* 2005. Molecular, structural, and functional characterization of Alzheimer's disease: evidence for a relationship between default activity, amyloid, and memory. J. Neurosci. **25:** 7709–7717.
31. PETRELLA, J., S. KRISHNAN, M. SLAVIN, *et al.* 2006. Mild cognitive impairment: evaluation with 4-T functional MR imaging. Radiology **240:** 177–186.
32. RAICHLE, M.E., A.M. MACLEOD, A.Z. SNYDER, *et al.* 2001. A default mode of brain function. Proc. Natl. Acad. Sci. USA **98:** 676–682.
33. KLUNK, W.E., H. ENGLER, A. NORDBERG, *et al.* 2004. Imaging brain amyloid in Alzheimer's disease with Pittsburgh Compound-B. Ann. Neurol. **55:** 306–319.
34. MELTZER, C.C., J.K. ZUBIETA, J. BRANDT, *et al.* 1996. Regional hypometabolism in Alzheimer's disease as measured by positron emission tomography after correction for effects of partial volume averaging. Neurology **47:** 454–461.
35. SILVERMAN, D.H., G.W. SMALL, C.Y. CHANG, *et al.* 2001. Positron emission tomography in evaluation of dementia: regional brain metabolism and long-term outcome. JAMA **286:** 2120–2127.
36. ALEXANDER, G.E., K. CHEN, P. PIETRINI, *et al.* 2002. Longitudinal PET evaluation of cerebral metabolic decline in dementia: a potential outcome measure in Alzheimer's disease treatment studies. Am. J. Psychiatry **159:** 738–745.
37. REIMAN, E.M., K. CHEN, G.E. ALEXANDER, *et al.* 2004. Functional brain abnormalities in young adults at genetic risk for late-onset Alzheimer's dementia. Proc. Natl. Acad. Sci. USA **101:** 284–289.
38. SMALL, G.W., L.M. ERCOLI, D.H. SILVERMAN, *et al.* 2000. Cerebral metabolic and cognitive decline in persons at genetic risk for Alzheimer's disease. Proc. Natl. Acad. Sci. USA **97:** 6037–6042.

39. JAGUST, W., A. GITCHO, F. SUN, *et al.* 2006. Brain imaging evidence of preclinical Alzheimer's disease in normal aging. Ann. Neurol. **59:** 673–681.

40. ALSOP, D.C., J.A. DETRE & M. GROSSMAN. 2000. Assessment of cerebral blood flow in Alzheimer's disease by spin-labeled magnetic resonance imaging. Ann. Neurol. **47:** 93–100.

41. JOHNSON, N.A., G.H. JAHNG, M.W. WEINER, *et al.* 2005. Pattern of cerebral hypoperfusion in Alzheimer disease and mild cognitive impairment measured with arterial spin-labeling MR imaging: initial experience. Radiology **234:** 851–859.

42. CELONE, K., V. CALHOUN, B. DICKERSON, *et al.* 2006. Alterations in memory networks in mild cognitive impairment and Alzheimer's disease: an independent component analysis. J. Neuroscience. **26(40):** 10222–10231.

43. BOOKHEIMER, S.Y., M.H. STROJWAS, M.S. COHEN, *et al.* 2000. Patterns of brain activation in people at risk for Alzheimer's disease. N. Engl. J. Med. **343:** 450–456.

44. SMITH, C.D., A.H. ANDERSEN, R.J. KRYSCIO, *et al.* 2002. Women at risk for AD show increased parietal activation during a fluency task. Neurology **58:** 1197–1202.

45. DICKERSON, B.C., D.H. SALAT, J.F. BATES, *et al.* 2004. Medial temporal lobe function and structure in mild cognitive impairment. Ann. Neurol. **56:** 27–35.

46. JOHNSON, S.C., L.C. BAXTER, L. SUSSKIND-WILDER, *et al.* 2004. Hippocampal adaptation to face repetition in healthy elderly and mild cognitive impairment. Neuropsychologia **42:** 980–989.

47. JOHNSON, S.C., T.W. SCHMITZ, C.H. MORITZ, *et al.* 2005. Activation of brain regions vulnerable to Alzheimer's disease: the effect of mild cognitive impairment. Neurobiol. Aging **27(11):** 1604–1612.

48. BASSETT, S.S., D.M. YOUSEM, C. CRISTINZIO, *et al.* 2006. Familial risk for Alzheimer's disease alters fMRI activation patterns. Brain **129:** 1229–1239.

49. MORRIS, J.C. 1993. The Clinical Dementia Rating (CDR): current version and scoring rules. Neurology **43:** 2412–2414.

# Quantitative EEG and Electromagnetic Brain Imaging in Aging and in the Evolution of Dementia

LESLIE S. PRICHEP[a,b]

[a]Brain Research Laboratories, Department of Psychiatry, New York University School of Medicine, New York, New York, USA

[b]Nathan S. Kline Institute for Psychiatric Research, NYS Department of Mental Health, Orangeburg, New York, USA

ABSTRACT: Electroencephalographic (EEG) changes with normal aging have long been reported. Departures from age-expected changes have been observed in mild cognitive impairment and dementia, the magnitude of which correlates with the degree of cognitive impairment. Such abnormalities include increased delta and theta activity, decreased mean frequency, and changes in coherence. Similar findings have been reported using magnetoencephalography (MEG) at rest and during performance of mental tasks. Electrophysiological features have also been shown to be predictive of future decline in mild cognitive impairment (MCI) and Alzheimer's disease (AD). We have recently reported results from initial quantitative electroencephalography (QEEG) evaluations of normal elderly subjects (with only subjective reports of memory loss), predicting future cognitive decline or conversion to dementia, with high prediction accuracy (approximately 95%). In this report, source localization algorithms were used to identify the mathematically most probable underlying generators of abnormal features of the scalp-recorded EEG from these patients with differential outcomes. Using this QEEG method, abnormalities in brain regions identified in studies of AD using MEG, MRI, and positron emission tomography (PET) imaging were found in the premorbid recordings of those subjects who go on to decline or convert to dementia.

KEYWORDS: electromagnetic imaging; QEEG; prediction; dementia; MCI

## INTRODUCTION

Information derived from brain electrical activity has contributed to the understanding of normal brain function and to a better understanding of the pathophysiology of brain dysfunction seen in neuropsychiatric disorders. Both

Address for correspondence: Leslie Prichep, Brain Research Laboratories, Old Bellevue Admin. Bldg., 8th Fl., 462 First Avenue, New York, NY 10016. Voice: 212-263-6288; fax: 212-263-6457. leslie.prichep@med.nyu.edu

Ann. N.Y. Acad. Sci. 1097: 156–167 (2007). © 2007 New York Academy of Sciences. doi: 10.1196/annals.1379.008

the electroencephalogram (EEG) and the magnetoencephalogram (MEG) are measures of brain electrical activity. MEG records the magnetic field generated by the electrical activity, using superconductive quantum interference devices (SQUID) placed over the head in arrays of 100 or more sensors. EEG records the electrical field, using electrodes pasted on the scalp in standard arrays of 19 or more placements. MEG selectively detects tangential fields from activity arising from pathways parallel to the surface of the brain (sulci) and therefore is most sensitive to cortical sources. Conversely, EEG measures both radial and tangential activity, with radial more dominant, from activity in the gyri and is therefore more sensitive to deep sources. Both EEG and MEG have ≤ 1 msec time resolution enabling them to provide neurophysiological data not obtainable from other neuroimaging techniques.

There is a vast literature spanning the past 30 years reporting EEG changes in the pattern of brain electrical activity associated with aging and noting relationships between specific changes in the EEG and degree of clinical deterioration in the elderly.[1-22] Space does not permit a review of these numerous studies, but it is noteworthy that they consistently demonstrate the relationship of particular features to the severity and progression of dementia. These features include: increased delta (1.5 to 3.5 Hz) and/or theta (3.5 to 7.5 Hz) power; decreased mean frequency of the total spectra; decreased frequency of the dominant occipital rhythm; and changes in coherence or synchronization patterns.

Researchers have used selected features of the quantitative electroencephalography (QEEG) to accurately discriminate between normal elderly controls, MCI elderly, and DAT patients, as well as between types of dementia and between dementia and depression. TABLE 1 summarizes results of representative recent QEEG studies.

A literature reporting MEG findings in dementia has begun to appear over the last 10 years. TABLE 2 below summarizes selected recent MEG studies that are the counterpart to the EEG studies in TABLE 1 above. These studies are in much smaller populations and present comparisons between two conditions. Since no normative data are currently available for the MEG, differences can only be reported relative to age-matched controls. None of these studies report sensitivity and specificity. It is of note, however, that both the QEEG and MEG studies of dementia report a significant relationship between temporal–parietal slowing (especially theta), slowing of the mean spectra, and degree of dementia and extent of hippocampal atrophy.

Further clinical utility of QEEG has been demonstrated in longitudinal studies of progression in MCI or DAT, showing a relationship between EEG features at baseline (BL) and future decline. Features reported to be related to future decline include: presence of QEEG slow wave at BL in patients with "probable" Alzheimer's disease (AD) (Soininen 1991, 1-year FU);[27] baseline relative power in alpha (8 to 12 Hz), relative power in theta, and mean frequency of EEG from left temporo–occipital regions predict further decline in MCI

TABLE 1. Summary of selected recent studies using QEEG to classify AD patients and to distinguish them from other patient and normal (NL) groups

| Reference | Groups [Ns] | Accuracy of separation/ prediction [%] (statistical method) | Sensitivity/ specificity [%] |
|---|---|---|---|
| Anderer et al. (1994)[23] | Mild–Mod AD (n = 80, train), Mild–Mod AD, Normal Control (56) | Test MID vs. Control = 88 AD vs. Control = 87 (neural network) | 82.0/90.0 84.0/90.0 |
| Besthorn et al. (1997)[24] | Possible AD (n = 18), Probable AD (n = 32), Normal controls (n = 42) | Probable vs. Control = 95.9 Possible vs. Control = 85.0 (discriminant function) | 96.8/95.3 84.6/93.0 |
| Deslandes et al. (2004)[25] | Dementia (n = 74) vs. Depression (n = 51) | Training = 91.2 Jackknife = 90.4 (discriminant function) | 91.9/92.2 |
| Huang et al. (2000)[12] | AD (n = 38) vs. normal controls, NC (n = 24) vs. MCI (n = 31). MCI who progress, PMCI (n = 14) vs. MCI stable, SMCI (n = 17) | AD vs NC = 85 AD vs. MCI = 78 PMCI vs. SMCI = 87 (discriminant function) | 87.0/83.0 87.0/68.0 79.0/94.0 |
| Lindau et al. (2003)[26] | FTD (n = 19) vs. AD (n = 16) vs. normal controls (n = 19) | AD vs. Control = 80 FTD vs. Control = 79 FTD vs. AD = 71 (logistic regression) | Not available |

patients (Jelic 2000, 21-month follow-up [FU]);[28] decreased alpha global field power (GFP) and anteriorization of sources predict decline in MCI (Huang 2000, 25-month FU);[12] high delta dipole density in MEG predicted increased risk of conversion in MCI in a 2-year follow-up.[29]

## Background Study

Almost all existing studies included only patients already diagnosed as MCI or DAT, none included normal elderly or those with only subjective complaints. In a recent publication we have reported results of a longitudinal study evaluating the predictive utility of BL QEEG in normal elderly subjects with only subjective complaints of memory loss, but no objective evidence of memory dysfunction. Diagnosis of MCI or AD was ruled out in all subjects, who were therefore clinically considered to be normal elderly with memory complaints. All study subjects were GDS 2s according to the Global Deterioration Scale.[36,37] All study subjects were electrophysiologically evaluated (BL) and were then followed for 5–7 years with clinically/cognitively restaging of GDS at intervals during this time period. Retrospectively, subjects were divided into those who showed no decline throughout the follow-up period (remaining at

**TABLE 2. Summary of selected recent studies using MEG to classify AD patients and to distinguish them from other patient and normal (NL) groups**

| | Groups studied | Task | Findings |
|---|---|---|---|
| Fernandez *et al.* (2003)[30] Fernandez *et al.* (2002)[31] | $n = 15$ AD vs. $n = 16$ NL | Eyes open fixated resting | Correl bet L temp–parietal slow waves and L hippocampal vol; L hipp vol with L temp theta 87.1% classif of AD pts |
| Fernandez *et al.* (2006)[32] | $n = 22$ AD. $n = 22$ MCI, $n = 22$ NL | Eyes closed resting | Mean freq tot spectrum NL>MCI>AD Noted dec MF with age in NL |
| Franciotti *et al.* (2005)[33] | $n = 8$ mod/7sev AD, $n = 7$ LBD, $n = 9$ NL | Eyes open vs. eyes closed; simple mental task | Reactivity: NL>Mod AD >Sev AD >LBD Alpha coh ↓ AD and LBD, especially long connections |
| Maestu *et al.* (2003)[34] | $n = 8$ AD vs. 8 NL | Probe letter memory ERP | Relationship bet hippocampal atrophy and activity in L temporal lobe at 400 ms |
| Puregger *et al.* (2003)[35] | $n = 10$ MCI vs. 10 NL | Non-semantic and semantic word encoding | Max diff 250–450 ms over L frontal and L temporal, ↑ differnce in MCI |

GDS stage 2) and those who declined to MCI or AD (changed to GDS stage 3 or higher).

The neurometric QEEG method was used.[38] Quantitative features were extracted, log transformed to obtain normal (Gaussian) distributions,[39,40] age-regressed, and Z-transformed relative to age-appropriate population norms. These population norms have been repeatedly confirmed to be independent of ethnic or cultural bias[41] and to have extremely high test–retest replicability over long intervals.[42] This method allows the statistical assessment of the significance of departure from age-expected normal values, thus taking into account (correcting for) the normal effects of aging. This was particularly important in this study, which included normal elderly subjects, since it allowed identification of those features of the EEG that did not reflect changes normally expected with aging.

Using only the BL QEEG evaluations, significant differences were found between *"Nondecliners"* and *"Decliners,"* ($F[12,31] = 5.08$, $P < 0.0001$). Features entered into the multivariate analysis of variance (MANOVA) included: theta relative power in the left lateral regions (F7, T3, T5); mean frequency of theta in the left dorsolateral prefrontal region; coherence across all bands between C4 and P4 regions; and absolute power in theta in right medial regions (FP2, F4, C4, P4, O2) and posterior temporal regions. All power features showed increases in *"Decliners,"* who had decreased coherence compared with *"Nondecliners."*

In a second analysis, the decliners were further divided into those who declined to MCI and those who converted to AD and compared to those subjects who did not decline. Using a logistic regression, the overall prediction accuracy was 90%, with an $R^2$ of 0.93, $P < 0.0001$. Variables with the highest significance included: total spectra mean frequency (right central region), decreasing in decliners and further in converters; delta mean frequency (left bipolar temporal and parietal–occipital regions), slowing in decliners and further in converters; absolute power across all frequency bands diffusely on the right hemisphere, especially on the right dorsolateral frontal region, increased in decliners and greatly increased in converters; and absolute power in the theta frequency band across the right frontal regions, greatly increased in decliners. Considering only those who in fact converted to dementia (GDS $\geq$ 4), the sensitivity was 96.3% and the specificity was 94.1% and considering only those who decline to MCI, the sensitivity was 95% and specificity was 94.1%.

This article describes the source localization within the brain of the putative generators of the predictive BL QEEG data in this population of normal elderly with differential prognosis.

## EEG METHOD

### Acquisition

A 20-min EEG was collected from each subject in an eyes closed resting state, from the 19 standardized locations of the International 10/20 placement system. A differential eye channel (diagonally placed above and below the eye orbit) was used for the detection of eye movement. All electrode impedances were below 5,000 Ohms. The EEG amplifiers had a bandpass from 0.5 to 70 Hz (3 dB points), with a 60-Hz notch filter. Data were sampled at a rate of 200 Hz with a 12-bit resolution.

### Frequency Analysis

From the 20-min raw EEG data, 2-min artifact-free data were selected for analysis. Artifact detection included visual inspection by a trained, experienced EEG technician, aided by the use of a computerized artifact detection algorithm. Artifact-free data were subjected to very narrow band spectral analysis (0.39 Hz increments from 0.39 to 19 Hz). As in the neurometric analysis of the EEG, transforms of the spectral power were applied to achieve Gaussian distributions. Using norms for narrow band spectral power,[43,44] regression equations for each frequency were calculated to correct for age-dependent sources of variance in the source log spectra. Using these normative data, Z-transformed spectra were computed.

## Source Localization

The Z score, which was most significantly abnormal in the narrow band frequency analysis (maxima) in the domain of the theta band (3.5–7.5 Hz), was selected as input for the source localization. Variable resolution electromagnetic tomography (VARETA) source localization method was used.[43] Using VARETA, the mathematically most probable source generators of scalp-recorded EEG are localized and anatomically identified by coregistration and superimposition upon brain slices from a probabilistic brain atlas (PBA) developed at the Montreal Neurological Institute.[45] Sources are restricted to gray matter by the use of a probabilistic mask that prohibits solutions in white matter and intraventricular regions where the mask is zero. A three-concentric sphere model was fitted to the MNI mean head by a least square procedure. When 19 electrodes have been used to record the EEG as in this study, the brain volume is divided by VARETA into 3,500 voxels.

Three-dimensional color-coded tomographic images are generated for the selected very narrow band, with source distributions superimposed upon transaxial, coronal, and sagittal slices of the PBA, which correspond to the loci of the inverse solutions. In each case, the frequency at which the maximum significance was found is taken as the frequency of the main source. Assessment of the statistical significance must take into consideration the large number of measurements and their intercorrelations. In this work, the corrections suggested by Worsley and colleagues[46] have been applied, and the color palette encodes excess or deficit of spectral activity above the threshold probability level.

## RESULTS

Figure 1 shows the VARETA images derived from the BL QEEG at levels that include the regions of interest, for those subjects who do not decline longitudinally (top row), those who decline to MCI (middle), and those who convert to AD (bottom row), for axial views (top panel) and coronal views (bottom panel). Clear differences between the groups can be seen with successively more regions of abnormality from the top to bottom of the figure and involvement of additional regions of interest in those groups that go on to show decline in the future. Note in particular the increasing significant abnormalities in the hippocampus, parahippocampal gyrus, amygdala, and parieto–temporal cortex, in the *Converters* as compared with *Decliners*.

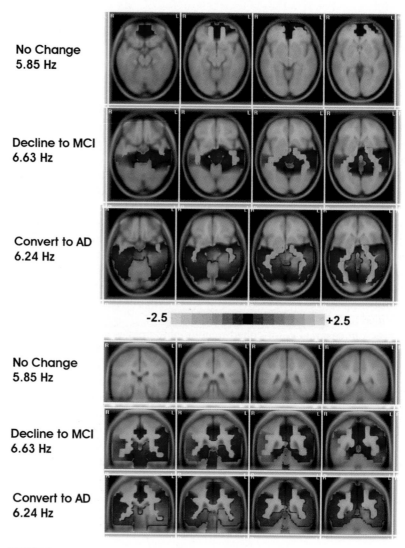

**FIGURE 1.** Images in this figure follow radiological convention, with the right side of the head depicted on the left side of the slice. Each row is a group average (*n* = 5) from a sample of subjects who show *No Change* (*top rows of both panels*), subjects who *Decline* to MCI (*middle rows*), and subjects who *Convert* to dementia (*bottom rows*) over the longitudinal follow-up period. Images are Z scores of the sources in every voxel viewed in transaxial views (*top panel*) and coronal views (*bottom panel*) superimposed upon slices taken from the probabilistic MRI Atlas constructed at the Montreal Neurological Institute.[45] The sources were identified using VARETA for most abnormal narrow band (VNB) theta peak in the QEEG, (actual value in Hz shown in label). Images are color coded in standard deviation units with excesses shown as increasing from red to yellow and deficits ranging from blue to turquoise, across the range of ± 2.5, which would be equivalent to the probability of *P* < 0.01 for a group of five subjects.

# DISCUSSION

The significance of abnormalities in the theta frequency band should be considered with respect to the known relationships between theta and brain functions assessed using other imaging modalities. In studies of dementia patients, theta power has been shown to be negatively correlated with perfusion, especially in temporo–parietal and central regions[14,47] and a substantial literature has reported high inverse correlations between theta excesses, cerebral ischemia, and cerebral blood flow.[41,48] Theta has also been negatively correlated with positron emission tomography (PET) glucose metabolism in temporo–parietal[49] and frontal regions[50] and positively correlated with hippocampal atrophy.[18,29,51] Thus, regions with excess of theta can be expected to be under perfused, have decreased glucose metabolism, and correlate with hippocampal atrophy.

A number of imaging studies have reported that abnormalities in the hippocampus and entorhinal cortex,[52–54] and the temporal neocortex,[55–57] may predict conversion to dementia in MCI patients. De Leon[58] reported reduced glucose metabolism in the entorhinal cortex of normal elderly who go on to decline. Rusinek[59] reported high predictive accuracy of rate of medial temporal lobe atrophy in prediction of decline of normal elderly.

One of the critical factors contributing to the sensitivity demonstrated in this study is the existence of norms for the QEEG measures and sources, across the human life span. Abnormalities can thus be identified and quantified as statistical deviations from age-expected normal values. The abnormalities reported in this study in the BL QEEG of normal elderly who go on to decline to MCI or convert to dementia demonstrate sensitivity of QEEG to the earliest manifestations of subcortical as well as cortical changes (with most probable sources in the hippocampus, amygdala, parahippocampal gyrus, and parieto–temporal cortex). EEG may represent a cost-effective, noninvasive brain imaging tool capable of identifying the earliest signs of brain dysfunction in subjects with evolving MCI or dementia.

## ACKNOWLEDGMENT

The author wishes to acknowledge Drs. Steven Ferris and Barry Reisberg of the Silberstein Aging and Dementia Research Center, NYU School of Medicine for their collaboration in identification and staging of the subject population. This work was supported in part by grants from Cadwell Laboratories and Cordis Corporation.

## REFERENCES

1. BRESLAU, J., A. STARR, N. SICOTTE, et al. 1989. Topographic EEG changes with normal aging and SDAT. Electroencep. Clin. Neurophysiol. **72:** 281–289.

2. BRUNOVSKY, M., M. MATOUSEK, A. EDMAN, *et al.* 2003. Objective assessment of the degree of dementia by means of EEG. Neuropsychobiology **48:** 19–26.
3. CANTER, N.L., M. HALLETT & J.H. GROWDON 1982. Lecithin does not affect EEG spectral analysis or P300 in Alzheimer's disease. Neurology **32:** 1260–1266.
4. COBEN, L.A., D. CHI, A.D. SNYDER, *et al.* 1990. Replication of a study of frequency of the resting awake EEG in mild probable Alzheimer's Disease. EEG Clin. Neurophysiol. **75:** 148–154.
5. COBEN, L.A., W.L. DANZIGER & L. BERG 1983. Frequency analysis of the resting awake EEG in mild senile dementia of Alzheimer type. EEG Clin. Neurophysiol. **55:** 372–380.
6. COBEN, L.A., W. DANZINGER & M. STORANDT 1985. A longitudinal EEG study of mild senile dementia of Alzheimer type: changes at 1 year and at 2.5 years. EEG Clin. Neurophysiol. **61:** 101–112.
7. DIERKS, T., I. PERISIC, L. FROLICH, *et al.* 1991. Topography of the quantitative electroencephalogram in dementia of the Alzheimer type: relation to severity of dementia. Psychiat. Res. **40:** 181–194.
8. DUFFY, F.H., M.S. ALBERT & G. MCNULTY 1984. Brain electrical activity in patients with presenile and senile dementia of the Alzheimer type. Ann. Neurol. **16:** 439–448.
9. GERSON, I.M., E.R. JOHN, F. BARTLETT, *et al.* 1976. Average evoked response (AER) in the electroencephalographic diagnosis of the normally aging brain: a practical application. Clin. EEG **7:** 77–90.
10. HELKALA, E.L., V. LAULUMAA, R. SOIKKELI, *et al.* 1991. Slow wave activity in the spectral analysis the electroencephalogram is associated with cortical dysfunction in patients with Alzheimer's disease. Behav. Neurosci. **105:** 409–415.
11. HIER, D.B., C.A. MANGONE, R. GANELLEN, *et al.* 1991. Quantitative measurement of delta activity in Alzheimer's disease. Clin EEG **22:** 178–182.
12. HUANG, C., L.O. WAHLUND, T. DIERKS, *et al.* 2000. Discrimination of Alzheimer's disease and mild cognitive impairment by equivalent EEG sources: a cross-sectional and longitudinal study. Clin. Neurophysiol. **111:** 1961–1967.
13. LEUCHTER, A.F., J.E. SPAR, D.O. WALTER, *et al.* 1987. Electroencephalographic spectra and coherence in the diagnosis of Alzheimer's-type and multi-infarct dementia. Arch. Gen. Psychiat. **44:** 993–998.
14. MATTIA, D., F. BABILONI, A. ROMIGI, *et al.* 2003. Quantitative EEG and dynamic susceptibility contrast MRI in Alzheimer's disease; a correlative study. Clin. Neurophysiol. **114:** 1210–1216.
15. PENTTILA, M., V.J. PARTANEN, H. SOININEN, *et al.* 1985. Quantitative analysis of occipital EEG in different stages of Alzheimer's Disease. EEG Clin. Neurophysiol. **60:** 1–6.
16. RAE-GRANT, A., W. BLUME, C. LAU, *et al.* 1987. The electroencephalogram in Alzheimer-type dementia: a sequential study correlating the electroencephalogram with psychometric and quantitative pathologic data. Arch. Neurol. **44:** 50–54.
17. RICE, D.M., M.S. BUCHSBAUM, A. STARR, *et al.* 1990. Abnormal EEG slow activity in left temporal areas in senile dementia of the Alzheimer's type. J. Gerontology **45:** 145–151.
18. SALETU, B., P. ANDERER, E. PAULUS, *et al.* 1991. EEG brain mapping in diagnostic and therapeutic assessment of dementia. Alzheimer Dis. Assoc. Disord. **5:** S57–S75.

19. Soininen, H., J. Partanen, V. Laulumaa, *et al*. 1989. Longitudinal EEG spectral analysis in early stage of Alzheimer's disease. EEG Clin. Neurophysiol. **72:** 290–297.

20. Soininen, H., V.J. Partanen, E.L. Helkala, *et al*. 1982. EEG findings in senile dementia and normal aging. Acta Neurol. Scand. **65:** 59–70.

21. Streletz, L.J., P.F. Reyes, M. Zolewska, *et al*. 1990. Computer analysis of EEG activity in dementia of the Alzheimer type and Huntington's disease. Neurobiol. Aging **11:** 15–20.

22. Williamson, P.C., H. Merskey, S. Morrison, *et al*. 1990. Quantitative electroencephalographic correlates of cognitive decline in normal elderly subjects. Arch. –Neurol. **47:** 1185–1188.

23. Anderer, P., B. Saletu, B. Klöppel, *et al*. 1994. Discrimination between patients and normals based on topographic EEG slow wave activity: comparison between Z statistics, discriminant analysis and artificial neural network classifiers. EEG Clin. Neurophysiol. **91:** 108–117.

24. Besthorn, C., R. Zerfass, C. Geiger-Kabisch, *et al*. 1997. Discrimination of Alzheimer's disease and normal aging data. EEG Clin. Neurophysiol. **103:** 241–248.

25. Deslandes, A., H. Veiga, M. Cagy, *et al*. 2004. Quantitative electroencephalography (QEEG) to discriminate primary degenerative dementia from major depressive disorder (depression). Arq Neuro-Psiquiatr **62:** 44–50.

26. Lindau, M., V. Jelic, S.E. Johansson, *et al*. 2003. Quantitative EEG abnormalities and cognitive dysfunctions in frontotemporal dementia and Alzheimer's disease. Dement. Geriatr. Cogn. Disord. **15:** 106–114.

27. Soininen, H., J. Partanen, A. Paakkonen, *et al*. 1991. Changes in absolute power values of EEG spectra in the follow-up of Alzheimer's disease. Acta Neurol. Scand. **83:** 133–136.

28. Jelic, V., S.E. Johansson, O. Almkvist, *et al*. 2000. Quantitative electroencephalography in mild cognitive impairment: longitudinal changes and possible prediction of Alzheimer's disease. Neurobiol. Aging **21:** 533–540.

29. Fernandez, A., A. Turrero, P. Zuluaga, *et al*. 2006. Magnetoencephalographic parietal dipole density in mild cognitive impairment. Arch. Neurol. **63:** 427–430.

30. Fernandez, A., J. Arrazola, F. Maestu, *et al*. 2003. Correlations of hippocampal atrophy and focal low-frequency magnetic activity in Alzheimer disease: Volumetric MR Imaging- Magnetoencephalographic Study. AJNR Am. J. Neuroradiol. **24:** 481–487.

31. Fernandez, A., F. Maestu, C. Amo, *et al*. 2002. Focal temporoparietal slow activity in Alzheimer's disease revealed by magnetoencephalography. Soc. Biol. Psychiatry **2:** 764–770.

32. Fernandez, A., R. Hornero, A. Mayo, *et al*. 2006. MEG spectral profile in Alzheimer's disease and mild cognitive impairment. Clin. Neurophysiol. **117:** 306–314.

33. Franciotti, R., D. Iacono, D. Penna, *et al*. 2006. Cortical rhythms reactivity in AD, LBD and normal subjects: a quantitative MEG study. Neurobiol. Aging. **27:** 1100–1109.

34. Maestu, F., J. Arrazola, A. Fernandez, *et al*. 2003. Do cognitive patterns of brain magnetic activity correlate with hippocampal atrophy in Alzheimer's disease? J. Neurol. Neurosurg. Psychiatry **74:** 208–212.

35. Puregger, E., P. Walla, L. Deecke, *et al*. 2003. Magnetoencephalographic— features related to mild cognitive impairment. Neuroimage **20:** 2235–2244.

36. REISBERG, B., S.H. FERRIS, M.J. DE LEON, et al. 1988. The global deterioration scale (GDS). Psychoparmacol. Bull. **24:** 699–702.
37. REISBERG, B., S.H. FERRIS, M.J. DE LEON, et al. 1982. The global deterioration scale for assessment of primary degenerative dementia. Am. J. Psychiatry **139:** 165–173.
38. JOHN, E.R., L.S. PRICHEP, J. FRIEDMAN, et al. 1988. Neurometrics: computer-assisted differential diagnosis of brain dysfunctions. Science **293:** 162–169.
39. JOHN, E.R., H. AHN, L.S. PRICHEP, et al. 1980. Developmental equations for the electroencephalogram. Science **210:** 1255–1258.
40. GASSER, T., P. BACHER & J. MOCHS 1982. Transformation towards the normal distribution of broad band spectral parameters of the EEG. EEG Clin Neurophysiol. **53:** 119–124.
41. HUGHES, J.R. & E.R. JOHN. 1999. Conventional and quantitative electroencephalography in psychiatry. J. Neuropsychiat. Clin. Neurosci. **11:** 190–208.
42. KONDACS, A. & M. SZABO 1999. Long-term intra-individual variability of the background EEG in normals. Clin. Neurophysiol. **110:** 1708–1716.
43. BOSCH-BAYARD, J., P. VALDES-SOSA, E. VIRUES-ALBA, et al. 2001. 3D statistical parametric mapping of EEG source spectra by means of variable resolution electromagnetic tomography (VARETA). Clin. EEG **32:** 47–61.
44. VALDES-SOSA, P., J. BOSCH, F. GRAY, et al. 1992. Frequency domain models of the EEG. Brain Topog. **4:** 309–319.
45. EVANS, A.C., D.L. COLLINS, S.R. MILLS, et al. 1993. 3D statistical neuroanatomical models from 305 MRI volumes. Proc. IEEE-Nuc. Sci. Symp. Med. Imag. Conf. **95:** 1813–1817.
46. WORSLEY, K.J., S. MARRETT, P. NEELIN, et al. 1995. A unified statistical approach for determining significant signals in images of cerebral activation. Hum. Brain Map. **4:** 58–73.
47. RODRIGUEZ, G., F. NOBILI, F. COPELLO, et al. 1999. 99mTc-HMPAO regional cerebral blood flow and quantitative electroencephalography in Alzheimer's disease: a correlative study. J. Nucl. Med. **40:** 522–529.
48. JONKMAN, E.J., D.C.J. POORTVLIET, M.M. VEERING, et al. 1985. The use of neurometrics in the study of patients with cerebral ischemia. EEG. Clin. Neurophysiol. **61:** 333–341.
49. SZELIES, B., M. GROND, K. HERHOLZ, et al. 1992. Quantitative EEG mapping and PET in Alzheimer's disease. J. Neurol. Sci. **110:** 46–56.
50. VALLADARES-NETO, D.C., M.S. BUCHSBAUM, W.J. EVANS, et al. 1995. EEG delta, positron emission tomography, and memory deficit in Alzheimer's disease. Neuropsychobiology **31:** 173–181.
51. HELKALA, E.L., T. HANNINEN, M. KONONEN, et al. 1996. Slow wave activity in the spectral analysis of the electroencephalogram and volumes of hippocampus in subgroups of Alzheimer's disease patients. Behav. Neurosci. **110:** 1235–1243.
52. DE LEON, M.J., G. SMITH, A. CONVIT, et al. 1992. The early detection of brain pathology in Alzheimer's Disease. *In* Neurophysiology and Alzheimer's Disease. Y. Christen, Ed.: 131–143. Springer-Verlag. Berlin.
53. DETOLEDO-MORRELL, L., T.R. STOUB, M. BULGAKOVA, et al. 2004. MRI-derived entorhinal volume is a good indicator of conversion from MCI to AD. Neurobiol. Aging **25:** 1197–1203.
54. KILLIANY, R.J., T. GOMEZ-ISLA, M. MOSS, et al. 2000. Use of structural magnetic resonance imaging to predict who will get Alzheimer's disease. Ann. Neurol. **47:** 430–439.

55. ARNAIZ, E., V. JELIC, O. ALMKVIST, *et al.* 2001. Impaired cerebral glucose metabolism and cognitive functioning predict deterioration in mild cognitive impairment. [abstract]. Neuroreport **12:** 851–855.
56. BERENT, S., B. GIORDANI, N. FOSTER, *et al.* 1999. Neuropsychological function and cerebral glucose utilization in isolated memory impairment and Alzheimer's disease. J. Psychiatric Res. **33:** 7–16.
57. CONVIT, A., J. DE ASIS, M.J. DE LEON, *et al.* 2000. Atrophy of the medial occipitotemporal, inferior, and middle temporal gyri in non-demented elderly predict decline to Alzheimer's disease. Neurobiol. Aging **21:** 19–26.
58. DE LEON, M., A. CONVIT, O. WOLF, *et al.* 2001. Prediction of cognitive decline in normal elderly subjects with 2-[18F]fluoro-2-deoxy-D-glucose/positron-emission tomography (FDG/PET). PNAS **98:** 10966–10971.
59. RUSINEK, H., S. DE SANTI, D. FRID, *et al.* 2003. Regional brain atrophy rate predicts future cognitive decline: 6-year longitudinal MR imaging study of normal aging. Radiology **229:** 691–696.

# [$^{123}$I]5-IA-85380 SPECT Imaging of β$_2$-Nicotinic Acetylcholine Receptor Availability in the Aging Human Brain

EFFIE M. MITSIS,[a,b] KELLY P. COSGROVE,[a] JULIE K. STALEY,[a,b] ERIN B. FROHLICH,[a] FREDERIC BOIS,[a] GILLES D. TAMAGNAN,[c] KRISTINA M. ESTOK,[a] JOHN P. SEIBYL,[c] AND CHRISTOPHER H. VAN DYCK[a]

[a]Department of Psychiatry, Yale University School of Medicine, New Haven, Connecticut, USA

[b]Veteran's Affairs Connecticut Healthcare System, West Haven, Connecticut, USA

[c]Institute for Neurodegenerative Disorders, New Haven, Connecticut, USA

ABSTRACT: Human postmortem studies have reported decreases with age in high-affinity nicotine binding in brain. We have been investigating *in vivo* the availability of the β$_2$-containing nicotinic acetylcholine receptor (β$_2$-nAChR) in healthy nonsmokers (18–85 years of age) using [$^{123}$I]5-IA-85380 SPECT imaging. Age and regional β$_2$-nAChR availability (V$_T$') have been observed to be inversely correlated in all brain regions analyzed, with decline ranging from 21% (cerebellum) to 36% (thalamus), or by up to 5% per decade of life. Preliminary results have confirmed postmortem reports of age-related decline in high-affinity nicotine binding with age and may elucidate the role of β$_2$-nAChRs in the cognitive decline associated with aging.

KEYWORDS: nicotinic receptors; aging; [$^{123}$I]5-IA-85380; SPECT imaging

## INTRODUCTION

Human postmortem studies have reported decreases with age in high-affinity nicotine binding in brain, although there have been some discrepant findings.[1] Few studies have investigated aging effects on nicotinic acetylcholine receptors in living subjects. We have been investigating *in vivo* the availability of the β$_2$-containing nicotinic acetylcholine receptor (β$_2$-nAChR) in healthy,

Address for correspondence: Christopher H. van Dyck, M.D., Department of Psychiatry, Yale University School of Medicine, Alzheimer's Disease Research Unit, One Church St., Suite 600, New Haven, CT 06510. Voice: 203-764-8100; fax: 203-764-8111.
christopher.vandyck@yale.edu

Ann. N.Y. Acad. Sci. 1097: 168–170 (2007). © 2007 New York Academy of Sciences.
doi: 10.1196/annals.1379.015

nonsmokers who ranged in age from 18 to 85 years (average age $= 46 \pm 22$ years).

Participants with no significant medical, neurological, or psychiatric illness were imaged with iodine-123-5-IA-85380 ([$^{123}$I]5-IA, [$^{123}$I]-5-iodo-3-[2(S)-2-azetidinylmethoxy] pyridine), and single photon emission computed tomography (SPECT) using a bolus plus constant infusion paradigm.[2] [$^{123}$I]5-IA demonstrates many of the properties necessary for *in vivo* imaging of $\beta_2$-nAChR with SPECT including high-affinity ($K_D = 11$ pM), rapid entry into brain, low nonspecific binding, and minimal toxicity.[3,4] Female subjects of childbearing potential were required to have a negative pregnancy test at screening and on the day of the SPECT scan immediately before tracer injection. Subjects $\geq 50$ years of age were also required to have no evidence of significant cognitive impairment, as indicated by Folstein Mini-Mental State Examination (MMSE)[5] score of $>26$, Clinical Dementia Rating Scale score of zero, and a delayed recall score on a complex verbal memory task (NYU Paragraph) of $\geq 9$ for $\geq 16$ years of education, $\geq 5$ for 8–15 years of education, and $\geq 3$ for 0–7 years of education. No subjects were taking medication that would potentially interfere with tracer uptake (i.e., cholinesterase inhibitors, antidepressants, antipsychotics, anticholinergics, anticonvulsants, or anxiolytics). Subjects were excluded if they had a pacemaker or other ferrous material in the body that would prevent them from having an MRI scan for purposes of co-registration.

Living human nonsmokers were imaged as described previously.[2] In brief, subjects were pretreated with stable supersaturated potassium iodide (SSKI, 800 mg) prior to radiotracer injection. Two antecubital venous catheters were placed and [$^{123}$I]5-IA was administered by a bolus (average $154 \pm 18$ MBq) followed by continuous infusion (average $22 \pm 2$ MBq/h) at a constant rate using a computer-controlled pump (IMED pump, Gemini PC-1, San Diego, CA, USA) for a bolus to infusion ratio of 7 h. Vital signs including blood pressure, and heart and respiration rates were measured 30–60 min before and between 30–60 min post [$^{123}$I]5-IA administration. Prior to scanning, five external fiducial markers containing 0.04–0.19 MBq of [$^{123}$I] were placed on the head along the canthomeatal line. One transmission scan (15 min) and three SPECT scans (30 min each) were obtained between 6 and 8 h of infusion, and plasma samples were collected immediately prior to and after the scan to quantify total parent and the free fraction of parent tracer in plasma ($f_1$, free fraction).[6] For the purposes of co-registration and to identify brain regions on the [$^{123}$I]5-IA SPECT scan, sagittal MR images were obtained on a separate day.

The effect of age on regional $\beta_2$-nAChR availability ($V_{T'}$, regional [$^{123}$I]5-IA activity/total plasma parent, a measure proportional to the binding potential) was analyzed using linear regression and Pearson product moment correlation ($r$). The brain regions analyzed were thalamus, frontal cortex, temporal cortex, parietal cortex, occipital cortex, anterior cingulate, striatum, and cerebellum.

$\beta_2$-nAChR availability has shown a significant inverse correlation with age in the eight brain regions analyzed. Rates of decline across the age range investigated have been greatest in thalamus (36%), frontal cortex (29%), parietal cortex (29%), and anterior cingulate (28%). Decline in receptor availability for the regions has ranged from 3% to 5% per decade of life. Pearson's correlation values for all regions investigated have ranged from $r = -0.38$ to $r = -0.62$ with $P$ values ranging from 0.01 to <0.0001.

These preliminary results in living human subjects have confirmed post-mortem reports of age-related decline in high-affinity nicotine binding with age. Given the well-documented importance of nicotinic mechanisms for learning and memory, these findings may elucidate the role of $\beta_2$-nAChRs in the cognitive decline associated with normal aging. Furthermore, loss of these receptors may be a diagnostic marker for individuals in presymptomatic stages of Alzheimer's disease.

## REFERENCES

1. NORDBERG, A. 1994. Human nicotinic receptors—their role in aging and dementia. Neurochem. Int. **25:** 93–97.
2. STALEY, J. et al. 2005. Iodine-123-5-IA-85380 SPECT measurement of nicotinic acetylcholine receptors in human brain by the constant infusion paradigm: feasibility and reproducibility. J. Nucl. Med. **46:** 1466–1472.
3. FUJITA, M. et al. 2000. Measurement of $\alpha_4\beta_2$ nicotinic acetylcholine receptors with [$^{123}$I]5-I-A85830 SPECT. J. Nucl. Med. **41:** 1552–1560.
4. FUJITA, M. et al. 2002. Whole-body biodistribution, radiation absorbed dose, and brain SPECT imaging with [$^{123}$I]5-I-A-85380 in healthy human subjects. Eur. J. Nucl. Med. Mol. Imaging **29:** 183–190.
5. FOLSTEIN, M.F., S.E. FOSTEIN & P.R. McHUGH. 1975. "Mini-mental state": a practical method for grading the cognitive state of patients for the clinician. J. Psychiatr. Res. **12:** 189–198.
6. ZOGHBI, S. et al. 2001. Measurement of plasma metabolites of (S)-5-[123I]iodo-3-(2-azetidinylmethoxy)pyridine (5-IA-85380), a nicotinic acetylcholine receptor imaging agent, in nonhuman primates. Nucl. Med. Biol. **28:** 91–96.

# Role of Aerobic Fitness and Aging on Cerebral White Matter Integrity

BONITA L. MARKS,[a,b] DAVID J. MADDEN,[a,c] BARBARA BUCUR,[a]
JAMES M. PROVENZALE,[d] LEONARD E. WHITE,[a,e]
ROBERTO CABEZA,[a,f] AND SCOTT A. HUETTEL[c,a,g]

[a] Center for the Study of Aging and Human Development, Duke University
Medical Center, Durham, North Carolina, USA

[b] Department of Exercise and Sport Science, University of North Carolina,
Chapel Hill, North Carolina, USA

[c] Department of Psychiatry, Duke University Medical Center, Durham,
North Carolina, USA

[d] Department of Radiology, Duke University Medical Center, Durham,
North Carolina, USA

[e] Department of Community and Family Medicine, Duke University Medical
Center, Durham, North Carolina, USA

[f] Center for Cognitive Neuroscience, Duke University, Durham,
North Carolina, USA

[g] Brain Imaging and Analysis Center, Duke University Medical Center, Durham,
North Carolina, USA

ABSTRACT: Neuroimaging research suggests that cerebral white matter
(WM) integrity, as reflected in fractional anisotropy (FA) via diffusion
tensor imaging (DTI), is decreased in older adults, especially in the prefrontal regions of the brain. Behavioral investigations of cognitive functioning suggest that some aspects of cognition may be better preserved
in older adults who possess higher levels of aerobic fitness. There are
only a few studies, however, investigating potential mechanisms for the
improvements in aerobic fitness. Our study suggests that greater aerobic
fitness may be related to greater WM integrity in select brain regions.

KEYWORDS: aging; aerobic fitness; exercise; white matter integrity;
older adults

Address for correspondence: Bonita L. Marks, Ph.D., Department of Exercise and Sport Science,
University of North Carolina at Chapel Hill, Fetzer Gym, CB 8700, Chapel Hill, NC 27599-8700.
Voice: 919-962-2260; fax: 919-962-0489.
marks@email.unc.edu

Ann. N.Y. Acad. Sci. 1097: 171–174 (2007). © 2007 New York Academy of Sciences.
doi: 10.1196/annals.1379.022

# INTRODUCTION

Executive functioning and the cortical volume of corresponding prefrontal brain regions have been shown to decline with aging. Although there is an emerging body of evidence suggesting that higher aerobic fitness ($VO_2$ max, maximal amount of oxygen consumed) may be related to improved executive functioning in older adults, there is a paucity of human-derived data regarding the potential mechanisms linking aerobic fitness to the functional anatomy of the brain.[1] Previous studies suggest that there is an age-related decline in cerebral white matter (WM) integrity, thus individual differences in aerobic fitness may be associated with differing levels of WM integrity, which may in turn have implications for preserved cognitive function. Diffusion tensor imaging can provide detailed delineation of WM pathways based on rates of microscopic water diffusion. A higher degree of WM integrity is reflected in a greater degree of fractional anisotropy (FA) of diffusion. Prior research has shown an age-related decline in FA, particularly in the prefrontal regions.[2] Therefore, the purpose of this study was to determine if individual differences in aerobic fitness would be associated with variations in WM integrity, independently of age and gender. Our hypothesis was that higher aerobic fitness would be positively associated with greater WM integrity (higher FA) in the prefrontal (executive function) areas of the brain (i.e., genu, pericallosal frontal).

# METHODS

This research was approved by Duke University Health System's Institutional Review Board. Twenty-eight healthy subjects (13 younger adults, $24 \pm 3$ years; 15 older adults, $69.6 \pm 4.7$ years) consented to participate. None were depressed or neurologically impaired (BDI Score: $2.4 \pm 2.3$; MMSE Score: $29.6 \pm 0.06$).

## *Aerobic Fitness Estimation*

Because exercise testing was not available, aerobic fitness was calculated from a nonexercise aerobic fitness regression equation using gender, age, body mass index (BMI), and a physical activity rating score (PAS) as predictors for estimated maximal oxygen consumption ($VO_2$ max in mL/kg/min). This equation was validated in a study sample of 2,009 men and women (18–70 years of age) at the Cooper Aerobic Clinic ($r = 0.78$; $P < 0.01$, SE = 5.6 mL/kg/min).[3] The PAS questionnaire required the subjects to rank their average level of physical activity/exercise on a 0–7 rating scale with a ranking of "0" representing little or no physical activity/exercise and a ranking of "7" representing running more than 10 miles a week or participating in 3 or more hours of heavy exercise weekly. Subjects were probed regarding the exact nature of their daily physical activity/exercise routine (mode, frequency, duration, and intensity of effort) by the telephone interviewer. The $VO_2$ max estimation formula was: $VO_2max$ $(mL/kg/min) \approx 56.363–(0.381 * age) + (1.951 * PAS)–(0.754 * BMI) + (gender * 10.987)$, where: PAS = physical activity rating score (0–7 scale); BMI = weight (kg) ÷ [height (m)]$^2$, and gender: 0 = women; 1 = men.

### Diffusion Tensor Imaging (DTI)

Magnetic resonance imaging was conducted at 4T with 30 contiguous near-axial slices parallel to the AC–PC, 3.8 mm thick; TR = 30,000; per slice, diffusion measured in six directions ($b = 1,000$ sec/mm$^2$) plus one image with no diffusion weighting ($b = 0$); five signal averages. Diffusion tensor eigenvalues were calculated from custom MATLAB scripts. Structural imaging consisted of 3D fast IRP SPGR sequence, 60 contiguous slices, parallel to AC–PC, 1.9 mm thick. For each subject, seven regions of interest were drawn on the diffusion tensor images on a slice-by-slice basis using the high-resolution SPGR images as a reference.

## RESULTS AND CONCLUSIONS

Analyses of aerobic fitness yielded significant, independent effects of age group ($t = -9.46$; $P < 0.0001$) and gender ($t = -5.88$; $P < 0.0001$), representing higher levels of fitness for younger adults and males, respectively. After covarying for age and gender, significant ($P < 0.05$) positive correlations remained between aerobic fitness and FA in two regions, the uncinate fasciculus (UNC) and the cingulum (CIN). Regression analyses revealed that the unique contribution of aerobic fitness to the FA variance was 15% for the UNC and 13% for the CIN. Although these preliminary findings suggest that increased aerobic fitness may be associated with greater WM integrity in select regions of the brain, independently of age and gender, the hypothesis that aerobic fitness is significantly related to specific prefrontal regions of the brain is not supported. These results should be viewed with caution due to potential influence of outliers and limitations with estimating $VO_2max$. Future research needs larger sample sizes and direct $VO_2$ assessments.

### ACKNOWLEDGEMENT

This research was funded in part by NIH Grants RO1 AG11622 and T32 AG000029.

# REFERENCES

1. COLCOMBE, S.J. *et al.* 2004. Cardiovascular fitness, cortical plasticity, and aging. PNAS **101:** 3316–3321.
2. MADDEN, D.J. *et al.* 2006. Adult age differences in the functional neuroanatomy of visual attention: A combined fMRI and DTI study. Neurobiol. Aging. Feb. 22 [E-pub ahead of print]. In press.
3. JACKSON, A.S. *et al.* 1990. Prediction of functional aerobic capacity without exercise testing. Med. Sci. Sports Exerc. **22:** 863–870.

# Age-Related Changes in Nociceptive Processing in the Human Brain

RAIMI L. QUITON,[a,b] STEVEN R. ROYS,[c] JIACHEN ZHUO,[c]
MICHAEL L. KEASER,[b] RAO P. GULLAPALLI,[c]
AND JOEL D. GREENSPAN[a,b]

[a]Program in Neuroscience, University of Maryland, Baltimore, Maryland, USA

[b]Department of Biomedical Sciences, Dental School, University of Maryland, Baltimore, Maryland, USA

[c]Department of Diagnostic Radiology, School of Medicine, University of Maryland, Baltimore, Maryland, USA

ABSTRACT: Functional magnetic resonance imaging (fMRI) was used to compare cortical nociceptive responses to painful contact heat in healthy young (ages 22–30, $n = 7$) and older (ages 56–75, $n = 7$) subjects. Compared to young subjects, older subjects had significantly smaller pain-related fMRI responses in anterior insula (aINS) ($P < 0.04$), primary somatosensory cortex (S1) ($P = 0.03$), and supplementary motor area ($P = 0.02$). Gray matter volumes in S1 and aINS were significantly smaller for the older group ($P = 0.02$ and $0.0001$, respectively), suggesting reduced processing capacity in these regions that might account for smaller pain-related fMRI responses.

KEYWORDS: aging; cortex; fMRI; nociception; pain

## INTRODUCTION

Normal aging is associated with complex changes in the pain experience. Elderly individuals often show higher pain thresholds[7] and report pain associated with acute pathologies, such as myocardial infarction[9] and appendicitis[1] less frequently than younger adults, suggesting that pain sensitivity declines with age. On the other hand, advancing age is associated with increased prevalence of several chronic pain disorders.[2,8,11] Despite the evidence for age-related changes in pain, little is known about how aging affects neural systems that process nociceptive information, particularly at the level of the cerebral cortex.

Address for correspondence: Raimi L. Quiton, Department of Biomedical Sciences, UMB Dental School, 650 W. Baltimore Street, 7th Floor, Baltimore, MD 21201. Voice: 410-706-2027; fax: 410-706-4172.
rquiton@umaryland.edu

Ann. N.Y. Acad. Sci. 1097: 175–178 (2007). © 2007 New York Academy of Sciences.
doi: 10.1196/annals.1379.024

A previous study reported reduced cortical electroencephalographic responses to painful stimulation in elderly compared to younger subjects;[6] however, studies using techniques with higher spatial resolution, such as functional magnetic resonance imaging (fMRI), are lacking and are needed to localize cortical regions where nociceptive processing differs with age.

The objective of this study was to characterize age-related changes in cortical processing of painful heat stimuli using fMRI in human volunteers. Healthy young (ages 22–30, $n = 7$) and older (ages 56–75, $n = 7$) subjects participated in three fMRI sessions (two scans per session) in which painful contact heat stimuli were delivered to the left dorsal forearm. Two temperatures of painful heat were delivered to each subject: (1) 48°C and (2) a subject-specific temperature perceived as moderately painful, which was defined as the temperature the subject rated between 50 and 60 on a 100-point computerized visual analog scale (VAS) for pain intensity. During each fMRI scan, the two temperatures were delivered six times each in a randomized order. After each stimulus, the subject rated peak pain intensity using the computerized VAS. Functional MR images were acquired using a single-shot echo planar imaging T2*-sensitive sequence (gradient echo time 35 ms, spatial resolution $1.875 \times 1.875 \times 6$ mm, temporal resolution 3 s, whole brain coverage in 24 axial slices). High-resolution T1-weighted volumetric scans were acquired for anatomical detail and segmentation analysis.

Using a regression model and cluster-thresholding approach, significant pain-related fMRI activation was identified in cortical regions of interest (ROI) involved in nociceptive processing: primary somatosensory cortex (S1), secondary somatosensory cortex, anterior cingulate cortex, anterior insula (aINS), posterior insula, supplementary motor area (SMA), and inferior frontal gyrus (IFG). For each ROI, two measures of pain-related fMRI activation were calculated: number of significantly active voxels (spatial extent) and signal change amplitude (amplitude). Age group differences were assessed for each measure in each ROI using a mixed-effects model, with age group as the between-subjects factor and session and scan as within-subjects factors.

Older subjects had significantly smaller pain-related fMRI responses than younger subjects in several ROIs. The spatial extent of pain-related activation was significantly smaller for older subjects in ipsilateral S1 ($P = 0.02$) and contralateral S1 ($P = 0.03$) for 48°C stimuli and in ipsilateral aINS ($P = 0.03$) and ipsilateral SMA ($P = 0.02$) for moderately painful stimuli. The amplitude of pain-related activation was significantly smaller for older subjects in ipsilateral aINS ($P = 0.04$) and contralateral aINS ($P = 0.005$) for 48°C stimuli and ipsilateral aINS ($P = 0.001$) for moderately painful stimuli. In addition, older subjects had a significantly smaller proportion of gray matter than young subjects in contralateral S1 ($P = 0.02$), contralateral aINS ($P = 0.0001$), ipsilateral aINS ($P = 0.003$), and contralateral IFG ($P = 0.03$).

This study is the first to identify regions of the human cerebral cortex where nociceptive processing is affected by age. Specifically, healthy older subjects (ages 56 to 75 years) had significantly smaller fMRI responses to painful contact heat in several brain regions (aINS, S1, and SMA) compared to young subjects (ages 22–30 years). The older group had significantly smaller proportions of gray matter in aINS and S1 than the younger group, a finding that suggests reduced processing capacity in these regions that might account for smaller pain-related responses. S1 has been implicated in coding intensity of painful stimuli.[3,10] Thus, age-related reductions in the S1 response to 48°C stimuli may reflect alterations in the ability to precisely gauge noxious stimuli, potentially explaining the clinical observation that elderly individuals report less intense and less frequent pain associated with acute pathology.[5] The aINS has been implicated in the affective component of interoception (generating emotions associated with the physical state of the body).[4] Thus, age-related reductions in the aINS response to pain may reflect impairments in the affective response to changes in physical homeostasis, potentially explaining the clinical observation that elderly individuals attach less importance to pain and symptoms from acute pathologies.[11] Overall, detection of significant age group differences in the small sample population used in this study is compelling evidence that advancing age has profound effects on cortical nociceptive processing. These effects may be related to the failure of many elderly individuals to detect and seek treatment for acute medical disorders.

## REFERENCES

1. ALBANO, W.A., C.M. ZIELINSKI & C.H. ORGAN 1975. Is appendicitis in the aged really different? Geriatrics **30**(1 Sz): 81–88.
2. BADLEY, E.M. & A. TENNANT. 1992. Changing profile of joint disorders with age: findings from a postal survey of the population of Calderdale, West Yorkshire, United Kingdom. Ann. Rheum. Dis. **51**: 366–371.
3. COGHILL, R.C., C.N. SANG, J.M. MAISOG & M.J. IADAROLA. 1999. Pain intensity processing within the human brain: a bilateral, distributed mechanism. J. Neurophysiol. **82**: 1934–1943.
4. CRAIG, A.D. 2002. How do you feel? Interoception: the sense of the physiological condition of the body. Nat. Rev. Neurosci. **3**: 655–666.
5. GAGLIESE, L. & R. MELZACK. 2005. Pain in the elderly. *In* Wall and Melzack's Textbook of Pain. Fifth edition. S.B. McMahon & M. Koltzenburg, Eds.: 1169–1180. Churchill Livingstone. Oxford, UK.
6. GIBSON, S.J., M.M. GORMAN & R.D. HELME. 1991. Assessment of pain in the elderly using event-related cerebral potentials. *In* Proceedings of the VIth World Congress on Pain. M.R. Bond, J.E. Charlton & C. Woolf, Eds.: 527–533. Elsevier Science Publishers BV. Amsterdam.
7. GIBSON, S.J. & M. FARRELL. 2004. A review of age differences in the neurophysiology of nociception and the perceptual experience of pain. Clin. J. Pain **20**: 227–239.
8. JUNG, B.F., R.W. JOHNSON, D.R. GRIFFIN & R.H. DWORKIN. 2004. Risk factors for postherpetic neuralgia in patients with herpes zoster. Neurology **62**: 1545–1551.

9. MEHTA, R.H., S.S. RATHORE, M.J. RADFORD, *et al.* 2001. Acute myocardial infarc-
    tion in the elderly: differences by age. J. Am. Coll. Cardiol. **38:** 736–741.
10. MOULTON, E.A., M.L. KEASER, R.P. GULLAPALLI, & J.D. GREENSPAN. 2005. Re-
    gional intensive and temporal patterns of functional MRI activation distinguish-
    ing noxious and innocuous contact heat. J. Neurophysiol. **93:** 2183–2193.
11. PICKERING, G. 2005. Age differences in clinical pain states. *In* Pain in Older Persons.
    S.J. Gibson & D.K. Weiner, Eds.: 67–85. IASP Press. Seattle, WA.

# Magnetic Resonance Spectroscopy and Environmental Toxicant Exposure

MARC G. WEISSKOPF

*Department of Environmental Health, Harvard School of Public Health, Occupational Health Program, Landmark Center, Boston, Massachusetts, USA*

ABSTRACT: The study of neurological impacts of toxicants has emphasized neuropsychological tests as important outcome variables. Direct assessment of neural substrates of environmental impacts could offer many advantages. I discuss our use of magnetic resonance spectroscopy (MRS) in the neurological assessment of adult lead poisoning of monozygotic twins as an example. Cognitive testing showed frontal lobe dysfunction in both twins, and more dramatic hippocampal dysfunction in the twin with higher lead exposure (JG). MRS showed lower N-acetylaspartate/creatine ratios in JG. The findings illustrate the potential utility of MRS in assessing impacts of not only lead, but other toxicants as well.

KEYWORDS: lead poisoning; nervous system; adult; psychological tests; monozygotic twins

## INTRODUCTION

The study of neurological impacts of environmental exposures has emphasized neuropsychological test results as important outcome variables. While the use of such tests has proven to be a valuable tool, there are certain drawbacks.[1] Neurobehavioral end points are highly integrative, serving as the final common pathways for the expression of the impacts of myriad factors, making them fertile ground for residual confounding. Additionally, redundancy in the underlying neural substrate may cause loss of sensitivity when measuring the environmental impact on nervous system function. The development of tests that directly assess the neurophysiologic substrates of different behaviors could provide a more objective and sensitive measure of the effects of

Address for correspondence: Marc G. Weisskopf, Department of Environmental Health, Harvard School of Public Health, Occupational Health Program, Landmark Center, 401 Park Dr., P.O. Box 15697, Boston, MA 02215. Voice: 617-384-8872; fax: 617-384-8994.
mweissko@hsph.harvard.edu

Ann. N.Y. Acad. Sci. 1097: 179–182 (2007). © 2007 New York Academy of Sciences.
doi: 10.1196/annals.1379.028

neurotoxicants on the brain. Furthermore, understanding the impact of environmental neurotoxicants at the level of the neural substrates of behavior could aid in the development of targeted interventions and therapies for prevention and/or remediation of any adverse health effects, particularly if that understanding allowed for an earlier detection of subtle, subclinical effects. Brain imaging techniques may provide just such a tool; one that has been practically unexplored to this point in the context of environmental health.

We set out to explore the use of magnetic resonance spectroscopy (MRS) in the context of environmental toxicant exposure, in particular exposure to lead. Despite the fact that the use of MRS in neurological disease has grown rapidly over the past decade, the use of MRS in the setting of environmental insult to the brain is quite new. In contrast, lead is one of the most extensively studied environmental toxicants. The adverse effect of lead exposure on neurobehavioral functioning is one of the most consistently reported impairments associated with lead exposure.[2] Despite this, little is known about the effects of lead on brain metabolism *in vivo,* or the structural and functional correlates of lead-related brain dysfunction. Only three published reports have examined the impact of lead exposure on brain metabolites as can be measured with MRS and all three of these studied children.[3-5]

As a first exploration of the use of MRS in the context of adult lead exposure, our group reported on 71-year-old identical twin brothers, identified with chronic lead poisoning from an occupational medicine clinic roster.[6] Besides being identical twins, the pair had extremely similar life experience: the two grew up together, went to the same high school, served in the Navy together, and worked together in the painting business. Both were retired, but when they had worked, one brother (JG) primarily performed paint removal, which entails a much higher risk of lead exposure than does the painting itself that his brother (EG) primarily did. We measured patella and tibia bone lead concentrations using K-shell-X-ray fluorescence.[7] Bone lead concentrations reflect cumulative exposure to lead as lead in circulation is laid down in bone where it has a half-life of about 7 years in trabecular bone (e.g., patella) and several decades in cortical bone (e.g., tibia). The twins' bone lead concentrations were 5–10 times that of nonoccupationally exposed adults,[8] and JG had concentrations approximately 2.5 times higher than his brother (JG: patella $= 343$ $\mu g/g$, tibia $=$ 189 $\mu g/g$; EG: patella $=119$ $\mu g/g$, tibia $= 79$ $\mu g/g$). MRS (1.5 T) showed lower N-acetylaspartate/creatine (NAA/Cr) ratios—a marker of neuronal density[9]— in JG than his brother in the hippocampus (1.30 vs. 1.60), frontal lobes (1.15 vs. 1.52), and the midbrain (1.47 vs. 1.65). On neurocognitive tests, working memory/executive function was found to be below expectation in both twins, while short-term memory function was dramatically worse in JG than his brother. These results are consistent with frontal lobe dysfunction in both twins, but with more dramatic hippocampal dysfunction in JG.

While we cannot infer causality from such a case study, there are unique aspects to the study of these painters that raise tantalizing questions. The identical genetic make up and the virtually identical life experiences make their differences in lead exposures stand out. The cognitive function findings are consistent with the toxic effects of lead and the difference in lead exposure between the two. The MRS results suggest a relation between chronic lead exposure and neuronal loss in the hippocampus and frontal cortex, but questions remain. Do the MRS changes contribute to the impairment in cognitive function? Why were cognitive differences between the twins dramatically more pronounced on hippocampal-based tests than frontal lobe-based tests while the differences in NAA/Cr ratio were similar in these regions? Could the NAA/Cr ratios found in the frontal lobes already have passed some threshold such that the associated cognitive deficits in both twins are similar? Or is the more reduced NAA/Cr ratio in JG picking up preclinical changes and the more dramatic cognitive effects are still to come? Such a possibility illustrates another tremendous potential for such imaging techniques: there is growing interest in the possible involvement of early life exposures in subsequent adult neurological disease.[10] A primary obstacle to meaningful results of such studies, though, is the long-time span between exposure and outcome. The identification and use of biomarkers of early, subclinical disease—MRS being one possibility—could shorten the time lag between exposure and outcome by providing an intermediate marker that could be separately linked with exposure and disease. Overall, the potential utility of MRS in determining impacts of, and mechanisms of neurotoxicity for, not only lead, but other toxicants as well is an exciting future path for environmental health research.

## REFERENCES

1. BELLINGER, D.C. 2002. Perspectives on incorporating human neurobehavioral end points in risk assessments. Risk Anal. **22:** 487–498.
2. AGENCY FOR TOXIC SUBSTANCES AND DISEASE REGISTRY. 2005. Toxicological profile for lead (Draft for Public Comment). US Department of Health and Human Services, Public Health Service. Atlanta, GA.
3. TROPE, I., D. LOPEZ-VILLEGAS & R.F. LENKINSKI. 1998. Magnetic resonance imaging and spectroscopy of regional brain structure in a 10-year-old boy with elevated blood lead levels. Pediatrics **101:** 1066–1067.
4. TROPE, I., D. LOPEZ-VILLEGAS, et al. 2001. Exposure to lead appears to selectively alter metabolism of cortical gray matter. Pediatrics **107:** 1437–1442.
5. MENG, X.M., D.M. ZHU, et al. 2005. Effects of chronic lead exposure on 1H MRS of hippocampus and frontal lobes in children. Neurology **64:** 1644–1647.
6. WEISSKOPF, M.G., H. HU, et al. 2004. Cognitive deficits and magnetic resonance spectroscopy in adult monozygotic twins with lead poisoning. Environ. Health Perspect. **112:** 620–625.
7. HU, H., M. RABINOWITZ & D. SMITH. 1998. Bone lead as a biological marker in epidemiologic studies of chronic toxicity: conceptual paradigms. Environ. Health Perspect. **106:** 1–8.

8. KIM, R., C. LANDRIGAN, *et al.* 1997. Age and secular trends in bone lead levels in middle-aged and elderly men: three-year longitudinal follow-up in the Normative Aging Study. Am. J. Epidemiol. **146:** 586–591.
9. ROSS, B.D., P. COLETTI & A. LIN. 2006. Magnetic resonance spectroscopy of the brain: neurospectroscopy. *In* Clinical Magnetic Resonance Imaging. Third edition. R.R. Edelman, J.R. Hesselink, M.B. Zlatkin & J.V. Crues, Eds.: 1840–1907. Saunders Elsevier. Philadelphia, PA.
10. WEISSKOPF, M.G., R.O. WRIGHT & H. HU. 2006. Early life environmental exposures and neurologic outcomes in adults. *In* Human Developmental Neurotoxicology. D. Bellinger, Ed.: 341–359. The Taylor and Francis Group, New York.

# Tracking Alzheimer's Disease

PAUL M. THOMPSON,[a] KIRALEE M. HAYASHI,[a] REBECCA A. DUTTON,[a] MING-CHANG CHIANG,[a] ALEX D. LEOW,[a,b] ELIZABETH R. SOWELL,[a] GREIG DE ZUBICARAY,[c] JAMES T. BECKER,[d,e,f] OSCAR L. LOPEZ,[d] HOWARD J. AIZENSTEIN,[e] AND ARTHUR W. TOGA[a]

[a]Department of Neurology, Laboratory of Neuro Imaging, UCLA School of Medicine, Los Angeles, California, USA

[b]Neuropsychiatric Institute, UCLA School of Medicine, Los Angeles, California, USA

[c]Centre for Magnetic Resonance, University of Queensland, Brisbane, Australia

[d]Department of Neurology, University of Pittsburgh, Pittsburgh, Pennsylvania, USA

[e]Department of Psychiatry, University of Pittsburgh, Pittsburgh, Pennsylvania, USA

[f]Department of Psychology, University of Pittsburgh, Pittsburgh, Pennsylvania, USA

ABSTRACT: Population-based brain mapping provides great insight into the trajectory of aging and dementia, as well as brain changes that normally occur over the human life span. We describe three novel brain mapping techniques, *cortical thickness mapping*, *tensor-based morphometry (TBM)*, and *hippocampal surface modeling*, which offer enormous power for measuring disease progression in drug trials, and shed light on the neuroscience of brain degeneration in Alzheimer's disease (AD) and mild cognitive impairment (MCI). We report the first time-lapse maps of cortical atrophy spreading dynamically in the living brain, based on averaging data from populations of subjects with Alzheimer's disease and normal subjects imaged longitudinally with MRI. These dynamic sequences show a rapidly advancing wave of cortical atrophy sweeping from limbic and temporal cortices into higher-order association and ultimately primary sensorimotor areas, in a pattern that correlates with cognitive decline. A complementary technique, TBM, reveals the 3D profile of atrophic rates, at each point in the brain. A third technique, *hippocampal surface modeling*, plots the profile of shape alterations across the hippocampal surface. The three techniques provide moderate to highly automated analyses of images, have been validated on hundreds of scans, and are sensitive to clinically relevant changes in individual patients and groups

Address for correspondence: Dr. Paul Thompson, Department of Neurology, Laboratory of Neuro Imaging, UCLA School of Medicine, 635 Charles E. Young Drive South, Suite 225E, Los Angeles, CA 90095-7332, USA. Voice: 310-206-2101; fax: 310-206-5518.
thompson@loni.ucla.edu

Ann. N.Y. Acad. Sci. 1097: 183–214 (2007). © 2007 New York Academy of Sciences.
doi: 10.1196/annals.1379.017

undergoing different drug treatments. We compare time-lapse maps of
AD, MCI, and other dementias, correlate these changes with cognition,
and relate them to similar time-lapse maps of childhood development,
schizophrenia, and HIV-associated brain degeneration. Strengths and
weaknesses of these different imaging measures for basic neuroscience
and drug trials are discussed.

KEYWORDS: MRI; Alzheimer's disease; aging; MCI; dementia; brain
degeneration; PET

# INTRODUCTION

Alzheimer's disease (AD) is arguably the greatest threat to public health in
the 21st century. Dementia doubles in frequency every 5 years after the age of
60, afflicting 1% of 60–64-year olds but 30–40% of those aged 85 years and
older.[1] With the size of the elderly population rising dramatically and incidence
of dementia also increasing, there are clear warning signs of an approaching
socioeconomic disaster. As novel, disease-modifying agents emerge, brain
imaging measures are vital to help demonstrate the effectiveness of pharmacologic treatments evidenced by any slowing of disease progression in the
brain. Brain imaging measures facilitate drug development in animal models
and patient studies,[2,3] and are also emerging as important tools for differential
diagnosis of dementia.[4]

MRI and PET studies allow visualization of brain structure and function in
three-dimensional detail. When performed repeatedly over time, they can be
used to visualize disease progression in living patients. Based on data from
many subjects, measures of regional brain volumes and rates of atrophy may
eventually aid in predicting who will suffer cognitive decline among those at
risk for dementia. These measures are already being used to gauge the effects
of therapy in drug trials. Imaging can also be used to track how different
degenerative diseases spread in the living brain, providing a better theoretical
understanding of how the various types of dementia differ (such as Alzheimer's
disease vs. vascular or semantic dementia). Imaging can also be used to explore
how the brain changes with normal aging,[5] pinpointing changes associated with
specific behavioral alterations, such as apathy or declining executive function.[6]

Brain imaging is also revealing important new information on other degenerative dementias, such as that resulting from HIV infection. Forty million
people are infected with HIV worldwide, and at least 40% of these patients
suffer from cognitive impairments ranging from minor cognitive motor disorders (MCMD) to HIV-associated dementia, often with a progressive trajectory
leading to death. The trajectory of brain degeneration in HIV is markedly different from that seen in Alzheimer's disease—the caudate, white matter, and
cortex degenerate progressively in a sequence that was recently visualized for
the first time.[7–10] As in Alzheimer's disease, maps of degeneration based on

MRI scans are increasingly needed to help gauge the success of neuroprotective therapies (e.g., memantine, CPI-1189, or NMDA-receptor antagonists in neuro-AIDS). As we describe later, MRI may also be combined with image analysis methods to track disease progression in individual patients.

Our understanding of degenerative disease has grown considerably due to rapid advances in brain imaging technologies. When combined with sophisticated analysis methods, structural MRI can now detect subtle, systematic brain volume changes on the order of 0.5% per year in individuals.[3,11] If the same group of subjects is scanned repeatedly as their disease progresses, the dynamic trajectory of cortical atrophy can be reconstructed as it spreads over time in the living brain.[12] New PET tracer compounds are being developed to visualize the profile of accumulating pathology.[13–17] Hailed as a breakthrough in the AD research community, these PET tracers visualize amyloid plaques and neurofibrillary tangles (NFT) in the living brain—hallmarks of AD previously only detectable at autopsy. These molecular probes are labeled with positron emitting isotopes—when they bind to the hallmark lesions of AD, their distribution in the brain can be determined using PET scanning. Both the UCLA and Pittsburgh compounds—respectively called [$^{18}$F]-FDDNP and [$^{11}$C]-PIB (Pittsburgh compound B)—show the expected pattern of accumulating pathology in initial studies of patients with AD and in small samples of mild cognitive impairment (MCI) subjects.[15,17] As PET and MRI measures track different aspects of the disease process, there is a race to determine which imaging measures are most sensitive to disease progression, which techniques are most accurate in predicting imminent degenerative changes, and which are best at discriminating pathological from healthy aging. Clearly, techniques with a relatively high *diagnostic* specificity (such as cerebro-spinal fluid [CSF] measures of β-amyloid levels) may not offer the greatest sensitivity to disease progression over time. The pace of analytic developments in computational anatomy is also high. Newer computational methods, such as tensor-based morphometry (TBM), can detect increasingly subtle brain changes in conventional MRI scans, and newer imaging techniques, such as diffusion tensor imaging (DTI), are providing new insight into the pattern of deteriorating fiber architecture.

### *Imaging of Alzheimer's Disease and MCI*

Imaging studies have become a priority in Alzheimer's disease research as they can be used to evaluate treatments that may slow or delay the disease process.[2,3] A major practical goal is shortening the minimum feasible follow-up interval in a drug trial, or reducing the sample size required to detect a given degree of slowing of brain degeneration. This would have immediate practical advantages as new drugs could be tested much more efficiently. Clinical testing is commonly combined with neuroimaging to determine how best to identify presymptomatic candidates for preventive treatments before the extensive neuronal damage of AD has set in. MCI, for example, is a transitional state between normal aging and dementia. MCI subjects have a cognitive complaint and test 1.5 standard deviations below age- and education-adjusted norms on one or more neuropsychological tests, but they are still capable of independent living.[18,19] MCI is defined using neuropsychiatric criteria, but many brain imaging studies aim to develop measures that are sensitive enough to distinguish MCI from healthy aging with high specificity.[20] Other studies attempt to differentiate between MCI subjects who will imminently convert to AD, over a specific follow-up interval, versus those who remain stable or even recover.[21,22]

Scientific interest in MCI is rising as MCI subjects convert to full-blown AD at a rate 3–6 times higher than normal subjects.[18,19] Alarmingly, *post mortem* studies have shown that most patients with MCI already have the pathological hallmarks of AD—neocortical senile plaques, NFT, atrophy, and neuronal loss in layer II of the entorhinal cortex.[23,24] Many imaging studies target individuals with MCI as they are more likely than the general elderly population to obtain diagnoses of AD later in life. Research efforts may ultimately be of greater benefit to those with MCI given that early intervention may eventually prevent progression to global cognitive decline. As the risk of AD increases exponentially with age, delaying disease onset, even by a couple of years, would vastly reduce the overall number of cases of AD.

### Statistical Power

Improved treatment is needed for patients at all stages of AD, but many drug trials focus on MCI subjects for pragmatic reasons. Cognitively normal elderly subjects convert to AD at a rate of only 1–2% per year, so trials to resist conversion from normality to MCI or AD would need to follow 3,000–6,000 subjects for 5 to 7 years to achieve sufficient clinical endpoints.[2] This is prohibitively expensive and too slow to be practical. On the other hand, MCI subjects convert to AD at a rate of 12%–15% per year. Secondary prevention studies (to prevent conversion from MCI to AD) typically need to assess only several hundred subjects, as a large proportion will convert to AD in 1–4 years (the duration of a typical research study). Even so, long time frames are necessary because of the high variability in clinical endpoints, and the relatively small degenerative changes that are barely detectable in brain images unless data from large numbers of subjects are combined (see Ref. 25, for studies of the detection limits of sequential MRI).

If any imaging method could demonstrate slowing, in a quantitative measure of the disease process, the hurdle for treatments to pass would be greatly lowered—drug evaluation would be greatly accelerated. For example, a treatment would be regarded as promising if it were shown to slow whole brain atrophic rates, in MCI, by as little as 10% over a 6-month interval. Many more clinical trials would be attempted, as the time required, costs, and associated economic risks, would be greatly reduced. With this in mind, developers of computational techniques now aim to extract the maximum amount of information from images of disease progression, often by compiling population-based repositories of statistical data on expected rates of atrophy. Other efforts are mathematically distilling new sources of contrast from images (using new tracer kinetic models for PET, or combining scans acquired at different magnetic field strengths to detect new features, such as iron (ferritin) accumulation in the brain.[26,27]

Here we review recent progress in the neuroimaging of dementia, focusing on structural brain mapping studies that track the disease as it spreads in the living brain. These imaging approaches are being used to map disease progression in individuals and populations, revealing group patterns of cortical thinning, gray and white matter atrophy, and shape changes in subcortical structures, such as the hippocampus. Functional and structural imaging methods may also be combined, relating anatomical deficits to plaque and tangle pathology observed *post mortem* or with new PET tracers. These brain mapping techniques show promise in identifying predictors of imminent decline and disease onset, which are valuable for identifying candidates for drug trials. An overarching goal of most brain mapping studies is to extract and analyze statistical data on the disease process and develop new mathematical methods to quantify how well treatments resist AD (see Ref. 12, for a review).

## THE TRAJECTORY OF ALZHEIMER'S DISEASE

Recent imaging studies have successfully tracked the emergence and spread of Alzheimer's disease pathology in the living brain (see e.g., Ref. 28). AD pathology progresses in a known, stereotypical sequence (FIG. 1), whether it is tracked with MRI, PET, SPECT, or in *post mortem* histologic studies of patients at different stages of the disease.

The time-course of disease progression varies substantially among individuals with AD, but neurofibrillary pathology typically starts in the transentorhinal cortex and quickly spreads to the entorhinal cortex before involving the hippocampus.[29-31] This temporal pathology persists for several years[11] before spreading cortically to engulf the rest of the temporal, frontal, and parietal lobes.[28,30-36]

Longitudinal 3D MRI scanning of groups of subjects can be used to map this process in detail. Time-lapse maps have been constructed from sequential brain MRI scans to reveal the anatomical sequence of cortical atrophy[28] (see http://www.loni.ucla.edu/~thompson/AD_4D/dynamic.html for movies of disease progression, that can be viewed over the Internet). Cortical regions

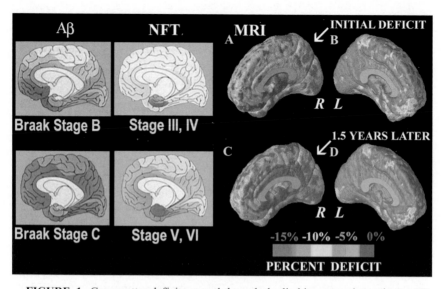

**FIGURE 1.** Gray matter deficits spread through the limbic system in moderate AD. Cortical atrophy occurring during the progression of AD is detected by comparing average profiles of gray matter between 12 AD patients (age: 68.4 ± 1.9 years) and 14 elderly matched controls (age: 71.4 ± 0.9 years). Average maps of gray matter density in patients and controls are subtracted at their first scan (when mean Mini-Mental State Exam (MMSE) score was 18 for the patients; [A] and [B]) and at their follow-up scan 1.5 years later (mean MMSE = 13; [C] and [D]). Colors show the average percentage loss of gray matter relative to the control average. Profound loss engulfs the left medial wall (>15%; [B] and [D]). On the right, however, the deficits in temporoparietal and entorhinal territory (A) spread forward into the cingulate gyrus 1.5 years later (C), after a 5-point drop in average MMSE. Limbic and frontal zones clearly show different degrees of impairment (C). The corpus callosum is indicated in white; maps of gray matter change are not defined here, as it is a white matter commissure. MRI-based changes, in living patients, agree strongly with the spatial progression of β-amyloid (Aβ) and NFT pathology observed *post mortem* (*Braak Stages B,C and III to VI; left four panels adapted from Braak and Braak, 1997*[30]). The deficit sequence also matches the trajectory of NFT distribution observed *post mortem*, in patients with increasing dementia severity at death.[30] Consistent with the deficit maps observed here, NFT accumulation is minimal in sensory and motor cortices, but occurs preferentially in entorhinal pyramidal cells, the limbic periallocortex (layers II/IV), the hippocampus/amygdala and subiculum, the basal forebrain cholinergic systems, and subsequently in temporoparietal and frontal association cortices (layers III/V).[37,38] Cortical layers III and V selectively lose large pyramidal neurons in association areas.[39,40] This figure appears in color online.

that myelinate first—and most heavily—in development are typically least vulnerable to AD pathology (e.g., primary sensorimotor and visual cortices). In contrast, NFT and neuropil threads in dendrites accumulate early in the late myelinating heteromodal association cortices, the posterior cingulate, and phylogenetically older limbic areas that remain highly plastic throughout life.[41]

## Why Does AD Progress in This Sequence?

It is not known why AD engulfs the brain in this limbic-to-frontal sequence. The sequence is well documented and is largely agreed upon by the AD research community. Essentially, the same degenerative sequence was observed *post mortem,* and in FDG-PET data, many years before MRI scanning had sufficient resolution to gauge how cortical atrophy progresses. More recently, PET ligands that track the molecular hallmarks of AD show that pathology accumulates in a similar spreading pattern. Cross-sectional studies at UCLA and the University of Pittsburgh, using the molecular probes [$^{18}$F]-FDDNP and [$^{11}$C]-PIB, suggest that amyloid plaques deposit sequentially in the brain, appearing first in cingulate cortex, progressing to temporal–parietal cortices and the caudate, and finally engulfing occipital and sensorimotor cortices.[15,17] This sequence agrees very closely with the *post mortem* Braak maps,[30] and with MRI-based maps of cortical degeneration.[28]

Why the changes occur in this sequence is the subject of debate. The term "retrogenesis" has been used to describe some of the regressive behavioral changes that occur in dementia, when behavior may regress to a form resembling childhood or infancy. The sequence of cortical atrophy in Alzheimer's disease is in some respects an "unraveling," or recapitulation in reverse, of the anatomical sequence of childhood brain maturation. Primary sensory areas myelinate first in early infancy, but offer greatest resistance to neurodegeneration, staying intact in late AD. We recently developed a time-lapse map of cortical maturation, based on serial brain MRI scans of 13 children aged 4 to 21 years, scanned every 2 years for 8 years[42] (see http://www.loni.ucla.edu/~thompson/DEVEL/dynamic.html for videos of these changes). In these images, a shifting pattern of gray matter loss appeared first (around ages 4–8 years) in dorsal parietal and primary sensorimotor regions near the interhemispheric margin, spreading laterally and caudally into temporal cortices and anteriorly into dorsolateral prefrontal areas. As expected from *post mortem* studies of cerebral myelination,[43,44] the first areas to mature were those with the most basic functions, such as processing the senses and movement. Areas involved in spatial orientation and language (parietal lobes) followed, around the age of puberty (11–13 years). Areas with more advanced functions—integrating information from the senses, reasoning and other "executive" functions (prefrontal cortex)— matured last (in late adolescence). Phylogenetically older cortical areas matured earlier than the more recently evolving higher-order association cortices, which integrate information from earlier maturing cortex. Provocatively, the last brain regions to develop in childhood are among the first to degenerate in dementia; and the earliest developing brain regions—subserving vision and sensation—are spared until the very latest stages of AD. As such, the age-related degenerative process progresses from late- to earlier myelinating regions.[43,44]

Bartzokis et al.[50] examined this myelination sequence and suggested that late myelinating regions are especially vulnerable in AD and other adult onset disorders, such as schizophrenia. In support of this, the frontal cortex in schizophrenia has been found to undergo derailed maturation in patients and in at-risk relatives who subsequently convert to full-blown psychosis.[45–48] If this is true, the anatomical trajectory of white matter maturation and degeneration has been comparatively overlooked in neuroimaging research. Recent work, with DTI, appears to support this view. In Kochunov et al.[143] we found that the most prominent age-related drop in diffusion anisotropy occurred in late myelinating white matter, such as the *genu* of the corpus callosum, which innervates the frontal lobes. The cognitive consequences of this drop need to be established, but this is consistent with prior reports that late myelinating regions are most vulnerable to age-related degeneration.[49–51]

## Other Dementias

Cortical changes do not follow the same trajectory in Alzheimer's disease as in other neurodegenerative diseases, or even other forms of dementia. In a recent study of Lewy body dementia (LBD), for example, we found that cortical gray matter in temporal and orbitofrontal cortices was comparatively preserved in 16 LBD patients (age: $76.4 \pm 6.7$ semantic dementia [SD]), compared with 29 AD patients matched for age and dementia severity. LBD patients showed severe anterior cingulate atrophy compared to 38 matched controls.[52] This was somewhat expected based on earlier neuropsychological studies of LBD, which suggested that temporal lobe degeneration and memory decline appear relatively late in LBD.[53,54]

We also compared the 3D profiles of cortical atrophy in frontotemporal dementia (FTD) and SD.[6] SD patients typically present with impoverished speech, but FTD patients show lack of empathy, disinhibition, and poor judgment. Congruent with these findings, we found predominantly posterior, left-sided gray matter (GM) atrophy in SD ($N = 5$) and more frontal, right-sided GM atrophy in FTD ($N = 10$). These studies, and others like them, suggest that pathophysiological differences underlying different forms of dementia are evident in brain images. Differential diagnosis based on MRI and PET is an active field.[4]

## Neurodegeneration in HIV/AIDS

Perhaps the most startling finding in comparing degenerative patterns with MRI was the observation of selective cortical neurodegeneration in patients with HIV/AIDS, with greatest deficits in sensorimotor and supplementary motor cortices, and in the underlying white matter, basal ganglia, and hippocampus (FIG. 2).[7,9]

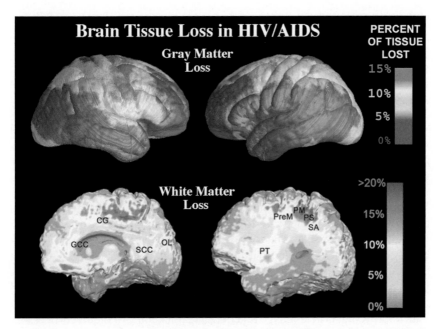

**FIGURE 2.** Visualizing brain tissue loss in HIV/AIDS. *(Top row):* In an MRI study of cortical thickness in 27 HIV/AIDS patients and 14 healthy controls, the primary sensory, motor, and premotor cortices were 15% thinner, and prefrontal and parietal tissue loss correlated with cognitive and motor deficits. Thinner frontopolar and language cortex also correlated with immune system deterioration measured via blood levels of CD4[+] T-lymphocytes. *(Bottom row):* When the same subjects were studied using TBM,[9] the pattern of white matter loss was in remarkable agreement with the cortical maps. The white matter volume was reduced in premotor areas where the cortex was significantly thinner, suggesting that cortical degeneration may be accompanied by degeneration in the underlying white matter pathways. Taken together, these and other studies support the notion that brain degeneration is present even in apparently healthy HIV-positive people on powerful drug regimens (HAART; highly active antiretroviral therapy). (Data in the top row are from Thompson *et al.*, 2005[7]; data in the bottom row are from Chiang *et al.*, 2006[9]).

The resulting maps provide a new approach to gauge the impact of HIV on the living brain (see also Refs. 9,10, for related maps of white matter degeneration). This unusual degenerative pattern is the opposite of that seen in common noninfectious dementias, such as AD, where the medial temporal, limbic, and association cortices are affected first, and primary sensorimotor and visual cortices only later. Clearly, different degenerative disorders may have quite different stereotypical patterns of atrophy and progression. Some have suggested the HIV virus migrates from the ventricles through the white matter to the cortex,[55] where HIV virus-encoded proteins overactivate NMDA-type glutamate receptors and the excess extracellular glutamate causes excitotoxic injury and cell death. Why specific brain systems are especially vulnerable to the neurotoxic effects of HIV is not yet understood, but brain mapping is providing vital information on the trajectory of the disease.

### Association with Specific Symptoms

If different forms of dementia progress in different ways, it is legitimate to ask whether different patterns of symptoms and functional decline are associated with different patterns of atrophy. In AD, we found that distinct cortical atrophy patterns were associated with apathy, versus language dysfunction, or versus global cognitive decline.[21,56,57] In a language study, we computed an individual average language domain Z-score from each subject's Z-scores on the Boston Naming Test and Animal Fluency test. Three-dimensional statistical maps then revealed that language performance was associated most strongly with left-sided gray matter loss in 19 AD and 5 MCI patients. More of the left hemisphere showed atrophy that linked with language function, suggesting that language abilities in AD are strongly influenced by cortical integrity in left perisylvian areas. A related study of healthy developing children revealed that thickening of language-related cortices, but not motor cortices, was linked with improvements in language function, and thickening of motor cortices, but not language cortices, was linked with improvements in motor function.[58] This type of double dissociation is remarkable, as a more simplistic model might predict that all functional domains would improve somewhat equally in concert with a generalized maturation of the cortex. In healthy adults, the quantity of gray matter overall and especially in the frontal lobes is associated with better performance on standardized IQ tests, and both of these measures are under strong genetic control.[59,60] This suggests a moderately strong linkage between regional brain volumes and intellectual ability. The association between brain volume and IQ has been replicated in numerous meta-analyses (e.g., Ref. 61), and may contribute to any detected association between cognitive performance and brain volumes in degenerative disease as well.

Mini-Mental State Exam (MMSE) scores offer a more general measure of overall cognitive decline in AD, and declining MMSE is associated with widely distributed atrophy in both hemispheres.[21,28] Anterior cingulate and supplementary motor cortices were more atrophied in 18 AD patients with apathy versus 18 without apathy but matched for dementia severity.[57] We also studied late-life depression in nondemented controls.[62] We found a regionally specific 5–20% gray matter deficit in the orbitofrontal cortex of 24 depressed patients compared to 19 age-matched nondepressed subjects. In a collaboration with the University of Brescia,[63] we compared cortical thinning in 10 late onset and 10 early onset AD patients of similar clinical severity (MMSE: 18.6 ± 3.5 vs. 19.2 ± 3.5). Early onset was defined as diagnosis before 65 years of age. Early onset AD primarily affected temporoparietal areas and late onset AD affected the medial temporal gray matter. These results may explain why early onset AD features primarily neocortical symptoms, while late onset AD generally features medial temporal symptoms.

These studies zero in on abnormal cortical systems contributing to specific functional deficits—revealing pathophysiological differences underlying the different symptoms of dementia or dementias with differences in the age of onset.

## METHODS TO TRACK BRAIN CHANGES IN ALZHEIMER'S DISEASE

Methods to track structural brain changes with conventional MRI fall into three main categories: (1) volumetric measurement of specific structures, such as the hippocampus or entorhinal cortex; (2) image processing techniques that estimate rates of whole brain atrophy as a percentage volume loss per year[11,64]; and (3) map-based techniques that visualize the 3D profile of group differences in gray matter loss,[65] atrophic rates,[66,67] white matter integrity,[68] or cortical gray matter thickness.[7,51,69,70] The main measures used in drug trials today are typically simpler ones that produce single numeric measures of disease burden, such as total hippocampal volume, or whole brain atrophic rates, which can all be expressed in cubic centimeters per year (or as a percentage change per year). The more exotic techniques that produce 3D maps of degenerative changes (reviewed below) have yielded substantial neuroscientific information on the disease trajectory, but have yet to gain acceptance in drug trials. Drug trials have not yet used these measures partly due to their complexity but also due to the pressure to express outcomes in a simple way, ideally using a small number of summary measures. Large-scale neuroimaging efforts (e.g., the Alzheimer's Disease Neuroimaging Initiative, www.loni.ucla.edu/ADNI) are now comparing the power of these map-based imaging measures, together with biomarkers and other clinical/functional measures, to differentiate MCI and AD from healthy aging, to predict future cognitive decline, and to predict conversion from MCI to AD. This is a vital effort—currently, given that in individual subjects assessed with MRI, MCI is not readily distinguished from AD or from normal aging, except when groups of subjects are compared in aggregate—individuals in each of these categories overlap substantially for all known MRI measures.

### *Hippocampal Volumes and Maps*

AD pathology emerges first in the entorhinal cortex and hippocampus, so most volumetric MRI studies of MCI and AD patients have focused on the medial temporal lobe structures. Neuronal atrophy, decreased synaptic density, and overt neuronal loss is evident on MRI as progressive cortical gray

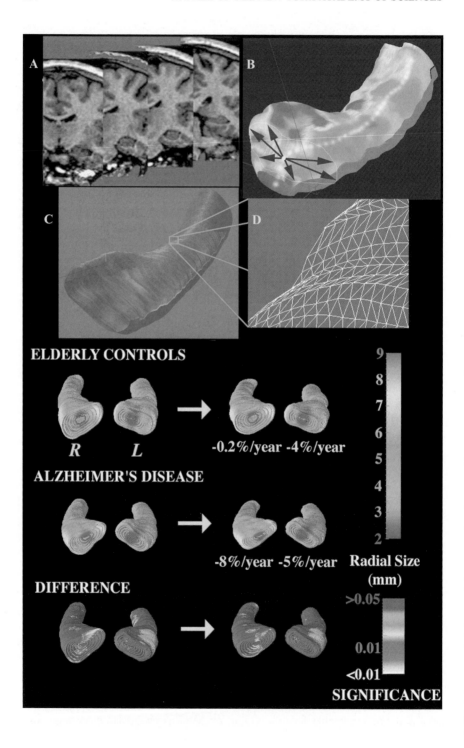

matter loss, reduced subcortical gray and white matter volumes, and expanding ventricular and sulcal CSF spaces.[71]

Patients with mild AD have roughly 25% smaller hippocampal volumes than matched healthy elderly controls,[72–74] whereas MCI patients show a mean reduction of around 11%.[74] Early studies by Jack *et al.*[144] found that 97.2% of the patients studied with very mild AD—that is, with Clinical Dementia Rating 0.5—had hippocampal volumes below the healthy normal average. In MCI, mean hippocampal volumes are variously reported as being roughly half way between AD and normals,[75–78] or as being more similar to AD patients.[79,80] Xu *et al.*[145] found that entorhinal cortex and hippocampal volume measures provided roughly equal intergroup discrimination ability in 30 control, 30 MCI, and 30 AD subjects; even though the entorhinal cortex typically atrophies earlier, it is harder to delineate reliably on MRI. Many groups have also used premorbid hippocampal atrophy, rated visually[81] or using volumetry,[82–84] to predict subsequent crossover to AD. Jack *et al.*[76] also found that hippocampal atrophy at baseline was associated with conversion from MCI to AD at a 33-month follow-up (relative risk: 0.69, $P = 0.01$; 27 of 80 MCI subjects had become demented).

Three-dimensional modeling techniques (FIG. 3) have localized specific regions of atrophy within the hippocampus in MCI. For example, Becker *et al.*[20] used 3D surface reconstruction techniques to model the shape of the hippocampus, creating average shape models for cohorts of subjects with amnestic MCI, nonamnestic MCI, AD, and healthy controls. These techniques can localize tissue atrophy or shape alterations[85] and can map the average pattern of hippocampal thickness reductions in millimeters.[71] Amnestic MCI patients showed diffuse hippocampal atrophy,[86] and reduced volumes in the mesial temporal lobe including the hippocampus, entorhinal cortex, and amygdala.[87] Nonamnestic MCI patients—who show cognitive impairments in single or multiple domains other than memory—typically have greater atrophy outside of the hippocampus, specifically in multimodal association cortices.

←——————————————————————————————————————————

**FIGURE 3.** Mapping hippocampal atrophy. The 3D profile of hippocampal atrophy in disease can be mapped using surface-based modeling methods.[71] The hippocampus is traced (**A**) either by hand or automatically, in serial coronal sections. After converting the traces to parametric surface mesh format (**C**) and (**D**), a medial core (i.e., a curve threading down the center of the hippocampus) is computed for each hippocampus. The distances from the medial core to each surface point are estimated and used to generate first individual and later average group distance maps. Here, group distance maps for elderly controls and patients with moderate Alzheimer's disease are compared at baseline (*left column*), and after an approximately 2-year follow-up interval (*right column*). The significance maps show regions with significant atrophy at each time point (white colors). Similar maps can be made to plot regions where there is evidence for progressive atrophy over time or changes that link with cognitive test performance or clinical outcomes.[92]

These methods provide, at each location on the hippocampal surface, a measure of how much radial atrophy there is, as either a proportion of average control values, or as a Z-score, or a significance map comparing one group with another. These methods have been used to detect structural differences in the hippocampus that are associated with Alzheimer's disease,[71,88] MCI,[20,21] schizophrenia,[89] normal development,[90] methamphetamine abuse,[91] epilepsy,[92] bipolar illness,[93] depression,[94] and HIV/AIDS.[86] Frisoni et al.[88] also used this method to compare a group of 28 AD patients and 40 elderly controls, and found significant tissue loss (20% or more) in the hippocampal CA1 fields and part of the subiculum. As expected from pathological studies,[95] regions corresponding to the CA2-3 fields were relatively spared. This atrophy distribution largely corresponds to the known selective involvement of hippocampal regions by AD pathology, and supports the possibility of carrying out *in vivo* macroscopic neuropathology of the hippocampus with MR imaging in the dementias.

*Predicting Outcomes in MCI*

Hippocampal surface maps have also been used to predict outcomes in MCI. In 20 MCI subjects followed neuropsychologically for 3 years, maps of hippocampal atrophy at the start of the study successfully differentiated the 7 patients who later converted to AD from 6 who stayed stable and 7 who improved. CA1 and subicular degeneration were associated with conversion to AD; these areas were intact in MCI patients who improved and no longer met MCI criteria at follow-up.[21]

*Accelerated Hippocampal Atrophy in Those at Genetic Risk*

The same hippocampal mapping technique has been used to detect accelerated atrophy in healthy elderly people at genetic risk for Alzheimer's disease. In a longitudinal study,[96] 3D hippocampal surface models were generated from volumetric brain MRI scans of 54 subjects (27 men, 27 women), scanned at two different time points (mean age at baseline = 68.6, mean interval: 1.6 years, 19 ApoE4 carriers: 2 homozygous, 17 heterozygous). We found a strong correlation ($P = 0.024$) between the left hippocampal rate of atrophy and the ApoE genotype, with E4 carriers showing a greater average atrophic rate than non-E4 carriers (left hippocampus:$-2.4\%$/year vs. $0.36\%$/year). Progressive hippocampal head atrophy occurred in healthy ApoE4 carriers, an atrophic pattern that is accelerated in AD. The maps showing greater average annualized loss and faster left hippocampal atrophy for ApoE4 carriers indicate that, in those at genetic risk for AD, abnormally accelerated structural changes are detectable prior to cognitive decline.

## *Automated Mapping of Gray Matter Changes: Voxel-Based Morphometry*

Conventional region-of-interest approaches, which use manual tracing to determine the volume of the structures, are ubiquitous but are gradually being replaced by more automated techniques for rapid large-scale processing of scans (see Ref. 97, for a review).[25,98] Automated image registration approaches can align groups of images into a common space and intergroup differences can be assessed using voxel-by-voxel statistics. Three-dimensional statistical maps of group differences in brain structure can be visualized, identifying regions where atrophy correlates with diagnosis, as well as clinical, therapeutic, genetic, or functional measures. Chetelat *et al.*[146] used an automated technique known as voxel-based morphometry (VBM)[99,100] to map gray matter changes in 18 amnestic MCI patients. In a follow-up scan 18 months later, subjects who had converted to Alzheimer's disease showed significantly greater GM loss— relative to nonconverters—in the hippocampus, inferior and middle temporal gyri, posterior cingulate, and precuneus. All of these regions show severe deficits in mild AD (see FIG. 1).

### *Optimized VBM*

Brief comment is warranted regarding a controversy that arose in the literature regarding the use of VBM.[100–104] This debate generated some confusion regarding the validity of VBM. VBM is an extremely popular approach for comparing structural brain images, partly due to its high automation, and it is implemented in the *Statistical Parametric Mapping* image analysis package (SPM; www.fil.ion.ucl.ac.uk/spm/). Prior to 2000, the most commonly used implementation of VBM involved warping all tissue class images (i.e., 3D maps of gray and white matter probabilities) to match the same standardized brain atlas, and preserving the probability values in the spatially transformed images. These data were typically then smoothed and statistical analyses performed. This approach was criticized by Bookstein[101] and Thacker[103] who noted that this method only detects registration errors, because if the warping was 100% exact, there would be no residual differences. Bookstein noted that the results of such studies depend heavily on the registration strategy used, and therefore VBM should not be used. In response to this criticism, the authors of VBM developed a modified approach, known as "modulated VBM."[100]This approach warps the tissue class images, but preserves information on the total volume of tissue by scaling the image intensities according to the amount of expansion or contraction. This approach was independently suggested by Davatzikos *et al.*[102] where it was termed "RAVENS" (Regional Analysis of Volumes Examined in Normalized Space); the same approach is known as "modulated VBM" by SPM users. Here the comparisons are volumetric, and the resulting "optimized" VBM approach is now similar in many respects to the "tensor-based morphometry" methods described below.

### Surface-Based Analysis of Cortical Thickness

Cortical modeling[12] may also be used to map the profile of gray matter thickness across the cortical mantle, providing better localization and statistical power by matching data from corresponding gyri, as far as possible, across subjects. These cortical modeling approaches can be considered as a variant of VBM, but offer several benefits. First, parameters, such as cortical thickness, can be computed in 3D, displayed on the cortical models, and averaged across subjects for group comparisons. Second, the explicit modeling of the cortical surface geometry allows one cortex to be precisely aligned with another before multisubject comparisons are made. This greatly reduces registration errors when comparing data across subjects and groups. An additional step known as *cortical pattern matching* can be used to fluidly match the entire gyral pattern from subject to subject, using a 3D deformation field to drive sulcal landmarks into correspondence.[12] This very high-order matching of anatomy can improve the power to detect subtle gray matter differences between groups or over time, and localizes effects relative to known cortical landmarks. In this process, clear anatomic divisions often emerge in the regions affected (e.g., the degree of cortical degeneration differs substantially on either side of the cingulate sulcus in (FIG. 1 C), a feature corroborated by the *post mortem* maps).

Composite maps of cortical thickness, based on MRI, have revealed a complex shifting pattern of cortical atrophy over the human life span, which is thought to primarily reflect neuronal shrinkage rather than overt neuronal loss ($N = 176$[105]; $N = 106$ subjects[51]). These cortical mapping techniques show great promise, but have yet to be applied in MCI.

Cortical gray matter thickness is a powerful neuroimaging marker of cortical integrity, and a reasonable question is: "What exactly is it measuring?" It is sensitive to subtle disease-related changes, and correlates with cognitive decline in Alzheimer's disease and schizophrenia.[28,45] Cortical thickness on MRI may be related to regional neuronal density in the cortical mantle,[106] but it may also depend on unknown vascular factors, glial cell numbers, and the extent and integrity of cortical myelination. We recently developed an approach to measure the thickness of the cortex from MRI, and mapped how it changes over the human life span. This approach has now been used in more than 30 studies, to compile composite maps of average cortical thickness and compare them between specific populations (see Ref. 12 for an overview; FIG. 4 shows the main steps). Regions with systematic differences in cortical thickness can be detected and displayed on the cortex, as can the trajectory of changes in development or disease.

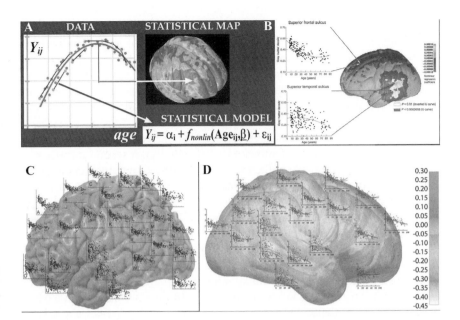

**FIGURE 4.** Mapping cortical changes. Several recent studies have examined the effects of age on the thickness of the cortex, measured in MRI scans of the brain.[5,7,70,109] This figure shows a general approach we developed to map cortical gray matter changes over time; it has also been used to produce time-lapse animations of the trajectory of cortical thinning with age, and to map the progression of diseases, such as childhood onset schizophrenia and Alzheimer's disease.[28,45,110] (**A**) First, measures ($Y_{ij}$) of gray matter thickness are obtained longitudinally (*green dots*) or once only (*red dots*) in a group of subjects at different ages. Fitting of statistical models to these data (*Statistical Model, lower right*) produces estimates of parameters that can be plotted onto the cortex, using a color code. These parameters can include age at peak (see arrow at peak of the curve), significance values, or estimated statistical parameters, such as rates of change, and effects of drug treatment or risk genes. (**B**) and (**C**): We estimated the trajectory of gray matter loss over the human life span in a cohort of 176 normal subjects.[5] After cortical pattern matching was used to associate data from corresponding cortical regions, we developed software to fit a general nonlinear statistical model to the gray matter data from the population. This revealed significant nonlinear (quadratic) effects of time on brain structure. To show that it is feasible to pick up very small systematic differences using this technique, Sowell *et al.* (2006) found a sex difference in the trajectory of cortical thinning (**D**). There was an absolute excess in cortical thickness in women relative to men, of around 0.3 mm, mainly in the perisylvian language areas (even without brain size adjustments). Our other cortical thickness studies provide evidence for this sex difference,[111] which is important to consider if cortical thickness is used to gauge degenerative brain changes. For full details of the approach, see Refs. 12,70. This figure appears in color online.

Cortical thickness can be defined in several different ways, but the simplest approach computes the 3D distance from the inner cortical gray–white matter boundary in tissue-classified brain volumes to the outer cortical surface (gray–CSF boundary) in each subject.[12] Neuroimaging and histological studies have found significant changes in cortical thickness in normal subjects.[5,42,107,108] In one study, we examined a large sample ($N = 176$) of normal individuals across the span of life between 7 and 87 years.[5,70] Cortical thickness decreased quadratically with age from an average thickness of ~2.6 mm at 20 years to less than 2 mm in the age range 80–90 years. Perhaps surprisingly, scatterplots of these effects revealed a dramatic decline in gray matter density between the ages of 7 and 60 years with a slower decline thereafter, in most brain regions (the most dramatic changes occurring in the frontal cortex during late adolescence, where gray matter thickness falls rapidly). A second surprise was that the most lateral aspects of the brain in the posterior temporal and inferior parietal lobes bilaterally showed a distinct pattern of gray matter change, one in which the nonlinear age effects were inverted relative to the age effects seen in more dorsal cortices, that is, cortical atrophy accelerated rather than remaining linear or slowing down with age.

Gender differences in other markers of cortical atrophy are also apparent. In Kochunov et al.,[147] we studied age-related trends for the width and the depth of major cortical sulci in 90 healthy subjects (47 males, 43 females) aged 20–82 years. The average sulcal width increased by ~0.7 mm/decade, while the average sulcal depth decreased by ~0.4 mm/decade. Greater age-related decline was found in men relative to women, and in multimodal relative to unimodal cortical areas.

The rate of cortical thickness reduction in abnormal aging and degenerative disorders has also been shown to be different from that in healthy aging, making it a useful biomarker of neurodegeneration in a variety of illnesses.[12,28,112] Our cortical mapping approach has been used to detect unsuspected alterations in gray matter distribution in Alzheimer's disease,[21,28,63] LBD,[52] MCI,[21] late-life depression,[62] HIV/AIDS,[7] methamphetamine users,[75] childhood and adult onset schizophrenia,[45,110,113] normally developing children,[42,114,115] fetal alcohol syndrome,[116] individuals at risk for schizophrenia,[48] adult and adolescent onset bipolar illness,[93,117] velocardiofacial syndrome (VCFS[118]), Williams syndrome,[8] epilepsy,[119] attention deficit hyperactivity disorder,[105] genetic influences on brain structure,[59,120] and lithium effects on brain structure.[93] The most general review of these methods is in Thompson et al.[12]

One of the most provocative recent findings is that significant cortical thinning is detectable in asymptomatic carriers of the high-risk allelic variant, apolipoprotein E ε4 (APOE ε4). This allele is quite prevalent in the general population, and results in a threefold increased risk of developing Alzheimer's disease. Using a technique to unfold the convoluted geometry of the hippocampus,[121] Burggen et al.[148] found that 9 (heterozygous) APOE ε4 carriers with normal memory performance showed significantly reduced cortical thickness compared to 14 noncarriers in entorhinal cortex and the subiculum (by 10.6% and 7.5% respectively; $P = 0.005, 0.003$), but not in the main body of the hippocampus or perirhinal cortex. Such a pattern of cortical thinning is consistent with the known progression of AD pathology and may reflect either a preexisting reduction in cortical thickness, or early dynamic changes in cortical structure that diminish the processing capacity of the cortex. These early changes may contribute to accelerated disease onset.

## Imaging White Matter with DTI

White matter changes in MCI and AD are also of interest. Conventional MRI has insufficient contrast to discriminate fiber tract organization within the white matter, but DTI, a newer MRI variant introduced in the mid 1990s,[122–124] is sensitive to myelin breakdown, as well as fiber integrity and orientation. Medina *et al.*[68] found that groups of MCI and AD subjects showed abnormal reductions in fractional anisotropy, a DTI-based measure of fiber integrity, in multiple posterior white matter regions. Rose *et al.*[149] found that relative to normal controls, AD patients showed a significant reduction in the integrity of the association white matter fiber tracts, including the splenium of the corpus callosum, the superior longitudinal fasciculus, and cingulum but not the pyramidal tracts. This is consistent with the typical clinical presentation of AD, that is, global cognitive decline but no motor disturbances. Other measures of water diffusion, such as the apparent diffusion coefficient (ADC), are abnormally elevated in the hippocampus in MCI,[125,126] and in broader areas—including the parietal white matter—in established AD.[127] Abnormal white matter changes can therefore be detected in MCI, prior to the development of dementia.

## Tensor-Based Morphometry

The best MRI measure to monitor disease progression in dementia depends, to some degree, on the follow-up interval after which patients are reassessed. At relatively short follow-up intervals (6 months), ventricular measures are three times more powerful than whole brain atrophic rates for distinguishing AD from controls; this advantage dissipates if the follow-up interval is extended to 1 year.[128]

Demonstration of *deteriorating* brain structure during the transition from MCI to AD has significant prognostic value as such changes over time almost certainly reflect the progression of underlying brain pathology. For tracking brain changes in exquisite detail, tensor-based morphometry (TBM)—also known as *deformation morphometry* or *voxel compression mapping*—has emerged as a powerful method to track brain change (Thompson *et al.*; Fox *et al.*; Janke *et al.*; Studholme *et al.*; Leow *et al.*; Chiang *et al.*)[25,66–132] TBM is a more complex image analysis approach; it quantifies tissue growth or atrophy throughout the brain, based on elastically warping sequentially collected MRI scans. It visually indicates the local rate at which tissue is being lost, or expanding, throughout the anatomy of the brain (see FIG. 5 for an illustration).

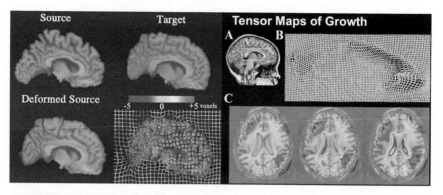

**FIGURE 5.** TBM maps rates of tissue gain or loss. Tensor-based morphometry, or TBM, can automatically map brain changes in large groups of subjects. Here, an example MRI image (*top left*) is aligned to a target image, and the shape of gyri, corpus callosum, and ventricles are well matched (data from Ref. 9). To better visualize the applied 3D deformation field, a colored grid is superimposed on the registered image—red and blue colors represent deformation orthogonal to the midsagittal plane (out of the page). (**A**) and (**B**): In Thompson *et al.* (2000), we used TBM to map growth rates (**B**) in the corpus callosum (**A**) of a young girl scanned at 3 years of age and again at 6 years—the anterior corpus callosum grows the fastest at this age (~20% local volume gain per year, most likely due to progressive myelination). Rates of tissue expansion are inferred from the derivatives of the warping field that aligns baseline to follow-up scans. (**C**): Progressive gray and white matter atrophy (*purple colors*) and ventricular expansion (*red and white colors*) are mapped in a patient with posterior cortical atrophy scanned 1, 1.5, and 2 years after diagnosis. After registering growth rate maps to a common neuroanatomical template, group differences in rates of brain change can be tested statistically (see Refs. 25 and 58, for examples of studies comparing groups cross-sectionally and longitudinally). This figure appears in color online.

It surveys the whole brain at once, but detects localized changes occurring at a regional level, without having to specify the regions of interest in advance. This approach may ultimately offer the greatest power for clinical trials. Deformation morphometry can detect subtle medication-related changes over a period of less than a month, such as effects of lithium on brain structure,[133] and is automated enough to apply to large cohorts of subjects efficiently, without the need for laborious interaction with images to identify regions of interest. The brain changes are then compared across subjects or groups. Correlations can be mapped between these changes and demographic or clinical measures, such as age, sex, diagnosis, cognitive scores, treatment outcomes, or biological serum measures (see Ref. 9, for examples of this approach in a study of HIV/AIDS).

*How TBM Detects Brain Changes*

If two brain images, acquired over time, are rigidly overlaid, brain changes cannot be localized: no information is available on exactly where atrophy is occurring. To localize changes within the brain, matching needs to be performed with a nonlinear "warping" algorithm. Over the last 15 years, many groups have developed nonlinear image warping techniques that align brain images with a compressible elastic or fluid model. This allows localized deformation. How well these approaches perform depends on the mathematical measure of image correspondence used to drive the alignment of the images, how flexible the deformation is (in terms of degrees of freedom), and whether steps are taken to ensure that the mappings are smooth and preserve the topology of the image.[134] In one approach (see Refs. 67,132, for mathematical details), the follow-up (repeat) image is globally aligned to the baseline scan, and then a 3D elastic or fluid image deformation is used to maximize the mutual information (or a related information–theoretic measure of correspondence) between the two consecutive scans. This fully 3D deformation reconfigures the baseline anatomy into the shape of the follow-up scan. The expansion or contraction at each image voxel is computed from the deformation field (using the Jacobian of the deformation field to produce a *"voxel compression map"* or *"tensor map"*). In this map, contraction implies atrophy; expansion implies local growth or dilation.[64] A color map then displays these changes on the follow-up scan. As shown in FIGURE 3, the method can be used to map patterns of brain changes in patients scanned longitudinally over short intervals,[25] in patients with semantic dementia,[135] and has been used to automatically map the profile of brain structural differences in cohorts with HIV/AIDS,[9,10] Fragile X syndrome,[136] Williams syndrome,[137] schizophrenia,[58] bipolar illness,[138] in healthy subjects treated with lithium,[133] and in twins imaged with DTI.[139] TBM has a relatively high throughput and sensitivity, making it attractive to use for gauging brain changes in large population studies and clinical trials. New statistical methods are also emerging to increase the sensitivity of TBM. For detecting degenerative brain changes, Lie group and Riemannian manifold methods can provide more statistical power than standard approaches, as they draw upon the full multidimensional information available in the deformation tensors.[10,139] Such an approach might be termed "generalized TBM."

### *Combining Fluid Registration with Anatomical Surface Modeling*

Fluid registration can also be combined with surface-based modeling to automatically create maps of anatomical surfaces in large numbers of images, and compare the resulting surfaces statistically. This approach combines the strengths of two very different methods, while providing automation and high throughput for large population studies. In the largest brain mapping study of MCI to date, Carmichael *et al.*[22] delineated the lateral ventricles on a single brain MRI data set, and fluidly deformed a surface model of these structures, using nonlinear image registration, to match the shape of the ventricles in other MRI scans from 74 MCI, 225 normal, and 40 AD subjects. The average ventricular shapes were compared using a surface-based modeling approach, which plots the regions with statistical shape differences on the surfaces using a color code.[12] MCI subjects showed significant, localized dilations relative to normal subjects in the atrium of the ventricles and in the occipital horns. AD subjects showed a greater extent of enlargement involving the frontal horns. In AD, temporal horn expansion progresses at a rate of 13–18% per year (compared with 2–4%/year in healthy controls[71]). In contrast, the mean annual rate of hippocampal volume loss on MRI is much more subtle: 1.73% in stable controls, 3.5% in AD, and 3.69% versus 2.55% in MCI subjects who decline or remain stable at 3-year follow-up.[140] Strictly speaking, this approach provides similar information to TBM, but surface models are used to constrain the search for significant effects to regions known to be implicated. This improves statistical power, as well as presenting results in a visually intuitive way.

## USE OF IMAGING IN DRUG TRIALS

Recent studies also suggest that imaging can be useful as a biomarker for therapeutic efficacy in AD. Refinements are occurring in the measures used, and large-scale projects, such as the Alzheimer's Disease Neuroimaging Initiative (www.loni.ucla.edu/ADNI/) are now comparing and cross-validating different imaging measures for detecting significant brain changes in AD. Even if only conventional volumetric measures are used, Jack et al.[2] estimated that in each arm of a therapeutic trial, only 21 subjects would be required to detect a 50% reduction in the rate of decline, if the hippocampal volume was used as the outcome measure. This compares with 241 subjects if MMSE scores were used, and 320 if the AD Assessment Scale Cognitive Subscale were used. Imaging measures are not likely to replace cognitive measures as outcome measures in clinical trials, but they are widely regarded as more stable and reproducible across sites. Significant work has been devoted to establishing imaging protocols that are reproducible across imaging centers and across time,[141] and the detection limits of image analysis techniques have been shown to be greatly improved if scanner-related factors, such as geometric stability, field homogeneity, RF coil type, and field strength are optimized.[25,141]

Automated measures of atrophy are also gaining acceptance in longitudinal studies, although not all studies have yielded the expected conclusions. Fox et al.[3] applied a powerful image analysis approach, known as the Brain Boundary Shift Integral, to estimate the overall brain volume decrease in registered serial images from 288 AD patients in a Phase IIa immunotherapy trial. Paradoxically, when assessed 11 months later, antibody responders ($N = 45$) had greater brain volume decreases (on average 3.1% vs. 2.0%), and greater ventricular enlargement than placebo patients ($N = 57$). Because this atrophy did not correlate with cognitive decline, the authors speculated that these volume changes may be attributed to amyloid removal and associated cerebral fluid shifts.

# CONCLUSION

Overall, structural brain scanning with MRI has yielded several measures that help to differentiate mildly impaired patients from controls. MRI can also be used to help predict who will imminently convert to suspected AD, and to gauge how well interventions resist atrophic brain changes, if at all, in clinical trials. Because therapeutic trials require sensitive biomarkers that track the disease process in detail, serial MRI scanning is often combined with powerful, automated analysis methods to compute maps of brain changes, and volumetric measures for brain regions that change early in AD, such as the hippocampus and entorhinal cortex. These efforts now use cutting-edge mathematics to map brain change on MRI and PET, as well as longitudinal data sets that track disease over multiyear time spans before and after disease onset.

Other innovations in neuroimaging include ongoing developments in DTI, MR relaxometry, imaging of iron deposition, and high-field MRI scanning. Each of these techniques aims to increase the repertoire of signals available for assessing tissue integrity in early neurodegenerative disease. Perhaps the most promising development is the recent advent of PET tracer compounds that visualize amyloid plaques and NFT in the living brain. These pathological features are the defining hallmarks of AD, previously only detectable at autopsy. New tracer compounds for plaque and tangle imaging ([$^{18}$F]-FDDNP and [$^{11}$C]-PIB) complement the now-standard PET measures (of perfusion and glucose metabolism) that are the mainstay of differential diagnosis in dementia. Many see in these new tracers the promise to track AD before it is clinically detectable—and assess how therapy resists it before symptoms become irreversible. Amyloid deposition gradually increases in the brain long before detectable symptoms of memory decline, so there is an expectation that amyloid plaque and/or tangle PET tracers can identify and monitor AD progression before any symptoms appear.[15,17] In addition, these tracers quantify pathology objectively, offering a direct means to evaluate antiamyloid therapies, such as secretase inhibitors.

It is not yet known whether these new PET markers correlate more tightly than MRI measures with observable clinical decline in MCI, although both distinguish AD and MCI from controls. A major effort in these analyses is to correlate the trajectory of pathology observed with new PET tracers with dynamic maps of cortical neurodegeneration on MRI. Initial studies in AD reveal a positive correlation between rates of whole brain atrophy and regional [$^{11}$C]-PIB uptake ($N = 9^{142}$). Each of these measures is tightly correlated with global cognitive function (MMSE[17,28]). It is of interest to relate the two views of the neurodegenerative process. A major goal is to develop joint measures of the disease process with far greater predictive power than either MRI or PET can provide on its own.

## ACKNOWLEDGMENTS

This research was supported by the National Institute on Aging, the National Library of Medicine, the National Institute for Biomedical Imaging and Bioengineering, the National Center for Research Resources, and the National Institute for Child Health and Development (AG016570, LM05639, EB01651, RR019771, and HD050735 to P.M.T.). E.R.S. was supported by the National Institute of Drug Abuse (NIDA R21 DA15878 and RO1 DA017831 to E.R.S.). Additional support was provided by a Taiwan government fellowship (to M.C.C.), and NCRR grants RR13642 and RR021813 (to A.W.T.).

## REFERENCES

1. JORM, A.F., A.E. KORTEN & A.S. HENDERSON. 1987. The prevalence of dementia: a quantitative integration of the literature. Acta Psychiatr. Scand. **76:** 465–479. Review.
2. JACK, C.R. JR, M. SLOMKOWSKI, S. GRACON, et al. 2003. MRI as a biomarker of disease progression in a therapeutic trial of milameline for AD. Neurology. **60:** 253–260.
3. FOX, N.C., R.S. BLACK, S. GILMAN, et al. AN1792(QS-21)-201 Study 2005. Effects of Abeta immunization (AN1792) on MRI measures of cerebral volume in Alzheimer disease. Neurology. **64:** 1563–1572.
4. SILVERMAN, D.H.S. & P.M. THOMPSON. 2006. Structural and functional neuroimaging: focusing on mild cognitive impairment. Appl. Neurol. **2:** 10–24.
5. SOWELL, E.R., B.S. PETERSON, P.M. THOMPSON, et al. 2003. Mapping cortical change across the human lifespan. Nat. Neurosci. **6:** 309–315.
6. APOSTOLOVA, L.G., D.G. CLARK, C. ZOUMALAN, et al. 2006. 3D mapping of gray matter atrophy in semantic dementia and frontal variant frontotemporal dementia, International Conference on Alzheimer's Disease (ICAD2006), Madrid, Spain.
7. THOMPSON, P.M., R.A. DUTTON, K.M. HAYASHI, et al. 2005. Thinning of the cerebral cortex in HIV/AIDS Reflects CD4+ T-lymphocyte decline. Proc. Natl. Acad. Sci. **102:** 15647–15652.
8. THOMPSON, P.M., A.D. LEE, R.A. DUTTON, et al. 2005. Abnormal cortical complexity and thickness profiles mapped in williams syndrome. J. Neurosci. **25:** 4146–4158.
9. CHIANG, M.C., R.A. DUTTON, K.M. HAYASHI, et al. 2006. Fluid registration of medical images using jensen-rényi divergence reveals 3D profile of brain atrophy in HIV/AIDS. IEEE Int. Symp. Biomed. Imag. (ISBI2006).
10. N. LEPORE, C.A. BRUN, Y.Y. CHOU, et al. 2006. Generalized tensor-based morphometry of HIV/AIDS using multivariate statistics on strain matrices and their application to HIV/AIDS, submitted to IEEE Transactions on Medical Imaging, Special Issue on Computational Neuroanatomy (Eds. Gee, J.C., Thompson, P.M.), to appear March 2007 [submitted, July 1, 2006].
11. SMITH, S.M., Y. ZHANG, M. JENKINSON, et al. 2002. Accurate, robust, and automated longitudinal and cross-sectional brain change analysis. Neuroimage. **17:** 479–489.

12. THOMPSON, P.M., K.M. HAYASHI, E.R. SOWELL, *et al.* 2004. Mapping cortical change in Alzheimer's disease, brain development, and schizophrenia, Special Issue on *Mathematics in Brain Imaging* (Thompson, P.M., Miller, M.I., Ratnanather, J.T., Poldrack, R., Nichols, T.E., Eds.), NeuroImage. **23**(Suppl 1): S2–S18.

13. BARRIO, J.R., S.-C. HUANG, G.M. COLE, *et al.* 1999. PET imaging of tangles and plaques in Alzheimer disease. J. Nucl. Med. **40**(Suppl): 70P–71P.

14. SHOGHI-JADID, K., G.W. SMALL, E.D. AGDEPPA, *et al.* 2002. Localization of neurofibrillary tangles and beta-amyloid plaques in the brains of living patients with Alzheimer disease. Am. J. Geriatr. Psychiatry **10**: 24–35.

15. KLUNK, W.E., B.J. LOPRESTI, M.D. IKONOMOVIC, *et al.* 2005. Binding of the positron emission tomography tracer Pittsburgh compound-B reflects the amount of amyloid-beta in Alzheimer's disease brain but not in transgenic mouse brain. J. Neurosci. **25**: 10598–10660.

16. V. KEPE, J.R. BARRIO, S.C. HUANG, *et al.* 2006. Serotonin 1A receptors in the living brain of Alzheimer's disease patients. Proc. Natl. Acad. Sci. USA. **103**: 702–707. Epub 2006 Jan 9

17. SMALL, G.W., V. KEPE, L. ERCOLI, *et al.* 2006. PET of brain amyloid and tau in mild cognitive impairment. N. Engl. J. Med. **355**(25): 2652–2663.

18. PETERSEN, R.C., G.E. SMITH, S.C. WARING, *et al.* 1999. Mild cognitive impairment: clinical characterization and outcome [erratum appears in Arch Neurol 1999 Jun;56(6):760]. Arch. Neurol. **56**: 303–308.

19. PETERSEN, R.C. 2000. Aging, mild cognitive impairment, and Alzheimer's disease. Neurol. Clin. **18**: 789–806.

20. BECKER, J.T., S.W. DAVIS, K.M. HAYASHI, *et al.* 2006. 3D patterns of hippocampal atrophy in mild cognitive impairment. Arch. Neurol. **63**: 97–101.

21. APOSTOLOVA, L.G., C.A. STEINER, G.G. AKOPYAN, *et al.* 2007. 3D gray matter atrophy mapping in mild cognitive impairment and mild Alzheimer's disease [submitted].

22. CARMICHAEL, O.T., P.M. THOMPSON, R.A. DUTTON, *et al.* 2006. Mapping ventricular changes related to dementia and mild cognitive impairment in a large community-based cohort, IEEE Int. Symp. Biomed. Imag. (ISBI2006).

23. PRICE, J.L. & J.C. MORRIS. 1999. Tangles and plaques in nondemented aging and "preclinical" Alzheimer's disease. Ann. Neurol. **45**: 358–368.

24. KORDOWER, J.H., Y. CHU, G.T. STEBBINS, *et al.* 2001. Loss and atrophy of layer II entorhinal cortex neurons in elderly people with mild cognitive impairment. Ann. Neurol. **49**: 202–213.

25. LEOW, A.D., A.D. KLUNDER, C.R. JACK, *et al.* 2006. Longitudinal stability of MRI for mapping brain change using tensor-based morphometry. Neuroimage **31**: 627–640. Epub 2006 Feb 15.

26. G. BARTZOKIS, D. SULTZER, J. MINTZ, *et al.* 1994. In vivo evaluation of brain iron in Alzheimer's disease and normal subjects using MRI. Biol.Psychiatry; **35**: 480–487.

27. G. BARTZOKIS, T.A. TISHLER, P.H. LU, *et al.* 2007. Brain ferritin iron may influence age- and gender-related risks of neurodegeneration. Neurobiol. Aging **28**: 414–423.

28. THOMPSON, P.M., K.M. HAYASHI, G. DE ZUBICARAY, *et al.* 2003. Dynamics of gray matter loss in Alzheimer's Disease. J. Neurosci. **23**: 994–1005.

29. BRAAK, H. & E. BRAAK. 1991. Neuropathological stageing of Alzheimer-related changes. Acta Neuropathol. **82**: 239–259.

30. BRAAK, H. & E. BRAAK. 1997. Staging of Alzheimer-related cortical destruction. Int. Psychogeriatr. **9**(Suppl 1): 257–261; discussion 269–272.
31. GOMEZ-ISLA, T., J.L. PRICE, D.W. MCKEEL, *et al.* 1996. Profound loss of layer II entorhinal cortex neurons occurs in very mild Alzheimer's disease. J. Neurosci. **16**: 4491–4500.
32. FRISONI, G.B., M.P. LAAKSO, A. BELTRAMELLO, *et al.* 1999. Hippocampal and entorhinal cortex atrophy in frontotemporal dementia and Alzheimer's disease. Neurology **52**: 91–100.
33. LAAKSO, M.P., K. PARTANEN, P. RIEKKINEN, *et al.* 1996. Hippocampal volumes in Alzheimer's disease, Parkinson's disease, with and without dementia, and in vascular dementia: an MRI study. Neurology **46**: 678–681.
34. LAAKSO, M.P., H. SOININEN, K. PARTANEN, *et al.* 1998. MRI of the hippocampus in Alzheimer's disease: sensitivity, specificity, and analysis of the incorrectly classified subjects. Neurobiol. Aging **19**: 23–31.
35. DICKERSON, B.C., I. GONCHAROVA, M.P. SULLIVAN, *et al.* 2001. MRI-derived entorhinal and hippocampal atrophy in incipient and very mild Alzheimer's disease. Neurobiol. Aging **22**: 747–754.
36. THAL, L.J. 2002. How to define treatment success using cholinesterase inhibitors. Int. J. Geriatr. Psychiatry. **17**: 388–390.
37. PEARSON, R.C.A., M.M. ESIRI, R.W. HIORNS, *et al.*1985. Anatomical correlates of the distribution of the pathological changes in the neocortex in Alzheimer's disease. Proc. Natl. Acad. Sci. USA **82**: 4531–4534.
38. ARNOLD, S.E., B.T. HYMAN, J. FLORY, *et al.* 1991. The topographical and neuroanatomical distribution of neurofibrillary tangles and neuritic plaques in the cerebral cortex of patients with Alzheimer's disease. Cereb. Cortex **1**: 103–116.
39. A. BRUN & E. ENGLUND. 1981. Regional pattern of degeneration in Alzheimer's disease: neuronal loss and histopathologic grading. Histopathology **5**: 549–564.
40. HYMAN, B.T., G.W. VAN HOESEN & A.R. DAMASIO. 1990. Memory-related neural systems in Alzheimer's disease: an anatomic study. Neurology **40**: 1721–1730.
41. MESULAM, M.M. 2000. A plasticity-based theory of the pathogenesis of Alzheimer's disease. Ann. N.Y. Acad. Sci. **924**: 42–52.
42. GOGTAY, N., J.N. GIEDD, L. LUSK, *et al.* 2004. Dynamic mapping of human cortical development during childhood and adolescence. Proc. Natl. Acad. Sci. **101**: 8174–8179.
43. YAKOVLEV, P.I. & A.R. LECOURS. 1967. The myelogenetic cycles of regional maturation of the brain. *In* Regional Development of the Brain in Early Life. A. Minkowski, Ed.: pp 3–70. Blackwell Scientific. Oxford.
44. BENES, F.M., M. TURTLE, Y. KHAN & P. FAROL. 1994. Myelination of a key relay zone in the hippocampal formation occurs in the human brain during childhood, adolescence, and adulthood. Arch. Gen. Psychiatry **51**: 477–484.
45. THOMPSON, P.M., C. VIDAL, J.N. GIEDD, *et al.* 2001. Mapping adolescent brain change reveals dynamic wave of accelerated gray matter loss in very early-onset schizophrenia. Proc. Natl. Acad. Sci. USA **98**: 11650–11655.
46. CANNON, T.D., P.M. THOMPSON, T. van ERP, *et al.* 2002. Cortex mapping reveals heteromodal gray matter deficits in monozygotic twins discordant for schizophrenia. Proc. Natl. Acad. Sci. USA **99**: 3228–3233.
47. PANTELIS C., D. VELAKOULIS, P.D. MCGORRY, *et al.* 2003. Neuroanatomical abnormalities before and after onset of psychosis: a cross-sectional and longitudinal MRI comparison. Lancet **361**: 281–288.

48. SUN, D., D. VELAKOULIS, A. YUNG, *et al.* 2007. Brain structural change during the development of psychosis: a longitudinal MRI study. submitted.

49. BARTZOKIS, G., J.L. CUMMINGS, D. SULTZER, *et al.*2003. White matter structural integrity in healthy aging adults and patients with Alzheimer disease: a magnetic resonance imaging study. Arch. Neurol. **60:** 393–398.

50. BARTZOKIS, G., D. SULTZER, P.H. LU, *et al.* 2004. Heterogeneous age-related breakdown of white matter structural integrity: implications for cortical "disconnection" in aging and Alzheimer's disease. Neurobiol. Aging **25:** 843–851.

51. SALAT, D.H., R.L. BUCKNER, A.Z. SNYDER, *et al.* 2004. Thinning of the cerebral cortex in aging. Cereb. Cortex **14:** 721–730. Epub 2004 Mar 28.

52. BALLMAIER, M., J.T. O'BRIEN, E.J. BURTON, *et al.* 2004a. Comparing gray matter loss profiles between dementia with Lewy bodies and Alzheimer's disease using cortical pattern matching: diagnosis and gender effects. Neuroimage **23:** 325–335.

53. HARVEY, G.T., J. HUGHES, I.G. MCKEITH, *et al.* 1999. Magnetic resonance imaging differences between dementia with Lewy bodies and Alzheimer's disease: a pilot study. Psychol. Med. **29:** 181–187.

54. MCKEITH, I.G., D.W. DICKSON, J. LOWE, *et al.* 2005. Diagnosis and management of dementia with Lewy bodies: third report of the DLB Consortium. Neurology **65:** 1863–1872. Epub 2005 Oct 19.

55. MASLIAH, E., R.M. DETERESA, M.E. MALLORY, & L.A. HANSEN. 2000. Changes in pathological findings at autopsy in AIDS cases for the last 15 years. AIDS **14:** 69–74.

56. APOSTOLOVA, L.G., P. LU, S. ROGERS, *et al.* 2007. 3D mapping of language networks in clinical and pre-clinical Alzheimer's disease [submitted].

57. CUMMINGS, J.L., L.G. APOSTOLOVA, G.G. AKOPYAN, *et al.* 2006. Structural correlates of apathy in Alzheimer's Disease. Annual Meeting of the American Academy of Neurology. San Diego, CA.

58. LU, A., A.D. LEOW, A.D. LEE, *et al.* 2006. Growth pattern abnormalities in childhood-onset schizophrenia visualized using tensor-based morphometry, 12th Annual Meeting of the Organization for Human Brain Mapping (OHBM), Florence, Italy, June 11–15.

59. THOMPSON, P.M., T.D. CANNON, K.L. NARR, *et al.* 2001. Genetic influences on brain structure. Nat. Neurosci. **4:** 1253–1258.

60. GRAY, J.R. & P.M. THOMPSON. 2004. Neurobiology of intelligence: science and ethics. Nat. Rev. Neurosci. **5:** 471–482.

61. MCDANIEL, M.A. & N.T. NGUYEN. 2002. A meta-analysis of the relationship between MRI-assessed brain volume and intelligence. Presented at Proc Int. Soc. Intel. Res., Nashville, TN.

62. BALLMAIER, M., A. KUMAR, P.M. THOMPSON, *et al.* 2004. Localizing gray matter deficits in late onset depression using computational cortical pattern matching methods. Am. J. Psychiatry **161:** 2091–2099.

63. PIEVANI, M., C. TESTA, F. SABATTOLI, *et al.* 2006. Structural correlates of age at onset in Alzheimer's disease: a cortical pattern matching study, 12th Annual Meeting of the Organization for Human Brain Mapping (OHBM), Florence, Italy, June 11–15.

64. FOX, N.C., S. COUSENS, R. SCAHILL, *et al.* 2000. Using serial registered brain magnetic resonance imaging to measure disease progression in Alzheimer disease: power calculations and estimates of sample size to detect treatment effects. Arch. Neurol. **57:** 339–344.

65. BARON, J.C., G. CHETELAT, B. DESGRANGES, et al. 2001. In vivo mapping of gray matter loss with voxel-based morphometry in mild Alzheimer's disease. Neuroimage **14**: 298–309.
66. FOX, N.C., W.R. CRUM, R.I. SCAHILL, et al. 2001. Imaging of onset and progression of Alzheimer's disease with voxel-compression mapping of serial magnetic resonance images. Lancet **358**: 201–205.
67. LEOW, A.D., S.C. HUANG, A. GENG, et al. 2005. Inverse Consistent Mapping in 3D Deformable Image Registration: its Construction and Statistical Properties, Information Processing in Medical Imaging (IPMI) 2005, Glenwood Springs, Colorado, July 11–15.
68. MEDINA, D., L. DETOLEDO-MORRELL, F. URRESTA, et al. 2006. White matter changes in mild cognitive impairment and AD: a diffusion tensor imaging study. Neurobiol. Aging **27**: 663–672.
69. FISCHL, B. & A.M. DALE. 2000. Measuring the thickness of the human cerebral cortex from magnetic resonance images. Proc. Natl. Acad. Sci. USA **97**: 11050–11055.
70. SOWELL, E.R., B.S. PETERSON, P.M. THOMPSON, et al. 2006. Sex differences in cortical thickness mapped in 176 healthy individuals between 7 and 87 years. [Epub ahead of print]
71. THOMPSON, P.M., K.M. HAYASHI, G. DE ZUBICARAY, et al. 2004. Mapping hippocampal and ventricular change in Alzheimer's Disease. Neuroimage. **22**: 1754–1766.
72. DE SANTI, S., M.J. DE LEON, H. RUSINEK, et al. 2001. Hippocampal formation glucose metabolism and volume losses in MCI and AD. Neurobiol Aging **22**: 529–539.
73. CALLEN, D.J., S.E. BLACK, F. GAO, et al. 2001. Beyond the hippocampus: MRI volumetry confirms widespread limbic atrophy in AD. Neurology **57**: 1669–1674.
74. DU, A.T., N. SCHUFF, D. AMEND, et al. 2001. Magnetic resonance imaging of the entorhinal cortex and hippocampus in mild cognitive impairment and Alzheimer's disease. J. Neurol. Neurosurg. Psychiatry **71**: 441–447.
75. SOININEN, H.S., K. PARTANEN, A. PITKANEN, et al. 1994. Volumetric MRI analysis of the amygdala and the hippocampus in subjects with age-associated memory impairment: correlation to visual and verbal memory. Neurology **44**: 1660–1668.
76. JACK, C.R., R.C. PETERSEN, Y.C. XU, et al. 1999. Prediction of AD with MRI-based hippocampal volume in mild cognitive impairment. Neurology **52**: 1397–1403.
77. VISSER, P.J., F.R.J. VERHEY, P.A.M. HOFMAN, et al. 2002. Medial temporal lobe atrophy predicts Alzheimer's disease in patients with minor cognitive impairment. J. Neurol. Neurosurg. Psychiatry **72**: 491–497.
78. PENNANEN, C., M. KIVIPELTO, S. TUOMAINEN, et al. 2004. Hippocampus and entorhinal cortex in mild cognitive impairment and early AD. Neurobiol. Aging **25**: 303–310.
79. DICKERSON, B.C., D.H. SALAT, J.F. BATES, et al. 2004. Medial temporal lobe function and structure in mild cognitive impairment. Ann Neurol. **56**: 27–35.
80. KILLIANY, R.J., B.T. HYMAN, T. GOMEZ-ISLA, et al. 2002. MRI measures of entorhinal cortex vs hippocampus in preclinical AD. Neurology **58**: 1188–1196.
81. DE LEON, M.J., J. GOLOMB, A.E. GEORGE et al. 1993. The radiologic prediction of Alzheimer disease: the atrophic hippocampal formation. AJNR Am. J. Neuroradiol. **14**: 897–906.

82. VISSER, P.J., P. SCHELTENS, F.R.J. VERHEY, *et al.* 1999. Medial temporal lobe atrophy and memory dysfunction as predictors for dementia in subjects with mild cognitive impairment. J. Neurol. **246:** 477–485.

83. LAAKSO, M.P., M. LEHTOVIRTA, K. PARTANEN, *et al.* 2000. Hippocampus in AD: a 3-year follow-up MRI study. Biol. Psychiatry **47:** 557–561.

84. KILLIANY, R.J., T. GOMEZ-ISLA, M. MOSS, *et al.* 2000. Use of structural magnetic resonance imaging to predict who will get Alzheimer's disease. Ann. Neurol. **47:** 430–439.

85. CSERNANSKY, J.G., L. WANG, S. JOSHI, *et al.* 2000. Early DAT is distinguished from aging by high dimensional mapping of the hippocampus. Neurology **55:** 1636–1643.

86. BECKER, J.T., K.M. HAYASHI, J.L. SEAMAN, *et al.* 2007. Alteration in Hippocampal and Caudate Nucleus Structure in HIV/AIDS Revealed by Three-Dimensional Mapping. [submitted].

87. BELL-MCGINTY, S., O.L. LOPEZ, C.C. MELTZER, *et al.* 2005. Differential cortical atrophy in subgroups of mild cognitive impairment. Arch. Neurol. **62:** 1393–1397.

88. FRISONI, G., F. SABATTOLI, A.D. LEE, *et al.* 2006. In vivo neuropathology of the hippocampal formation in AD: a radial mapping MR-based study. Neuroimage **32:** 104–110.

89. NARR, K.L., R.M. BILDER, A.W. TOGA, *et al.* 2005. Mapping cortical thickness and gray matter concentration in first episode schizophrenia. Cereb. Cortex **15:** 708–719.

90. GOGTAY, N., T.F. NUGENT, D. HERMAN, *et al.* 2006. Dynamic mapping of human hippocampal development during childhood and adolescence. Hippocampus **16:** 664–672.

91. THOMPSON, P.M., K.M. HAYASHI, S. SIMON, *et al.* 2004. Structural abnormalities in the brains of human subjects who use methamphetamine. J. Neurosci. **24:** 6028–6036.

92. LIN, J.J., N. SALAMON, A.D. LEE, *et al.* 2005. 3D pre-operative maps of hippocampal atrophy predict surgical outcomes in temporal lobe epilepsy. Neurology **65:** 1094–1097.

93. BEARDEN, C.E., P.M. THOMPSON, M. DALWANI, *et al.* 2007. Cortical gray matter density increases in lithium-treated patients with bipolar disorder. Biol. Psychiatry [In press].

94. BUTTERS, M.A., H.J. AIZENSTEIN, K.M. HAYASHI, *et al.* 2007. Three-dimensional mapping reveals decreased volume of the caudate nucleus in late-life depression. Biol. Psychiatry [submitted].

95. VAN HOESEN, G.W., J.C. AUGUSTINACK, J. DIERKING, *et al.* 2000. The parahippocampal gyrus in Alzheimer's disease. Clinical and preclinical neuroanatomical correlates. Ann. N. Y. Acad. Sci. **911:** 254–274.

96. ROYBAL, D.J., R.A. DUTTON, K.M. HAYASHI, *et al.* 2005. Mapping ApoE4 and Gender Effects on Hippocampal Atrophic Rates: A Longitudinal MRI Study of Normal Aging, 2005 Annual Scientific Meeting of the American Geriatric Society (AGS), Orlando, FL, May 11–15.

97. ASHBURNER, J., J.G. CSERNANSKY, C. DAVATZIKOS, *et al.* 2003. Computer-assisted imaging to assess brain structure in healthy and diseased brains. Lancet **2:** 78–88.

98. GOOD, C.D., I.S. JOHNSRUDE, J. ASHBURNER, *et al.* 2001. A voxel-based morphometric study of ageing in 465 normal adult human brains. Neuroimage **14:** 21–36.

99. ASHBURNER, J. & K.J. FRISTON. 2000. Voxel-based morphometry–the methods. Neuroimage **11:** 805–821.

100. ASHBURNER, J. & K.J. FRISTON. 2001. Why voxel-based morphometry should be used. Neuroimage **14:** 1238–1243.

101. BOOKSTEIN, F. 2001. Voxel-based morphometry should not be used with imperfectly registered images. Neuroimage **14:** 1454–1462.

102. DAVATZIKOS, C., A. GENC, D. XU & S.M. RESNICK. 2001a. Voxel-based morphometry using the RAVENS maps: methods and validation using simulated longitudinal atrophy. Neuroimage **14:** 1361–1369.

103. THACKER, N. 2003. 'Tutorial: A Critical Analysis of VBM,' http://www.tina-vision.net/docs/memos/2003-011.pdf, 2003.

104. CRUM, W.R., L.D. GRIFFIN, D.L. HILL & D.J. HAWKES. 2003. Zen and the art of medical image registration: correspondence, homology, and quality. Neuroimage. **20:** 1425–1437. Review.

105. SOWELL, E.R., P.M. THOMPSON, S.E. WELCOME, et al. 2003. Cortical abnormalities in children and adolescents with attention-deficit hyperactivity disorder. Lancet **362:** 1699–1707.

106. SELEMON, L.D., G. RAJKOWSKA & P.S. GOLDMAN-RAKIC. 1995. Abnormally high neuronal density in the schizophrenic cortex. A morphometric analysis of prefrontal area 9 and occipital area 17. Arch. Gen. Psychiatry **52:** 805–818; discussion 819–20.

107. RAZ, N. et al. 1997. Selective aging of the human cerebral cortex observed in vivo: differential vulnerability of the prefrontal gray matter. Cereb. Cortex **7:** 268–282.

108. MAGNOTTA, V.A. et al. 1999. Quantitative in vivo measurement of gyrification in the human brain: changes associated with aging. Cereb. Cortex **9:** 151–160.

109. SHAW, P., D. GREENSTEIN, J. LERCH, et al. 2006. Intellectual ability and cortical development in children and adolescents. Nature **440:** 676–679.

110. VIDAL, C.N., K.M. HAYASHI, J.A. GEAGA, et al. 2006. Dynamically spreading frontal and cingulate deficits mapped in adolescents with schizophrenia. Arch. Gen. Psychiatry **63:** 25–34.

111. LUDERS, E., K.L. NARR, P.M. THOMPSON, et al. 2005. Gender Effects on Cortical Thickness, 11th Annual Meeting of the Organization for Human Brain Mapping (OHBM), Toronto, Canada, 12–16.

112. LERCH, J.P., J.C. PRUESSNER, A. ZIJDENBOS, et al. 2004. Focal decline of cortical thickness in Alzheimer's disease identified by computational neuroanatomy. Cereb Cortex. **15:** 995–1001. Epub 2004 Nov 10.

113. NARR, K.L., A.W. TOGA, P. SZESZKO, et al. 2005. Cortical thinning in cingulate and occipital cortices in first episode schizophrenia. Biol. Psychiatry **58:** 32–40.

114. SOWELL, E.R., P.M. THOMPSON, C.M. LEONARD, et al. 2004. Longitudinal mapping of cortical thickness and brain growth in normal children. J. Neurol. Sci. **24:** 8223–8231.

115. LU, L.H., C.M. LEONARD, P.M. THOMPSON, et al. 2006. Normal developmental changes in inferior frontal gray matter are associated with improvement in phonological processing: a longitudinal MRI analysis. Cerebral Cortex. [June 16 Epub ahead of print.]

116. SOWELL, E.R., P.M. THOMPSON, S.N. MATTSON, et al. 2002a. Regional brain shape abnormalities persist into adolescence after heavy prenatal alcohol exposure. Cereb. Cortex **12:** 856–865.

117. GOGTAY, N., A. ORDONEZ, D.H. HERMAN, *et al.* 2007. Dynamic mapping of cortical brain development in pediatric bipolar illness. J. Child Psychol. Psychiatry [In press].

118. BEARDEN, C.E., R.A. DUTTON, T.G.M. VAN ERP, *et al.* 2006. Abnormal cortical thickness and cortical asymmetry mapped in children with 22q11.2 Microdeletions, 12th Annual Meeting of the Organization for Human Brain Mapping (OHBM), Florence, Italy, June 11–15.

119. LIN, J.J., N. SALAMON, A.D. LEE, *et al.* 2006. Reduced Cortical Thickness & Complexity Mapped in Mesial Temporal Lobe Epilepsy with Hippocampal Sclerosis. Cerebral Cortex [In press].

120. CANNON, T.D., W. HENNAH, T.G.M. VAN ERP, *et al.* 2005. DISC1/TRAX haplotypes associate with schizophrenia, reduced prefrontal gray matter, and impaired short- and long-term memory. Arch. Gen. Psychiatry **62**: 1205–1213.

121. ZEINEH, M.M., S.A. ENGEL, P.M. THOMPSON, & S. BOOKHEIMER. 2003. Dynamics of the hippocampus during encoding and retrieval of face-name pairs. Science **299**: 577–580.

122. LE BIHAN, D., E. BRETON, D. LALLEMAND, *et al.* 1986. MR imaging of intravoxel incoherent motions: application to diffusion and perfusion in neurologic disorders. Radiology **161**: 401–407.

123. MOSELEY, M.E., Y. COHEN, J. KUCHARCZYK, *et al.* 1990. Diffusion-weighted MR imaging of anisotropic water diffusion in cat central nervous system. Radiology **176**: 439–445.

124. BASSER, P.J., J. MATTIELLO, D. LEBIHAN. 1994. Estimation of the effective self-diffusion tensor from the NMR spin echo. J. Magn. Reson. B **103**: 247–254.

125. KANTARCI, K., C.R. JACK JR, Y.C. XU, *et al.* 2000. Regional metabolic patterns in mild cognitive impairment and Alzheimer's disease: A 1H MRS study. Neurology. **55**: 210–217.

126. KANTARCI, K., C.R. JACK JR, Y.C. XU, *et al.* 2001. Mild cognitive impairment and Alzheimer disease: regional diffusivity of water. Radiology. **219**: 101–107.

127. SANDSON, T.A., O. FELICIAN, R.R. EDELMAN, & S. WARACH. 1999. Diffusion-weighted magnetic resonance imaging in Alzheimer's disease. Dement. Geriatr. Cogn. Disord. **10**: 166–171.

128. SCHOTT, J.M., S.L. PRICE, C. FROST, *et al.* 2005. Measuring atrophy in Alzheimer disease: a serial MRI study over 6 and 12 months. Neurology **65**: 119–124.

129. THOMPSON, P.M., J.N. GIEDD, R.P. WOODS, *et al.* 2000. Growth patterns in the developing brain detected by using continuum-mechanical tensor maps. Nature **404**: 190–193.

130. JANKE, A.L., G.D. ZUBICARAY, S.E. ROSE, *et al.* 2001. 4D deformation modeling of cortical disease progression in Alzheimer's dementia. Magn Reson Med **46**: 661–666.

131. STUDHOLME, C., V. CARDENAS, N. SCHUFF, *et al.* 2001. Detecting Spatially Consistent Structural Differences in Alzheimer's and Fronto Temporal Dementia Using Deformation Morphometry. Conference Series on Medical Imaging Computing and Computer-Assisted Intervention (MICCAI) 2001, 41–48.

132. CHIANG, M.C., A.D. LEOW, R.A. DUTTON, *et al.* 2006. Fluid registration of diffusion tensor imaging using information theory. Submitted to IEEE Transactions on Medical Imaging, Special Issue on Computational Neuroanatomy (eds. Gee, J.C., Thompson, P.M.), to appear March 2007 [submitted, June 29, 2006].

133. LEOW, A.D., J.C. SOARES, K.M. HAYASHI, *et al.* 2006. Asymmetrical effects of lithium on brain structure mapped in healthy individuals, [submitted].

134. THOMPSON, P.M. & A.W. TOGA. 2003. Cortical diseases and cortical localization [Review Article]. Nature Encyclopedia of the Life Sciences (ELS), 2003.
135. LEOW, A.D., A.D. LEE, M.C. CHIANG, et al. 2005. Analysis of Regional Brain Atrophy in a Single Case of Semantic Dementia Using Serial MRI with Inverse-Consistent Non-Rigid Registration, 11th Annual Meeting of the Organization for Human Brain Mapping (OHBM), Toronto, Canada, June 12–16.
136. LEE, A.D., A.D. LEOW, A. LU, et al. 2006. Tensor-Based Morphometry Reveals 3D Profile of Altered Brain Structure in Fragile X Syndrome, 61st Annual Scientific Convention of the Society of Biological Psychiatry (SOBP), Toronto, Ontario, Canada, May 18–20.
137. CHIANG, M.C., A.L. REISS, R.A. DUTTON, et al. 2006. 3D Pattern of Brain Volume Reduction in Williams Syndrome Visualized using Tensor-Based Morphometry, 12th Annual Meeting of the Organization for Human Brain Mapping (OHBM), Florence, Italy, June 11–15.
138. FOLAND, L.C., L.L. ALTSHULER, A.D. LEOW, et al. 2006. A Tensor-Based Morphometric Study of Bipolar Disorder, 12th Annual Meeting of the Organization for Human Brain Mapping (OHBM), Florence, Italy, June 11–15.
139. LEPORE, N., Y.Y. CHOU, C.A. BRUN, et al. 2006. Genetic Influences on Brain Structure and Fiber Architecture Mapped Using Diffusion Tensor Imaging and Tensor-Based Morphometry in Twins, 12th Annual Meeting of the Organization for Human Brain Mapping (OHBM), Florence, Italy, June 11–15.
140. JACK, C.R. JR, R.C. PETERSEN, Y. XU, et al. 2000. Rates of hippocampal atrophy correlate with change in clinical status in aging and AD. Neurology. 55: 484–489.
141. BERNSTEIN, M.A., C. LIN, B.J. BOROWSKI, et al. 2005. Alzheimer's Disease Neuroimaging Initiative (ADNI): The MR Imaging Protocol. Presented at State-of-the-Art Cardiovascular and Neuro MRI, a Joint Workshop of the ISMRM and CSR, Beijing, China, September.
142. ARCHER, H.A., P. EDISON, D.J. BROOKS, et al. 2006. Amyloid load and cerebral atrophy in Alzheimer's disease: An (11)C-PIB positron emission tomography study. Ann Neurol. 60: 145–147 [Epub ahead of print].
143. KOCHUNOV, P.K. et al. 2007. Relationship among neuroimaging markers of merebral atrophy during normal aging. Human Brain Mapping. Feb 8 [Epub ahead of print].
144. JACK, C.R. JR., R.C. PETERSEN, Y.C. XU, et al. 1997. Medial temporal atrophy on MRI in normal aging and very mild Alzheimer's disease. Neurology 49: 786–794.
145. XU, Y. et al. 2000. Usefulness of MRI measures of entorhinal cortex versus hippocampus in AD. Neurology 54(9): 1760–1767.
146. CHETELAT, G., B. DESGRANGES, V. DE LA SAYETTE, et al. 2002. Mapping gray matter loss with voxel-based morphometry in mild cognitive impairment. Neuroreport. 13: 1939–1943.
147. KOCHUNOV, P. et al. 2005. Age-related morphology trends of cortical sulci. Human Brain Mapping 26(3): 210–220.
148. BURGGREN, A.C. et al. 2007. Reduced cortical thickness in hippocampal subregions in people at genetic risk for Alzheimer's disease. [submitted].
149. ROSE, S.E. et al. 2006. Diffusion indices on magnetic resonance imaging and neuropsychological performance in amnestic mild cognitive impairment. J. Neurol. Neurosurg. Psychiatry 77(10): 1122–1128.

# Shifting Paradigms in Dementia

## Toward Stratification of Diagnosis and Treatment Using MRI

WIESJE M. VAN DER FLIER,[a] FREDERIK BARKHOF,[b] AND PHILIP SCHELTENS[a]

[a] Alzheimer Center and Department of Neurology, Vrije Universiteit Medical Center, Amsterdam, The Netherlands

[b] Alzheimer Center and Department of Radiology, Vrije Universiteit Medical Center, Amsterdam, The Netherlands

ABSTRACT: Atrophy and cerebrovascular disease are the two most important magnetic resonance imaging (MRI) characteristics in the evaluation of dementia. On MRI, atrophy is the primary hallmark of neurodegenerative dementias including Alzheimer's disease (AD), while vascular dementia is characterized by the presence of ischemic vascular damage, such as territorial infarcts, lacunes, and white matter hyperintensities. Evidence is accumulating that vascular factors play an important role in the development of cognitive decline at old age and clinical AD. In the present article we present results of four recent MRI studies suggesting the additional involvement of small vessel disease in neurodegenerative disorders. Atrophy in the medial temporal lobe, as typically observed in AD, and small vessel disease often coincide. In terms of clinical significance, their effects may even be synergistic. The strict distinction between AD and vascular dementia is often artificial, as most patients suffer from both disorders to some extent. For the future, we see an important role for MRI in identifying those different compartments, regardless of clinical classification. Treatment could be directed by (and evaluated through) MRI patterns, rather than a diagnostic label.

KEYWORDS: Alzheimer's disease; dementia; neurodegenerative disorders; cerebrovascular disease; small vessel disease; white matter hyperintensities; atrophy; medial temporal lobe

One of the most important issues in the differential diagnosis of dementia is Alzheimer's disease (AD) versus vascular dementia, or in a broader way, neurodegenerative versus cerebrovascular disease. AD is characterized by memory deficits. On magnetic resonance imaging (MRI), atrophy can be observed,

Address for correspondence: W.M. van der Flier, Ph.D., Department of Neurology and Alzheimer Center, Vrije Universiteit Medical Center, PO Box 7057, 1007 MB Amsterdam, The Netherlands. Voice: +31-20-444-1079; fax: +31-20-444-0715.
wm.vdflier@vumc.nl

Ann. N.Y. Acad. Sci. 1097: 215–224 (2007). © 2007 New York Academy of Sciences.
doi: 10.1196/annals.1379.013

primarily in the medial temporal lobe. Vascular dementia, on the other hand, is caused by cerebrovascular tissue damage (large vessel infarcts or small vessel disease). Clinically, vascular dementia often presents with mental slowness and impaired executive functioning. In the present article, we describe recent evidence suggesting that the distinction between neurodegenerative and cerebrovascular disease is often neither valid, nor useful, since overlap is commonly observed. Rather than classifying all patients as either neurodegenerative or cerebrovascular, we propose to view both disorders as a continuum.

Pure vascular dementia—i.e., dementia purely caused by large vessel infarcts and/or small vessel disease (observed on MRI as white matter hyperintensities (WMH), lacunes)—is rare. In prevalence studies, 15–20% of dementia cases are attributed to vascular dementia, but postmortem studies show that less than 5% of dementia cases are based on vascular brain damage only.[1,2] AD is the most common type of dementia. Estimates of its prevalence vary between 50% and 80%. Again, it should be noted that postmortem studies have demonstrated that the prevalence of dementia caused by Alzheimer-type pathology only are far lower. These prevalences point to the main message of this article: mixed, rather than pure pathology seems to be the norm with respect to dementia, certainly at old age.[3]

A different story emerges when we evaluate cerebrovascular disease as the causative factor of cognitive decline in a broader perspective. It has even been suggested that cerebrovascular disease is the most common cause of dementia at old age.[4] Expressed in this way, cerebrovascular disease refers to both pure vascular dementia and the contribution of vascular pathology to other neurodegenerative disorders. Just as dementia based on cerebrovascular disease only is highly rare, it is almost equally rare to develop dementia with no addition of cerebrovascular disease at all. Cerebrovascular disease can also be involved in mild cognitive deficits, not sufficient for a diagnosis of dementia. In analogy with the term "mild cognitive impairment" (MCI)—mostly used to designate patients at risk to develop AD—the term "vascular cognitive impairment" (VCI) has been coined. VCI refers to patients with (risk factors for) cerebrovascular disease and cognitive impairment.[5] Intrinsic to the concept of VCI is the hope that cerebrovascular disease will be more amenable to treatment than brain damage caused by Alzheimer-type pathology. With cure for neurodegenerative disorders not yet available, treatment of vascular risk factors may be the best strategy to postpone the development of frank dementia.[6,7]

## POSTMORTEM

From postmortem studies we know that Alzheimer pathology (i.e., senile plaques and neurofibrillary tangles) and cerebrovascular disease not only often coexist, but may even amplify each other's effect. Individuals with both types of pathology during life more often suffered from dementia than individuals where only one type of pathology was observed.[3] Moreover, patients with dementia and both types of pathology had more severe cognitive deficits during life than patients with only one type of pathology.[8] Results of these and other studies suggest that Alzheimer-type pathology and cerebrovascular disease are both important correlates of cognitive decline at old age. Moreover, these two types of pathology may act in synergy to cause cognitive decline. Postmortem studies have several disadvantages. By definition the brain processes are studied *post hoc*. It is possible that the disease process started out as purely neurodegenerative, with the involvement of cerebrovascular disease only at a later stage. Ultimately, it is even conceivable that some of the abnormalities developed during the dying process, for example, due to oxygen deficiency. Ideally, brain abnormalities are studied *in vivo* at the same time, or even before, cognitive decline takes place. MRI offers the opportunity to study subtle brain changes in a noninvasive way. In the following, we present results of four recent MRI studies assessing the role of small vessel disease in AD and cognitive decline at old age.

## MEDIAL TEMPORAL LOBE AND WHITE MATTER HYPERINTENSITIES IN AD

To study the combined effect of Alzheimer-type pathology and cerebrovascular pathology, we measured volumes of medial temporal lobe[9] and white matter hyperintensities (WMH)[10] in a group of 58 patients with AD and 28 elderly controls.[11] Both MRI measures were medianized (atrophy of the medial temporal lobe present/absent, WMH mild/severe) and odds ratios were calculated with the group with no medial temporal lobe atrophy and mild WMH as reference group. Subjects with severe WMH had a nonsignificant modestly increased risk of AD, while atrophy of the medial temporal lobe (MTA) was clearly associated with AD (TABLE 1). However, patients in whom both abnormalities were observed on MRI all had a clinical diagnosis of AD, implying that the known association between hippocampal atrophy and AD is amplified by the additional presence of WMH. These results support the view that cerebrovascular disease contributes to the clinical syndrome of AD.

## MTA AND WMH IN NONDEMENTED ELDERLY

Having demonstrated that Alzheimer-type pathology and cerebrovascular disease, measured on MRI as MTA and WMH, amplify each other in AD, the next step was to study the effect of these abnormalities in individuals who are not (yet) demented. The multicenter European LADIS study offered an excellent opportunity. LADIS—which stands for Leukoaraiosis and Disability—studies the predictive value of WMH for the transition to disability in initially

**TABLE 1.** Odds ratios for AD dependent on medial temporal lobe volume and white matter hyperintensities[11]

| Medial temporal lobe white matter hyperintensities | Large mild | Large severe | Small mild | Small severe |
|---|---|---|---|---|
| AD (number) | 9 | 10 | 16 | 23 |
| control (number) | 14 | 10 | 4 | 0 |
| Odds ratio | 1.0 | 1.6 | 6.2 | infinity |
| (95% CI) | (Reference) | (0.4–6.2) | (1.3–32.7) | (6.3–inf.) |

NOTE: Data are presented as odds ratios (ORs) and their exact 95% confidence intervals (CIs). Note that, due to the zero cell, the accompanying OR is indeterminably high. However, using the exact method, the lower limit of the CI can be calculated.

nondisabled elderly.[12] At baseline, 639 subjects (age: 74 ± 5 years, 55% female) with some degree of WMH were included. All were living independently. They were allowed to have some degree of impairment, but only mild, so as not to interfere with their instrumental activities of daily living. MTA and WMH were both scored using a visual rating scale.[13,14] The entire group was divided into four groups, depending on the absence/presence of MTA and/or the presence of mild/severe WMH.[15] General cognitive function was assessed using the Mini-Mental State Examination (MMSE). On average, all four groups performed within normal limits (FIG. 1). Patients with either MTA or severe WMH did not have a significantly lower MMSE score than patients without either abnormality. However, patients with both MTA and severe WMH performed worse than patients with a single or no abnormality,

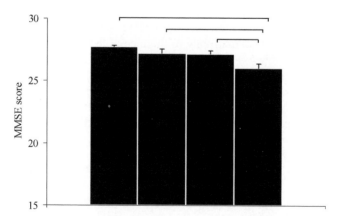

**FIGURE 1.** Average Mini Mental State Examination (MMSE) score according to the presence of medial temporal lobe atrophy (MTA) and/or white matter hyperintensities (WMH). The group with both MTA and severe WMH had a lower score on the MMSE than the groups with a single or no MRI abnormality ($P < 0.05$).[15]

suggesting an additive effect of both MRI abnormalities. These results suggest that Alzheimer-type pathology and cerebrovascular disease are both involved in the earliest stages of cognitive decline.

## SMALL VESSEL DISEASE: WMH AND LACUNES

In the same LADIS cohort, the effect of WMH and lacunes— two expressions of small vessel disease—on general cognitive function was studied.[16] WMH were scored as mild, moderate, or severe according to Fazekas' rating scale.[14] Lacunes were counted and recoded into none, few (1–3), or many (4 or more). There was a modest correlation between WMH and lacunes (Spearman $r = 0.25, P < 0.001$). After correction for age and sex, both lacunes and WMH were observed to be associated with general cognitive functioning, as measured using the MMSE and the Alzheimer's disease assessment scale (FIG. 2). Even when both measures of small vessel disease were entered in the regression model simultaneously, the association with cognitive function remained, although to a lesser extent for lacunes. These results suggest that when evaluating vascular damage on MRI in relation to cognitive decline at old age, it is important to evaluate both WMH and lacunes as separate indicators of small vessel disease (arteriosclerotic and embolic, respectively).

## MICROBLEEDS

Microbleeds are a third expression of small vessel disease. Microbleeds are small, dot-like lesions of low signal intensity in the brain that can be observed on T2*-weighted MRI sequences. Histologically, they represent focal leakage of hemosiderin from abnormal small blood vessels affected by lipohyalinosis or arising from arteries affected by amyloid deposition.[17] Microbleeds are highly prevalent among patients with a stroke,[18] but prevalence is low in population-based studies.[19–21] We studied the prevalence of microbleeds in almost 772 patients who visited our memory clinic in the past few years.[22] The overall prevalence of at least one microbleed was 17%, and differed according to diagnostic group ($\chi^2 = 59.0; P < 0.001$, see FIG. 3). The majority (65%) of patients with vascular dementia had one or more microbleeds. Patients with AD or MCI showed at least one microbleed in 20% and 18%, respectively. By contrast, only 10% of patients with subjective memory complaints had one or more microbleeds. The presence of microbleeds was associated with other expressions of cerebrovascular disease on MRI. However, within diagnostic groups, an association with cognitive impairment was not observed. Further study is needed to assess the prognostic value of microbleeds for the course of the disease, and possible treatment implications.

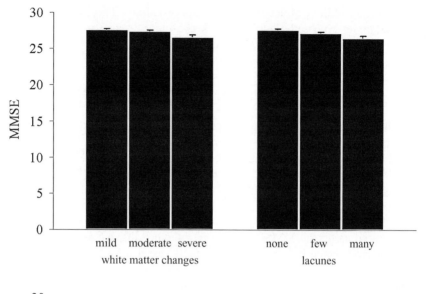

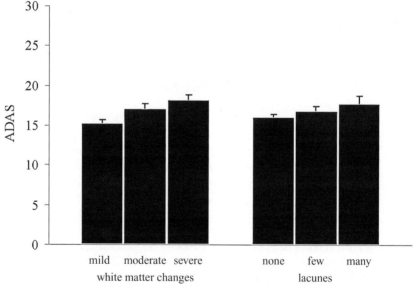

**FIGURE 2.** Bars represent estimated means (corrected for age and sex) with estimated standard errors. General linear models were performed for white matter hyperintensities (WMH) and lacunes separately, correcting for age and sex and with Mini-Mental State Examination (MMSE) and Alzheimer Disease Assessment Scale (ADAS) as dependent variable, respectively.[16] In these models, WMH and lacunes each were associated with scores on the MMSE and ADAS (MMSE-WMH: $\beta(SE) = -0.48\,(0.12)$, $P < 0.001$; MMSE-lacunes: $\beta(SE) = -0.62\,(0.14)$, $P < 0.001$, ADAS-WMH: $\beta(SE) = 1.31\,(0.35)$, $P < 0.001$; ADAS-lacunes: $\beta(SE) = 1.12\,(0.41)$, $P = 0.007$).

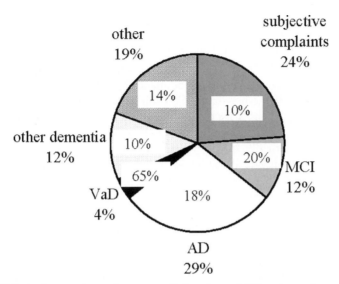

**FIGURE 3.** Among the total memory clinic cohort of 772 patients, there were 184 (24%) patients with subjective memory complaints, 90 (12%) patients with mild cognitive impairment (MCI), 223 (29%) patients with Alzheimer's disease (AD), 31 (4%) patients with vascular dementia (VaD), 94 (12%) patients with any other type of dementia, and 150 (19%) patients with some other disorder, including psychiatric disorders and neurological disorders other than dementia.[22] Within each wedge, the prevalence of microbleeds is shown. The prevalence of microbleeds differed by diagnostic group ($\chi^2 = 59.0$; $P < 0.001$).

## PROPOSING A NEW DIAGNOSTIC PARADIGM

The studies described above build on a growing body of evidence showing the involvement of cerebrovascular disease in the development of clinical AD and cognitive decline at old age. With respect to the brain damage involved in cognitive decline at old age, mixed rather than pure pathology seems to be the norm. On MRI, different types of pathology can be discerned that seem to be contributing to the clinical picture independently. This observation leads us to suggest that diagnostic labeling of subtypes of dementia, as is customary in clinical practice, may not be the most fruitful approach. Accumulating evidence suggests that patients do not have *either* AD *or* vascular dementia; rather, they may have aspects of both. Instead of exclusively labeling all patients as either neurodegenerative or cerebrovascular, both disorders could be viewed as a continuum, with purely neurodegenerative disease at one end and purely cerebrovascular disease at the other end of the spectrum.

To date, the role of MRI is undisputed in the diagnosis of dementia. Neuroimaging is recommended at least once during the diagnostic work-up.[23] In addition to the exclusion of surgical disorders such as tumors or hematomata, MRI may also add positive evidence for the presence of specific types of neuropathology. More specifically, MTA is generally viewed as supportive of a diagnosis of AD. If sufficient vascular abnormalities are observed, the diagnosis of vascular dementia can be made.[24] However, MTA may also be observed in disorders other than AD, while cerebrovascular disease is also observed in neurodegenerative disorders. For example, MTA and small vessel disease are often observed together in clinical AD.[25,26]

It is conceivable that the role of MRI in dementia will change in the future. We propose a new diagnostic paradigm where—irrespective of specific diagnostic labels—MRI is used both as a starting point for treatment choice, and as a means of monitoring disease progression and treatment effect. In this paradigm, where a diagnosis would be more than just a label, treatment and management of the patient would directly follow observations of markers on MRI. For example, observation of MTA might be a reason to start cholinesterase inhibitors (currently allowed for AD and dementia with Lewy bodies only, while MTA is also frequently observed in vascular dementia). Evidence of cerebrovascular disease would lead to treatment of vascular risk factors and lifestyle modification (e.g., quit smoking and increase physical activity), even when the clinical diagnosis is probable AD only. Observation of multiple types of abnormalities would lead to a multifaceted treatment approach. By stratification of treatment based on MRI findings, effectiveness of treatment may be improved. Moreover, with repeated imaging, the MRI markers may be used to evaluate treatment effect and to monitor disease progression.[27] In fact, this is happening already, and increasingly clinical trials in dementia are using MRI measures as inclusion criteria, stratifiers, and outcome measures. Similarly, one could think of a trial on the treatment of hypertension in AD to influence both clinical and MRI endpoints (e.g., WMH). Earlier trials did not include MRI and missed the opportunity to document the underlying mechanisms of the beneficial effect.[28] It has been estimated that a total number of 227 patients with early confluent and confluent WMH per treatment arm would suffice to show a 30% therapeutic effect on WMH in a 3-year study.[29] Using MRI markers as surrogate endpoints not only increases our knowledge of the disease process, but may also provide cost-effective ways of identifying those therapies that slow specific neuropathological processes as opposed to providing temporary symptomatic benefit. Ideally, a surrogate marker of disease progression should relate directly to the extent of the underlying pathology, i.e., senile plaques, neurofibrillary tangles, and synaptic loss. Such measures, however, to date are not available *in vivo*. Cerebral atrophy as measured on MRI is secondary to neuronal destruction, and therefore can serve as an *in vivo* marker of progression of neurodegeneration. Other biomarkers, such as cerebrospinal fluid biomarkers and positron emission tomography, may have added value in combination with the use of MRI.

# REFERENCE

1. LOBO, A., L.J. LAUNER, L. FRATIGLIONI, *et al.* 2000. Prevalence of dementia and major subtypes in Europe: a collaborative study of population-based cohorts. Neurologic Diseases in the Elderly Research Group. Neurology **54**(Suppl 5): S4–S9.
2. BARKER, W.W., C.A. LUIS, A. KASHUBA, *et al.* 2002. Relative frequencies of Alzheimer disease, Lewy body, vascular and frontotemporal dementia, and hippocampal sclerosis in the State of Florida Brain Bank. Alzheimer Dis. Assoc. Disord. **16:** 203–212.
3. NEUROPATHOLOGY GROUP OF THE MEDICAL RESEARCH COUNCIL COGNITIVE FUNCTION AND AGEING STUDY (MRC CFAS). 2001. Pathological correlates of late-onset dementia in a multicentre, community-based population in England and Wales. Lancet **357:** 169–175.
4. ROMAN, G.C. 2003. Stroke, cognitive decline and vascular dementia: the silent epidemic of the 21st century. Neuroepidemiology **22:** 161–164.
5. ERKINJUNTTI, T. & S. GAUTHIER. Eds. 2002. Vascular Cognitive Impairment. Martin Dunitz. London.
6. FORETTE, F., M.L. SEUX, J.A. STAESSEN, *et al.* 2002. The prevention of dementia with antihypertensive treatment: new evidence from the Systolic Hypertension in Europe (Syst-Eur) study. Arch. Intern. Med. **162:** 2046–2052.
7. WOLOZIN, B., W. KELLMAN, P. RUOSSEAU, *et al.* 2000. Decreased prevalence of Alzheimer disease associated with 3-hydroxy-3-methyglutaryl coenzyme A reductase inhibitors. Arch. Neurol. **57:** 1439–1443.
8. SNOWDON, D.A., L.H. GREINER, J.A. MORTIMER, *et al.* 1997. Brain infarction and the clinical expression of Alzheimer disease. The Nun Study. JAMA **277:** 813–817.
9. GOSCHE, K.M., J.A. MORTIMER, C.D. SMITH, *et al.* 2002. Hippocampal volume as an index of Alzheimer neuropathology: findings from the Nun Study. Neurology **58:** 1476–1482.
10. PANTONI, L. & J.H. GARCIA. 1997. Pathogenesis of leukoaraiosis: a review. Stroke **28:** 652–659.
11. VAN DER FLIER, W.M., H.A. MIDDELKOOP, A.W. WEVERLING-RIJNSBURGER, *et al.* 2004. Interaction of medial temporal lobe atrophy and white matter hyperintensities in AD. Neurology **62:** 1862–1864.
12. PANTONI, L., A.M. BASILE, G. PRACUCCI, *et al.* 2005. Impact of age-related cerebral white matter changes on the transition to disability—the LADIS study: rationale, design and methodology. Neuroepidemiology **24:** 51–62.
13. SCHELTENS, P., L.J. LAUNER, F. BARKHOF, *et al.* 1995. Visual assessment of medial temporal lobe atrophy on magnetic resonance imaging: interobserver reliability. J. Neurol. **242:** 557–560.
14. FAZEKAS, F., J.B. CHAWLUK, A. ALAVI, *et al.* 1987. MR signal abnormalities at 1.5 T in Alzheimer's dementia and normal aging. AJR Am. J. Roentgenol. **149:** 351–356.
15. VAN DER FLIER, W.M., E.C. VAN STRAATEN, F. BARKHOF, *et al.* 2005. Medial temporal lobe atrophy and white matter hyperintensities are associated with mild cognitive deficits in non-disabled elderly people: the LADIS study. J. Neurol. Neurosurg. Psychiatry **76:** 1497–1500.

16. VAN DER FLIER, W.M., E.C. VAN STRAATEN, F. BARKHOF, et al. 2005. Small vessel disease and general cognitive function in nondisabled elderly: the LADIS study. Stroke **36:** 2116–2120.

17. FAZEKAS, F., R. KLEINERT, G. ROOB, et al. 1999. Histopathologic analysis of foci of signal loss on gradient-echo T2*-weighted MR images in patients with spontaneous intracerebral hemorrhage: evidence of microangiopathy-related microbleeds. AJNR Am. J. Neuroradiol. **20:** 637–642.

18. ROOB, G., A. LECHNER, R. SCHMIDT, et al.. 2000. Frequency and location of microbleeds in patients with primary intracerebral hemorrhage. Stroke **31:** 2665–2669.

19. ROOB, G., R. SCHMIDT, P. KAPELLER, et al. 1999. MRI evidence of past cerebral microbleeds in a healthy elderly population. Neurology **52:** 991–994.

20. TSUSHIMA, Y., Y. TANIZAKI, J. AOKI & K. ENDO. 2002. MR detection of microhemorrhages in neurologically healthy adults. Neuroradiology **44:** 31–36.

21. JEERAKATHIL, T., P.A. WOLF, A. BEISER, et al. 2004. Cerebral microbleeds: prevalence and associations with cardiovascular risk factors in the Framingham Study. Stroke **35:** 1831–1835.

22. CORDONNIER, C., W.M. VAN DER FLIER, J.D. SLUIMER, et al. 2006. Prevalence and severity of microbleeds in a memory clinic setting. Neurology **66:** 1356–1360.

23. KNOPMAN, D.S., S.T. DEKOSKY, J.L. CUMMINGS, et al. 2001. Practice parameter: diagnosis of dementia (an evidence-based review): Report of the Quality Standards Subcommittee of the American Academy of Neurology. Neurology **56:** 1143–1153.

24. VAN STRAATEN, E.C., P. SCHELTENS, D.L. KNOL, et al. 2003. Operational definitions for the NINDS-AIREN criteria for vascular dementia. An interobserver study. Stroke **34:** 1907–1912.

25. DE LEEUW, F.E., F. BARKHOF & P. SCHELTENS. 2004. White matter lesions and hippocampal atrophy in Alzheimer's disease. Neurology **62:** 310–312.

26. WU, C.C., D. MUNGAS, C.I. PETKOV, et al. 2002. Brain structure and cognition in a community sample of elderly Latinos. Neurology **59:** 383–391.

27. SCHELTENS, P. & F. BARKHOF. 2006. Structural neuroimaging outcomes in clinical dementia trials, with special reference to disease modifying designs. J. Nutr. Health Aging **10:** 123–130.

28. BIRKENHAGER, W.H., F. FORETTE & J.A. STAESSEN. 2004. Dementia and antihypertensive treatment. Curr. Opin. Nephrol. Hypertens. **13:** 225–230.

29. SCHMIDT, R., P. SCHELTENS, T. ERKINJUNTTI, et al. 2004. White matter lesion progression: a surrogate endpoint for trials in cerebral small-vessel disease. Neurology **63:** 139–144.

# Imaging-Guided Microarray

## Isolating Molecular Profiles That Dissociate Alzheimer's Disease from Normal Aging

ANA CAROLINA PEREIRA, WILLIAM WU, AND SCOTT A. SMALL

*Department of Neurology, Taub Institute for Research on Alzheimer's Disease and the Aging Brain, Columbia University College of Physicians and Surgeons, New York, New York, USA*

ABSTRACT: Although both Alzheimer's disease (AD) and normal aging contribute to age-related hippocampal dysfunction, they are likely governed by separate molecular mechanisms. In principle, gene expression profiling can offer molecular clues about underlying mechanisms, but in practice techniques like microarray present unique analytic challenges when applied to disorders of the brain. Imaging-guided microarray is an approach designed to address these analytic challenges. Here, we will first review findings applying variants of functional magnetic resonance imaging (fMRI) to AD and normal aging, establishing the spatiotemporal profiles that dissociate one from the other. Then, we will review preliminary findings applying imaging-guided microarray to AD and normal aging, in an attempt to isolate molecular profiles that dissociate the two main causes of age-related hippocampal dysfunction.

KEYWORDS: Alzheimer's disease (AD); microarray; functional magnetic resonance imaging (fMRI)

## IMAGING-GUIDED MICROARRAY

The last two decades have been characterized by a remarkable success in isolating the molecular defects underlying monogenic diseases of the brain. The combination of technologies formed the basis of this success.[1] First, molecular techniques were developed that could generate an array of genetic markers, establishing large-scale genetic profiles of patients and controls. Second, analytic techniques were developed, which were required for analyzing these large-scale genetic datasets. By relying on statistical models, based on assumptions of Mendelian inheritance, these analytic techniques were able to pinpoint candidate genes among thousands of possibilities.

Address for correspondence: Scott A. Small, M.D., Department of Neurology, Taub Institute for Research on Alzheimer's Disease and the Aging Brain, Columbia University College of Physicians and Surgeons, New York, NY 10032. Voice: 212-305-9194; fax: 212-305-2426.
sas68@columbia.edu

Ann. N.Y. Acad. Sci. 1097: 225–238 (2007). © 2007 New York Academy of Sciences.
doi: 10.1196/annals.1379.005

With this success as a backdrop, the persistent difficulty in isolating the molecular defects that underlie complex brain processes, such as Alzheimer's disease (AD) and cognitive aging, is particularly glaring. Complex disorders emerge from an interplay between genes and the environment, and constitute by far the vast majority of diseases. It was no surprise, therefore, that when microarray was introduced in the late1990s,[2] a technique that simultaneously profiles the levels of thousands of mRNA transcripts, this technical advance was enthusiastically met by clinical neuroscientists. Because mRNA expression profiles are anatomically specific, and because expression levels are influenced by both genetic and epigenetic factors, microarray held great promise for uncovering the pathogenic molecules underlying complex disorders.

Despite a number of interesting and potentially important findings, this promise has not yet been fully realized. Molecular heterogeneity can be invoked to account for this lack of success, in which defects in many separate molecular pathways produce overlapping disease phenotypes. Nevertheless, we believe that molecular parsimony should still be assumed—that AD and cognitive aging are driven primarily by relatively few molecular pathways—and that the difficulty in pinpointing pathogenic molecules with microarray is more likely a reflection of its analytic challenges. As illustrated with monogenic diseases, generating a wealth of molecular information is by itself insufficient for successful molecular discovery. What is required is a statistical model to address the analytic challenges presented by microarray in order to isolate candidate molecules.

With this in mind, we have recently introduced an approach designed to isolate pathogenic molecules underlying complex disorders of the brain.[3] As with monogenic diseases, this approach is based on a combination of technologies. The first is microarray, which can be used to generate large-scale molecular profiles from selective regions of the brain. The second is brain imaging techniques, whose findings can potentially be used to generate statistical models predicting *a priori* how a pathogenic molecule should behave.

In constructing the statistical models used to analyze monogenic diseases, Mendelian patterns of inheritance are relied on to make assumptions on how a pathogenic gene should behave—across family and nonfamily members. In contrast, when constructing a statistical model for AD and cognitive aging, we propose that findings from brain imaging can be used to make assumptions about how a pathogenic molecule should behave—spatially and temporally within the brain. Specifically, brain imaging can, in principle, identify regions that are differentially vulnerable and resistant to AD and aging. This spatial pattern can then be used in designing and analyzing a microarray experiment, whose goal is to isolate candidate molecules. According to the spatial pattern, microarray data can be generated from both vulnerable and resistant regions, harvested from both affected and from control brains. Then, guided by the spatial pattern, a "double-subtraction" statistical model can be constructed to identify molecules whose expression patterns are different between vulnerable and resistant regions, between affected and control brains. In statistical terms, the spatial information provided by brain imaging allows a mixed-factorial ANOVA to be designed, including both within-group (vulnerable vs. resistant regions) and between-group (affected vs. control brains) variables. On theoretical grounds, this statistical model is effective in addressing the inherently low effect-size and high interindividual variance that must be anticipated when microarray is applied to disorders of the brain.[3]

Besides poor signal-to-noise, high false-positivity—the type I error that naturally occurs with thousands of comparisons—is the other analytic limitation presented by microarray. Relying on temporal information is an approach that has proven effective for addressing the type I error. For example, in microarray studies applied to simpler organisms,[2] the most relevant molecules have been successfully isolated by requiring that expression profiles match the temporal pattern of a phenotype under investigation. In principle, the same logic can be applied to brain disorders, and brain imaging is particularly well suited to establish a disease's temporal pattern of dysfunction—over time or across age groups. Then, guided by the temporal pattern, a statistical model can be designed, so that when applied to a microarray dataset it will act as an analytic filter against false-positive findings.

To summarize, if brain imaging can establish a precise spatiotemporal pattern of dysfunction associated with AD and cognitive aging, then this information can be used to construct biologically meaningful statistical models. When forward applied onto a microarray dataset, these models will naturally address two of the main analytic limitations presented by microarray—poor signal-to-noise and the high false-positivity rate.[3]

### *Imaging Requirements for Imaging-Guided Microarray*

For imaging-guided microarray to work the imaging technique upon which the statistical model is based must fulfill two requirements. First, the technique must be able to visualize anatomically meaningful regions of the brain. From a clinical perspective, a "region" is best defined as a brain area that houses a distinct population of neurons, unique in their molecular expression profiles. In accordance with basic tenets in clinical neuroscience, it is this molecular uniqueness that accounts for why regions of the brain are differentially vulnerable to separate diseases. The hippocampal formation, a structure targeted by both AD and aging illustrates this point (FIG. 1). Many disorders cause hippocampal-dependent memory loss. However, because the hippocampal formation is divided into separate and molecularly-distinct hippocampal subregions different diseases target different hippocampal regions.[4]

Besides the ability to visualize molecularly distinct brain regions, a brain imaging technique must fulfill a second requirement as dictated by the

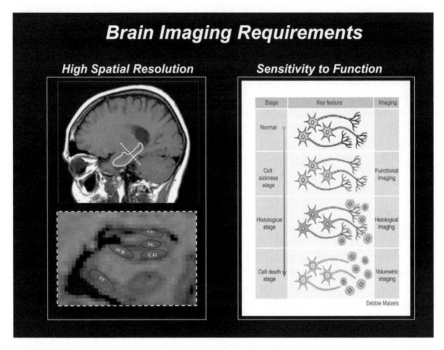

**FIGURE 1.** Brain imaging requirements. Spatial resolution (*left panel*). The neuronal population is the basic anatomical unit of disease. The hippocampal formation (blue highlight in sagital image) is made up of different neuronal populations, anatomically organized into separate hippocampal subregions. The subregions are best appreciated by slicing the hippocampus down its tranverse axis (stippled line in sagital image) and viewing the slice on-end (bottom image). The hippocampal subregions include the EC, the SUB, the CA1 and CA3 subfields, and the DG. Sensitivity to function (*right panel*). AD progresses through different pathological stages. The first "cell sickness" stage of AD, characterized by synaptic failure in relatively intact neurons, is most informative in pinpointing the hippocampal subregions most vulnerable and resistant to the disease. Normal aging never progresses out a "cell sickness" stage. (Reprinted with permission from Small.[33]) This figure is shown in color online.

pathophysiology of AD and cognitive aging. AD begins by causing "cell sickness"—characterized by metabolic and physiologic dysfunction—before the aggregation of amyloid plaques and neurofibrillary tangles, and before the emergence of wholesale cell death. Pathophysiologically, it is the cell-sickness stage of AD that is most informative in localizing the disease, because the distribution of protein aggregates do not necessarily mark the sites of greatest physiologic dysfunction, and patterns of cell death might reflect differential vulnerability to apoptosis than metabolic failure. Sensitivity to physiologic dysfunction is even more important for cognitive aging, because normal aging is characterized by a notable absence of cell death or telltale histological markers (FIG. 1).

Thus, to establish the spatiotemporal pattern of AD and cognitive aging a brain imaging technique should: (i) be sensitive to cell sickness and not just cell death and (ii) possess sufficient spatial resolution in order to visualize molecularly distinct hippocampal subregions.

*In vivo* imaging has been subdivided into *structural imaging*, such as magnetic resonance imaging (MRI) or computerized axial tomography (CT) imaging, versus *functional imaging*—single photon emission tomography (SPECT), positron emission tomography (PET), or functional magnetic resonance imaging (fMRI). Of course, in principle, functional imaging techniques are more likely to be sensitive to cell sickness. What exactly is meant by the "function" in functional imaging? Since the early studies performed by Kety and Schmidt as reviewed in Small,[5] functional brain imaging has come to imply a method that detects changes in regional energy metabolism. Energy metabolism is best defined as the rate with which cells produce adenosine $5'$-triphosphate (ATP), which in neurons requires the consumption of oxygen and glucose from the blood stream. Visualizing ATP directly is challenging, but imaging techniques have been developed that can visualize correlates of oxygen and glucose consumption. With the use of radiolabeled glucose, PET can quantify the regional rates of glucose uptake. In contrast, MRI-based techniques have typically relied on the second ingredient of ATP production, oxygen consumption, to visualize correlates of energy metabolism. Because of hemodynamic coupling, oxygen consumption is correlated with cerebral blood flow (CBF), cerebral blood volume (CBV), and deoxyhemoglobin content (dHB), and all these correlates can be estimated with MRI (FIG. 2).

The cell-sickness stage of any disease typically affects the basal metabolic rate of oxygen consumption, and relying on the basal state to map anatomical sites of dysfunction enhances parametric quantification and spatial resolution. Indeed, the basal changes of energy metabolism associated with disease have been detected relying on all metabolic correlates—glucose uptake, CBF, CBV, and dHB. Among these variables, however, only MRI measures of CBV and dHB can achieve the spatial resolution required to visualize individual hippocampal subregions. Studies have used MRI measures of basal CBV or dHB to investigate the hippocampal circuit in aging and AD, and this will be reviewed in the next section.

## *Imaging the Spatiotemporal Profile of Alzheimer's Disease and Normal Aging*

By quantifying cell loss in postmortem tissue of AD patients, studies have suggested that either the entorhinal cortex (EC) or the CA1 subfield is the hippocampal subregion most vulnerable to AD.[6–11] In many of these studies, the EC and the CA1 subfield were not assessed simultaneously, accounting in part for the reported inconsistencies. More generally, however, isolating the

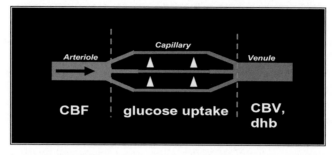

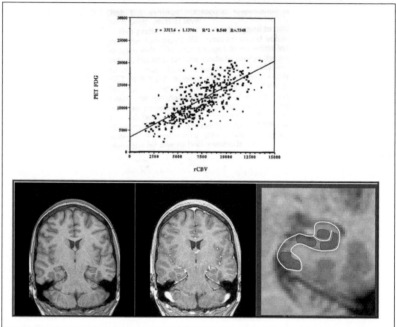

**FIGURE 2.** Functional imaging measures correlates of energy metabolism. Correlates of energy metabolism (*upper panel*). Energy metabolism is best defined as the rate at which a neuron consumes ATP. Measuring ATP directly has proven difficult, and so the field of functional imaging has identified four correlates of energy metabolism, correlates that can be visualized with imaging "cameras": CBF, glucose update, CBV, and dHB. MRI-generated CBV maps of the hippocampal formation (*lower panel*). Imaging glucose uptake with PET is the "gold standard" approach for mapping metabolic dysfunction in disease. PET, however, does not possess sufficient spatial resolution to visualize individual hippocampal subregions. MRI techniques can be used to image CBF, dHB, and CBV. Among these, CBV turns out to be the variable that is best suited for detecting metabolic changes in small areas of the brain. CBV measured with MRI tightly correlates with glucose uptake measured with PET (upper graph) (reprinted with permission from Gonzalez *et al.* [20]). CBV maps with MRI are generated by imaging the brain with (lower left image) and without (lower middle image) a contrast agent, thereby deriving CBV maps of the hippocampal subregions (lower right image). This figure is shown in color online.

hippocampal subregion most vulnerable to AD is difficult relying on post-mortem studies alone. Not only are postmortem series biased against the earliest and most discriminatory stages of disease, but these studies are limited in assessing the cell-sickness stage of AD.[12]

As discussed above, variants of fMRI sensitive to basal correlates of neuronal function are well suited to aid in resolving this debate. In one study, an MRI measure sensitive to basal levels of deoxyhemoglobin was used to assess the hippocampal subregions in patients with AD dementia compared to age-matched controls.[13] This MRI measure has proven capable to detect cell sickness in individual hippocampal subregions. Univariate analysis revealed that normalized signal intensity was reduced in all hippocampal subregions in patients compared to controls. Nevertheless, when the hippocampus was analyzed as a circuit—namely, using a multivariate model to analyze signal from all hippocampal subregions simultaneously—the EC was found to be the primary site of dysfunction in AD.[13]

This study suggests that the EC, not the CA1 subfield, is the hippocampal subregion most vulnerable to AD—agreeing with some, though not all, postmortem studies. Nevertheless, the patients assessed in this study already had full-blown dementia indicating that they had already progressed from the cell-sickness to the cell-death stage of AD. Furthermore, this study does not inform us about the hippocampal subregions most vulnerable to normal aging.

Both of these issues were addressed in a second study, in which 70 subjects across the age span—from 20 to 88 years of age—were imaged with the same MRI measure.[14] Importantly, all subjects were healthy. The older age groups in particular were carefully screened against any evidence of dementia. The starting assumption made in this study was that some of the older subjects were in the earliest stage of AD and some subjects were aging normally. The question was how to make this distinction. Remember, there is no independent indicator to determine who had early AD or not. This is true even if the hippocampal formation of all subjects could be examined postmortem, because, as mentioned, the earliest stages of AD may be invisible to the microscope. Instead, formal parametric criteria were used to distinguish a "pathological pattern" of decline (i.e., related to AD) versus a "normal pattern" of decline. Specifically, because the effect of normal aging on the brain is, by definition, a stochastic process, the variance of signal intensity among an older age group should be equal to the variance among a younger age group, although a shift in the mean is expected. In contrast, because it is a disease, AD should affect a subgroup within an older age group, which should significantly broaden the variance of signal intensity compared to a younger age group.

Applying this and other criteria, the results of this study showed that age-related changes in the EC fulfilled criteria for pathological decline; in contrast, age-related changes in the dentate gyrus (DG), and to a lesser extent in the subiculum (SUB), fulfilled criteria for normal aging.[14] These findings not only confirm but also extend the results of the previous study. First, the EC indeed appears to be the hippocampal subregion most vulnerable to AD, even during the early cell-sickness stage. Second, these findings provided evidence that the DG might be the hippocampal subregion most vulnerable to normal aging.

This study had a number of limitations. First, despite the strict criteria independent verification of which older subjects did or did not have early AD was not possible. Second, although the MRI measure used is sensitive to basal deoxyhemoglobin levels, these images are also sensitive to other, nonmetabolic, tissue constituents that are potential confounds.[15,16]

These potential limitations were addressed in a third study. First, a cohort of aging individuals was needed that indisputably were free of AD. Because this cohort is difficult, or even impossible, to identify in human subjects, we turned to aging nonhuman primates instead. Like all mammals, monkeys develop age-related hippocampal dysfunction, yet they do not develop the known molecular or histological hallmarks of AD. Second, because of the stated limitations of imaging techniques sensitive to dHB, we relied on MRI to generate regional measures of CBV. Previous studies have established that CBV is a hemodynamic variable tightly correlated with brain metabolism, capable of detecting brain dysfunction in the hippocampus and other brain regions.[17–20]

In the third study, the hippocampal subregions of 14 rhesus monkeys were imaged across the age span from 7 to 31 years of age.[21] In a remarkable parallel to the previous human study, age-related decline in CBV was observed only in the DG, and to a lesser extent in the SUB. Notably, CBV measured from the EC and the CA1 subregion remained stable across the lifespan. Indeed, when all subregions were analyzed simultaneously—in accordance with the circuit organization of the hippocampus—the DG was the primary subregion that declined with age. Furthermore, because all monkeys were assessed cognitively, we found that a decline in DG CBV was the only subregion that correlated with a decline in memory performance.[21]

Despite the reliance on CBV to investigate aging monkeys this third study also had a number of limitations. The first limitation applies to all functional imaging: As derived from Fick's principle,[5] all hemodynamic variables— deoxyhemoglobin, CBV, or CBF—are correlates of oxygen metabolism; nevertheless, they are only *indirect* correlates. The possibility always exists that these measures are confounded by changes in vascular physiology, and not underlying neuronal physiology. Thus, we cannot exclude the possibility that there is something unique to the vascular system within the DG that caused shrinkage of CBV, independent of DG physiologic dysfunction. The second limitation of the monkey MRI study has to do with the cellular complexity of any brain subregion, including the DG. Although the granule cells are the primary neurons of the DG, the DG contains other types of neurons as well as glial cells. Even if the CBV measure does reflect underlying cellular function MRI cannot be relied on to isolate the cells that govern this observed effect.

A fourth study was designed to address these concerns. Here, *in vitro* imaging was used, directly visualizing correlates of neuronal physiology. Aging rats were investigated, who like humans and monkeys develop age-related hippocampal dysfunction. Immunocytochemisty was used to visualize the behaviorally induced expression of *Arc* in the hippocampal subregions of aging rats. *Arc* is an immediate early gene whose expression has been shown to correlate with spike activity and with long-term plasticity in hippocampal neurons.[22] Rats of different ages were allowed to explore a novel place and sacrificed and processed for *Arc* staining. *Arc* expression was quantified in the granule cells of the DG and in the pyramidal neurons of the CA1 and CA3 subregions. The DG was the only hippocampal subregion whose neurons were found to have a significant age-related decline in *Arc* expression.[21] Thus, this study confirms and extends the prior studies, showing that it is in fact neuronal, not vascular, physiology that underlies the aging effect. Moreover, this study established that aging primarily targets the granule cells of the DG.

## *Isolating the Molecular Profiles of Alzheimer's Disease and Normal Aging*

Guided by the imaging studies reviewed above we generated an *a priori* model predicting how a pathogenic molecule associated with AD should behave, spatially and over time (FIG. 3). Specifically, the model predicts that a pathogenic molecule should be differentially expressed in the EC versus the DG; and that the differences between AD and controls should be age independent. On theoretical grounds, focusing on the EC as the subregion of greatest vulnerability enhances the "signal amplitude" of the microarray analysis, while relying on the DG as a within-subject control subregion reduced sources of noise. Thus, the spatial profile of the model naturally enhances the signal-to-noise of the microarray analysis. The temporal profile of the model is used as an analytic filter against false positivity.

Our analysis revealed five molecules whose expression levels conformed to the spatiotemporal model, of which VPS35 was the molecule whose expression best conformed to the spatiotemporal model.[23] VPS35 is the core of the retromer trafficking complex, a newly described coat complex that transports type-I transmembrane proteins from the endosome back to the trans-golgi network (TGN). Because many Alzheimer's-related molecules are type-I transmembrane proteins (notably, amyloid precursor protein [APP] and its cleaving enzyme, β-amyloid cleaving enzyme [BACE]), it is easy to begin hypothesizing how retromer dysfunction might be relevant to AD. Nevertheless, because of its correlational nature, any microarray finding must be independently validated in "true" experimental paradigms—that is, by systematically manipulating a molecule of interest and measuring a relevant readout. Accordingly, we turned to cell culture studies in which we could use molecular techniques to

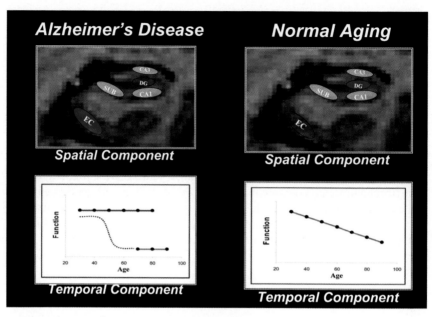

**FIGURE 3.** Spatiotemporal profiles of AD and aging used in imaging-guiding microarray. Alzheimer' disease (*left panel*). Spatially, functional imaging studies have suggested that the EC is the hippocampal subregion most vulnerable to AD while the DG is relatively resistant. Temporally, functional imaging studies have suggested that once EC dysfunction begins it does not worsen across age groups or over time. Normal aging (*right panel*). Spatially, functional imaging studies have suggested that the DG is the hippocampal subregion most vulnerable to normal aging while the EC is relatively resistant. Temporally, functional imaging studies have suggested that DG dysfunction progresses linearly across the age span.

systematically increase or decrease VPS35 levels and measure Aβ levels—a peptide whose levels are elevated in AD and that represents a biochemical "smoking gun" of the disease. As predicted, we found that decreasing VPS35 led to an increase in Aβ levels, while increasing VPS35 led to a decrease in Aβ levels, thereby validating that the retromer plays a role in APP processing.

Identifying the type-I transmembrane proteins that are transported by the neuronal retromer would mechanistically inform on how retromer dysfunction causes an increase in Aβ. Although the retromer is highly expressed in the brain, the type-I transmembrane proteins transported by the neuronal retromer have remained unknown. As a first step, we relied on an analytic approach that has successfully been applied to microarray data, screening for molecules that are candidates for interacting with one another.[24] Underlying this approach is the assumption that molecules that interact with each other are likely to have expression levels that cross-correlate. Guided by this approach, we returned to our microarray data and determined which type-I transmembrane molecule had expression levels that significantly correlated with VPS35. Among a list of possible retromer cargo molecules, this study demonstrated that sorLA and BACE were among the type-I transmembrane molecules whose expression levels cross-correlated most strongly with levels of neuronal VPS35.[25,26] Direct evidence that the retromer plays a role in BACE sorting has recently emerged from a study that used siRNA to knock down VPS26 in cell culture.[27] This manipulation, which was originally used in the studies implicating the retromer in mannose-6-phosphate receptor sorting, reduces both VPS26 and VPS35 levels causing retromer dysfunction.[28–30] By knocking down VPS26, retromer dysfunction was shown to missort BACE as manifested by an increase in endosomal BACE.[27] Experimental confirmation regarding interaction of VPS35 with sorLA has not yet been provided. Nevertheless, because sorLA has close homologies to sortilin, its VPS10-containing family member, one would plausibly speculate that sorLA is also sorted by the neuronal retromer. Interestingly, a number of studies have shown that sorLA binds APP, so that if future studies confirm that if sorLA is the cargo of the neuronal retromer, this would suggest that the retromer might also be involved in APP sorting.

Taken together, a model can be generated predicting how retromer dysfunction might lead to accelerated Aβ production. We hypothesize that the retromer directly or indirectly via sorLA transports APP and/or BACE from the endosome to the TGN. Retromer dysfunction, therefore, is predicted to increase the colocalization of APP and BACE, thereby increasing the cleavage of APP and resulting in increased production of Aβ.

We are currently in the process of applying imaging-guided microarray to cognitive aging. In contrast to the AD spatiotemporal pattern, our imaging studies suggest that a pathogenic molecule underlying cognitive aging should be differentially expressed in the DG versus the EC, and that temporally the expression should change linearly across the age span (Fig. 3). Accordingly, we hope to find molecules whose levels decline linearly across age span, differentially in the DG but not the EC, harvested from healthy brains.

Once we have isolated candidate molecules, we will need to validate that they are truly related to cognitive aging. Simply establishing a correlation between molecular expression and age or between molecular expression and memory performance does not establish a causal relationship. Rather, what is required is an experimental paradigm in which we can systematically manipulate the expression levels of a given molecule and measure a meaningful readout.

In the case of AD we were able to rely on cell cultures because measuring shifts in Aβ levels is a readout reflective of the actual disease. Unfortunately, normal cognitive aging does not have a commensurate cellular readout. Thus, we will need to turn to genetic engineering and generate transgenic mice that molecularly phenocopy the expression changes we find in the aging human DG, and test these genetically manipulated mice for hippocampal-dependent dysfunction.

# SUMMARY

Isolating pathogenic molecules, among thousands of possibilities, is obviously an analytic challenge. When attempting to isolate pathogenic molecules that underlie monogenic disorders of the brain it is the genome that represents the basic unit of investigation, and extracting genetic material from any cell is sufficient for these purposes. In contrast, when attempting to isolate pathogenic molecules that underlie complex disorders of the brain—namely, disorders that are not necessarily caused by genetic mutations—the neurons in the targeted brain region represent the basic unit of investigation. Once the neuronal population most vulnerable to a disease process is identified, then a molecular analysis of these neurons is likely to provide clues about pathogenesis.

Although obvious from an analytic perspective, it is not always clear how to identify the one brain region most vulnerable and affected by disease. This issue is particularly problematic for physiologic rather than structural disorders, where telltale histological or structural lesions cannot be used as landmarks. Even in neurodegenerative diseases—such as Alzheimer's,[12] Parkinson's,[31] and Huntington's disease[32]—it is generally agreed that the histological distribution of protein aggregates does not necessarily mark the sites of greatest physiologic dysfunction. Furthermore, although cells do eventually degenerate after many years of sublethal injury, patterns of cell death might reflect differential sensitivity to apoptosis rather than to synaptic dysfunction.

Pinpointing sites of physiologic dysfunction in the early stages of a disease is one of the great promises of fMRI. Nevertheless, as discussed, conventional functional imaging approaches do not possess sufficient spatial resolution to visualize individual neuronal populations, or the "signal" measured with these approaches is difficult to interpret in the context of brain disease. Motivated by these concerns, we have dedicated the last few years to optimizing a variant of fMRI that can detect physiologic dysfunction in individual hippocampal subregions—each housing a distinct population of neurons. As discussed, guided by the results from our imaging studies identifying the subregions differentially vulnerable and resistant to AD and establishing the temporal pattern of dysfunction, we have found that the retromer trafficking pathway is implicated in AD. We are currently in the process of applying imaging-guided microarray to normal aging and hope to identify molecular pathways linked to cognitive aging.

## ACKNOWLEDGMENTS

This work was supported in part by the NIH federal grant AG025161, the McKnight Neuroscience of Brain Disorders Award, and the James S. McDonnell Foundation.

# REFERENCES

1. TERWILLIGER, J.D. & H.H. GORING. 2000. Gene mapping in the 20th and 21st centuries: statistical methods, data analysis, and experimental design. Hum. Biol. **72:** 63–132.
2. DERISI, J.L., V.R. IYER & P.O. BROWN. 1997. Exploring the metabolic and genetic control of gene expression on a genomic scale. Science **278:** 680–686.
3. LEWANDOWSKI, N.M. & S.A. SMALL. 2005. Brain microarray: finding needles in molecular haystacks. J. Neurosci. **25:** 10341–10346.
4. SMALL, S.A. 2001. Age-related memory decline; current concepts and future directions. Arch. Neurol. **58:** 360–364.
5. SMALL, S.A. 2004. Quantifying cerebral blood flow: regional regulation with global implications. J. Clin. Invest. **114:** 1046–1048.
6. PRICE, J.L., A.I. KO, M.J. WADE, *et al.* 2001. Neuron number in the entorhinal cortex and CA1 in preclinical Alzheimer disease. Arch. Neurol. **58:** 1395–1402.
7. FUKUTANI, Y., N.J. CAIRNS, M. SHIOZAWA, *et al.* 2000. Neuronal loss and neurofibrillary degeneration in the hippocampal cortex in late-onset sporadic Alzheimer's disease. Psychiatry Clin. Neurosci. **54:** 523–529.
8. GIANNAKOPOULOS, P., F.R. HERRMANN, T. BUSSIERE, *et al.* 2003. Tangle and neuron numbers, but not amyloid load, predict cognitive status in Alzheimer's disease. Neurology **60:** 1495–1500.
9. BRAAK, H. & E. BRAAK. 1996. Evolution of the neuropathology of Alzheimer's disease. Acta Neurol. Scand. Suppl. **165:** 3–12.
10. SHOGHI-JADID, K., G.W. SMALL, E.D. AGDEPPA, *et al.* 2002. Localization of neurofibrillary tangles and beta-amyloid plaques in the brains of living patients with Alzheimer disease. Am. J. Geriatr. Psychiatry **10:** 24–35.
11. SCHONHEIT, B., R. ZARSKI & T.G. OHM. 2004. Spatial and temporal relationships between plaques and tangles in Alzheimer pathology. Neurobiol. Aging **25:** 697–711.
12. SELKOE, D.J. 2002. Alzheimer's disease is a synaptic failure. Science **298:** 789–791.
13. SMALL, S.A., A.S. NAVA, G.M. PERERA, *et al.* 2000. Evaluating the function of hippocampal subregions with high-resolution MRI in Alzheimer's disease and aging [In Process Citation]. Microsc. Res. Tech. **51:** 101–108.
14. SMALL, S.A., W.Y. TSAI, R. DELAPAZ, *et al.* 2002. Imaging hippocampal function across the human life span: is memory decline normal or not? Ann. Neurol. **51:** 290–295.
15. SMALL, S., E. WU, D. BARTSCH, *et al.* 2000. Imaging physiologic dysfunction of individual hippocampal subregions in humans and genetically modified mice. Neuron. **28(3):** 653–664.
16. SMALL, S.A. 2003. Measuring correlates of brain metabolism with high-resolution MRI: a promising approach for diagnosing Alzheimer disease and mapping its course. Alzheimer Dis. Assoc. Disord. **17:** 154–161.
17. HARRIS, G.J., R.F. LEWIS, A. SATLIN, *et al.* 1998. Dynamic susceptibility contrast MR imaging of regional cerebral blood volume in Alzheimer disease: a promising alternative to nuclear medicine. AJNR Am. J. Neuroradiol. **19:** 1727–1732.
18. BOZZAO, A., R. FLORIS, M.E. BAVIERA, *et al.* 2001. Diffusion and perfusion MR imaging in cases of Alzheimer's disease: correlations with cortical atrophy and lesion load. AJNR Am. J. Neuroradiol. **22:** 1030–1036.

19. WU, R.H., R. BRUENING, S. NOACHTAR, et al. 1999. MR measurement of regional relative cerebral blood volume in epilepsy. J. Magn. Reson. Imaging 9: 435–440.
20. GONZALEZ, R.G., A.J. FISCHMAN, A.R. GUIMARAES, et al. 1995. Functional MR in the evaluation of dementia: correlation of abnormal dynamic cerebral blood volume measurements with changes in cerebral metabolism on positron emission tomography with fludeoxyglucose F 18. AJNR Am. J. Neuroradiol. 16: 1763–1770.
21. SMALL, S.A., M.K. CHAWLA, M. BUONOCORE, et al. 2004. From the cover: imaging correlates of brain function in monkeys and rats isolates a hippocampal subregion differentially vulnerable to aging. Proc. Natl. Acad. Sci. USA 101: 7181–7186.
22. GUZOWSKI, J.F., G.L. LYFORD, G.D. STEVENSON, et al. 2000. Inhibition of activity-dependent arc protein expression in the rat hippocampus impairs the maintenance of long-term potentiation and the consolidation of long-term memory. J. Neurosci. 20: 3993–4001.
23. SMALL, S.A., K. KENT, A. PIERCE, et al. 2005. Model-guided microarray implicates the retromer complex in Alzheimer's disease. Ann. Neurol. 58: 909–919.
24. BHARDWAJ, N. & H. LU. 2005. Correlation between gene expression profiles and protein-protein interactions within and across genomes. Bioinformatics 21: 2730–2738.
25. SMALL, S.A., A.L. PEIRCE, K. KENT, et al. 2003. Combining functional imaging with microarray; identifying an unexplored cellular pathway implicated in sporadic Alzheimer's disease. Annual Meeting of the Society for Neuroscience. New Orleans, LO.
26. SMALL, S.A. & T.W. KIM. 2003. Vps35-based assays and methods for treating Alzheimer's disease. U.S. patent 20050176668.
27. HE, X., F. LI, W.P. CHANG & J. TANG. 2005. GGA proteins mediate the recycling pathway of memapsin 2 (BACE). J. Biol. Chem. 280(12): 11696–11703.
28. ARIGHI, C.N., L.M. HARTNELL, R.C. AGUILAR, et al. 2004. Role of the mammalian retromer in sorting of the cation-independent mannose 6-phosphate receptor. J. Cell Biol. 165: 123–133.
29. SEAMAN, M.N. 2004. Cargo-selective endosomal sorting for retrieval to the Golgi requires retromer. J. Cell Biol. 165: 111–122.
30. VERGES, M., F. LUTON, C. GRUBER, et al. 2004. The mammalian retromer regulates transcytosis of the polymeric immunoglobulin receptor. Nat. Cell Biol. 6: 763–769.
31. DAUER, W. & S. PRZEDBORSKI. 2003. Parkinson's disease: mechanisms and models. Neuron. 39: 889–909.
32. ARRASATE, M., S. MITRA, E.S. SCHWEITZER, et al. 2004. Inclusion body formation reduces levels of mutant huntingtin and the risk of neuronal death. Nature 431: 805–810.
33. SMALL, S.A. 2005. Alzheimer disease, in living color. Nat. Neurosci. 8: 404–405.

# Fibrillar and Oligomeric β-Amyloid as Distinct Local Biomarkers for Alzheimer's Disease

MICHAEL C. MONTALTO,[a] GILL FARRAR,[b] AND CRISTINA TAN HEHIR[a]

[a]Molecular Imaging and Diagnostics Advanced Technology Program, Biosciences, GE Global Research Center, Niskayuna, New York, USA

[b]Medical Diagnostics R and D, GE Healthcare, Little Chalfont, Bucks, United Kingdom

ABSTRACT: β-amyloid is a key component of Alzheimer's disease (AD) pathology. Researchers in both academic and industry are actively pursuing the development of imaging tracers and techniques to noninvasively measure local levels of β-amyloid in the Alzheimer's brain. This presentation summarizes recent data and discusses the opportunities and challenges of imaging plaques containing fibrillar β-amyloid for the early diagnosis and therapeutic monitoring of amyloid targeted therapies. Further, the value and feasibility of measuring the recently described soluble oligomeric form of β-amyloid as an alternative noninvasive biomarker is also discussed.

KEYWORDS: β-amyloid imaging; plaque; imaging; β-amyloid oligomers; soluble β-amyloid; biomarkers; Alzheimer's

## THE AMYLOID HYPOTHESIS

The β-amyloid peptide is the main constituent of senile plaques found in the brains of patients suffering from Alzheimer's disease (AD).[1,2] β-amyloid peptide is generated by the proteolytic cleavage of the amyloid precursor protein (APP). Cleavage is mediated by the transmembrane proteins beta and gamma secretases.[3,4] Depending on the exact cleavage site, a peptide may be generated that is 38 to 43 amino acids in length. The most common forms of β-amyloid contain either 40 or 42 amino acids and account for the majority of β-amyloid found *in vivo*.[5] Following cleavage, the β-amyloid peptide can self-aggregate by a complex process starting with self-dimerization, followed by oligomerization, protofibril formation, and eventual aggregation to

Address for correspondence: Michael C. Montalto, K1-5D63 One Research Circle, Niskayuna, NY 12309. Voice: 518-387-5409; fax: 518-387-7765.
montalto@crd.ge.com

Ann. N.Y. Acad. Sci. 1097: 239–258 (2007). © 2007 New York Academy of Sciences.
doi: 10.1196/annals.1379.023

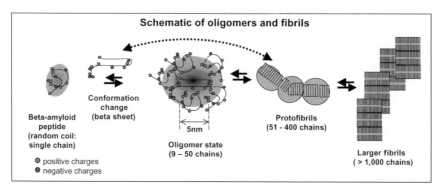

**FIGURE 1.** Aggregation states of β-amyloid. Aggregation begins with a random coiled single peptide changing conformation into a stable β-sheet, allowing for oligomerization and fibril formation. The exact number of chains and specific sizes per state are approximations.

large insoluble fibrillar structures (FIG. 1).[6–9] Due to its hydrophobic nature, β-amyloid$_{1-42}$ has a higher tendency to aggregate and is believed to be the culprit form of β-amyloid in the initiation of senile plaques.[10] However, the production of β-amyloid occurs even in healthy brains, and alone may not be sufficient to induce plaque formation. It has been suggested that elevated levels of β-amyloid peptide result from either a dysregulation of clearance out of the brain or increased rates of production that shift the normal delicate equilibrium of production and clearance. These elevated levels then lead to neuronal dysfunction and plaque build-up.[11–13] Thus, the complex dynamic of production and clearance, as well as the multiple forms of β-amyloid, are important factors when considering novel therapeutic and diagnostic approaches.

While there are many pathological hallmarks of AD, there is a wide support for the theory that deposited β-amyloid is the main pathological entity in the AD brain (FIG. 2). It is well known that exposure of neuronal cultures to insoluble aggregated β-amyloid results in significant cell death. These observations establish a potential role of aggregated β-amyloid in disease pathogenesis.[14–16] However, there are several phenomena that cannot be explained by fibrillar deposited β-amyloid alone. For example, the spatial location of affected neuronal circuits does not necessarily correlate with the location of β-amyloid plaques in the AD brain.[17] Similarly, plaque loads do not correlate well with cognitive function, as would be expected if plaques were the main neurotoxic entity in the AD brain.[18–21] Additionally, transgenic mice engineered to produce significant amounts of β-amyloid have cognitive deficits that precede the appearance of β-amyloid plaques indicating that a nonfibrillar β-amyloid-mediated mechanism contributes to cognitive changes seen in AD models.[22]

**The Beta-amyloid Cascade in
Alzheimer's Pathogenesis**

*Mutations in Amyloid Precursor
Protein, Presinilins, Epigenetic
Factors*

*Increased Beta-amyloid
Accumulation (decreased clearance,
enhanced production)*

*Beta-amyloid Oligomerization and
Aggregation*

*Effects on Synaptic Transmission*

*Inflammation, Oxidative Stress,
Plaques*

*Neuronal Insults and Dysfunction,
Tangle Formation*

*Clinical Symptoms:*
**Dementia**

**FIGURE 2.** The amyloid hypothesis.

## THE ROLE OF SOLUBLE β-AMYLOID OLIGOMERS

One explanation that appears to reconcile the discrepancy between deposited β-amyloid and lack of cognitive changes is suggested by recent data on soluble oligomers of β-amyloid. Soluble oligomers of β-amyloid are a distinct form of low molecular weight β-amyloid that have been demonstrated to exist in the AD brain.[20–27] Soluble oligomers of β-amyloid are approximately 40–200 kDa, which loosely correspond to small species containing 9 to 50 molecules of β-amyloid, although a consensus does not exist as to how many chains of β-amyloid constitute an oligomeric species. Nonetheless, exposure of neuronal cultures to soluble oligomers of β-amyloid result in significantly higher toxicity compared to fibrillar species.[16] Additionally, exposure of mouse brains to soluble β-amyloid oligomers results in significant neuronal dysfunction and inhibition of long-term potentiation.[18,28,29] Interestingly, preclinical studies in transgenic mice treated with agents that are capable of removing soluble β-amyloid from the brain can enhance cognitive function even in the absence of plaque reduction, confirming that plaques are not solely responsible for neuronal deficits *in vivo*.[13,30,31] These studies support earlier human clinical studies that showed soluble β-amyloid correlated significantly with cognitive decline and disease progression, whereas fibrillar β-amyloid did not.[20,21,32] More recent data by Lesne *et al.* demonstrate that the appearance of a distinct oligomeric β-amyloid in the brain of transgenic animals coincides temporally with observed decreases in memory function, further validating the claim that oligomers are responsible for the cognitive changes associated with β-amyloid accumulation.[33]

Interestingly, soluble β-amyloid has selective neurodegenerative effects on *ex vivo* hippocampal neurons as opposed to the cerebral neurons, suggesting a mechanism for selective neurodegeneration.[34] Lastly, antibodies that are reported to have favored selectivity toward soluble oligomers of β-amyloid have been used to identify β-amyloid oligomers in postmortem brain sections from AD patients.[25,27,35] Two of these studies independently found increased levels of soluble oligomers in AD versus normal aged matched controls,[25,27] confirming earlier studies that demonstrated a significant difference in soluble β-amyloid in normal versus control subjects.[20,21,32] Thus, it is clear that soluble β-amyloid, presumably in the form of small oligomers, are potent mediators of neuronal dysfunction both *in vitro* and *in vivo* models of AD. Further, soluble oligomers are elevated in the AD brain, suggesting that soluble oligomers of β-amyloid may be directly linked to the pathological mechanisms of disease associated with AD.

It is important to note that there have been several distinct species of β-amyloid oligomers reported in the literature (i.e., amyloid-derived diffusible ligands, globulomers, Aβ*, Aβ*56, and cell-derived oligomers).[27–29,33] With respect to exact neurotoxic assemblies, Klyubin *et al.* demonstrated that dimers and timers were sufficient to inhibit LTP when injected *in vivo* whereas Lesne *et al.* demonstrated that 12mers were the source of memory deficits in transgenic Tg2576 animals.[33,36] Such discrepant results have confounded the development of a unified theory as to the exact species of oligomers *in vivo* that may cause cognitive dysfunction. Additional research is warranted to examine the similarities and differences of different isolation and production techniques of β-amyloid oligomers such that clinically relevant diagnostic and therapeutic strategies can be developed.

## THE CLINICAL DIAGNOSIS OF AD: CONVENTIONAL IMAGING AND BIOMARKERS

The future success of anti-β-amyloid therapies depends on the ability to identify patients early and to measure the therapeutic efficacy of such approaches. Currently, the clinical diagnosis of AD includes symptomatic cognitive measures and is primarily achieved using a series of structural imaging tests to rule out gross abnormalities in conjunction with various cognitive tests, such as the Alzheimer's disease assessment scale (ADAS-cog) and the mini-mental state exam (MMSE).[37,38] Although the sensitivity and specificity are relatively high for these clinical measures to detect AD, a definitive diagnosis relative to other causes of dementia can only be made postmortem when the histopathological features of AD are identified.[39] It should be noted that the definitive clinical diagnosis of AD during the early stages of dementia is often difficult as symptoms have not yet manifested as overt cognitive dysfunction.

Recently, there has been great progress using conventional imaging approaches, such as 5-fluoro-deoxy-glucose (FDG) positron emission tomography (PET), which measures patterns of hypometabolism in the parietotemporal region in the AD brain and magnetic resonance imaging (MRI) to quantify global and regional brain atrophy.[40] FDG-PET can achieve 70–80% positive predictive values for predicting the conversion to AD from MCI.[40,41] More recently, visual inspection of the metabolism of FDG in the medial temporal lobe has been shown to have diagnostic accuracy similar to that achieved by quantitative region of interest (ROI) measurements.[42] However, FDG–PET imaging is ultimately aimed at measuring neuronal function and/or density, which is not necessarily specific to AD. More importantly, this approach will not be able to measure $\beta$-amyloid levels directly and thus monitoring future therapy targeted at APP processing may be unreliable.

A more direct approach for monitoring disease progression and therapeutic efficacy would be the measurement of $\beta$-amyloid itself. It has been shown that decreased levels of $\beta$-amyloid$_{1-42}$ in cerebrospinal fluid (CSF) is associated with AD and combined with measures of tau in CSF may be a reliable method for AD diagnosis.[43,44] However, it is unclear whether CSF sampling via lumbar puncture will be clinically feasible in patients suffering from dementia, and whether CSF levels can accurately reflect the local levels of $\beta$-amyloid being deposited in the AD brain, especially during early stages.[45,46] It is unknown if CSF levels will indicate any reliable response to therapies that reduce $\beta$-amyloid production in the brain.

As a result, there has been considerable interest in measuring local levels of $\beta$-amyloid in the brain using targeted imaging techniques, such as PET, single photon emission computed tomography (SPECT) or MRI.[40] Despite the overwhelming interest and great advances during the past several years in imaging amyloid, there remain huge challenges in the development and clinical acceptance of targeted imaging probes for AD.

## CURRENT APPROACHES TO IMAGING $\beta$-AMYLOID

There are several reports of potential imaging agents that bind to $\beta$-amyloid deposits, some of which have been tested in human studies (TABLE 1). The blood–brain barrier (BBB) presents special challenges when developing molecular imaging agents designed to target specific epitopes within the brain. In the absence of a compromised BBB, small molecules are the best candidates

TABLE 1. Representative approaches to plaque-imaging agents

| Modality | Probe | Species | Reference |
|---|---|---|---|
| PET | FDDNP | Human | 51,58,85 |
| | [$^{11}$C]-PIB | Human | 52,86,87 |
| | SB-13 | Human | 53 |
| | [$^{18}$F]-PIB | Human | 57 |
| | Benzoxazole | Mouse | 88,89 |
| SPECT | IMPY | Human | 54,60 |
| | IMPY | Mouse | 50,90 |
| | IBOX | Mouse | 90 |
| SPECT | Rhenium Oxo | in vitro | 91 |
| Optical | BSB | Mouse ex vivo | 92 |
| (Near-IR) | AOI987 | Mouse | 93 |
| MRI | Peptide | Mouse ex vivo | 48,49,94 |

for brain imaging due to their proven ability to penetrate the brain. Thus, the use of PET or SPECT to image β-amyloid in the brain is favored over other imaging modalities, such as MRI, that necessarily require large amounts of contrast agents to sufficiently generate reasonable signal to noise. Although there are non-PET approaches aimed at imaging β-amyloid, such as magnetically active peptides or SPECT agents, this review focuses primarily on PET approaches targeted at β-amyloid.[47–50]

There have been four successful compounds shown to have increased the uptake of radioactivity in the brains of AD patients compared to aged controls.[51–54] The approach that was first published used the [$^{18}$F]-labeled analogue of the aminonaphthalene ([fluoroethyl] [methyl] [aminol-2-napthylidene] [malononitrile]) (FDDNP), and has been developed by Barrio et al.[51] Another approach that has shown great promise and has been reproduced by many centers throughout the world is that using the radiolabeled Thioflavin analog OH-BTA-1 (N-Methylaminophenyl-6-hydroxybenzothiazole;).[52,55,56] The [$^{11}$C] version of this compound is commonly referred to as "Pittsburgh Compound B (PIB)," named by the Uppsala University PET Center who imaged the first AD patients. [$^{18}$F]-labeled benzothiazoles are currently in early development.[57] Other approaches include an [$^{123}$I]Iodine-labeled Thioflavin derivative ([$^{123}$I]-IMPY) and a [$^{11}$C]-labeled stilbene ([$^{11}$C]-SB-13).[53,54]

FDDNP has been shown to differentiate AD from controls and demonstrates an approximate 20% increase of signal in brain compared to normal controls.[51] In the initial study, nine Alzheimer's patients (seven were probable AD; two were possible AD) and seven non-AD healthy aged matched controls were selected. FDDNP binding to amyloid plaques was quantified using a relative residence time (RTT) approach that compares washout rates of the probe in various brain regions (hippocampus, amygdala, entorhinal cortex) to a reference region expected to have low plaque density and low nonspecific binding (pons). RTT values were estimated from a linear fit and extrapolation to integrals over

12–120 min post injection. It should be noted that it is well established that FDDNP binds to both β-amyloid plaques, as well as neurofibrillar tangles (NFTs).[58] Since NFTs are not necessarily specific to AD, it is unclear if FDDNP binding will be capable of achieving the necessary positive or negative predictive value that is needed for clinical use.

In the human study using the PIB compound, 16 AD patients and 9 normal controls (three young and six older subjects) were scanned following injection of the [11]C-labeled PIB compound. Images were acquired over a 60-min interval following injection.[52] Standard uptake values were computed for 40–60 min. Results showed that there was a significantly higher frontal, parietal, and temporal cortical uptake in AD patients versus controls, indicating that PIB may show promise as a specific imaging agent for AD diagnosis. PIB has also been detected in 80% of cases of dementia with Lewy Bodies. In frontotemporal cases, however, brain radioactivity was similar to that seen in aged normals.[59]

IMPY has recently been compared in four AD cases compared to three aged matched controls, with an approximate 40% increase in signal in AD patients compared to controls.[60] [11]C-SB-13 was shown in five AD cases and six healthy females to demonstrate target to background ratios, which were comparable with those seen with [11]C-PIB.[53]

## IDENTIFYING PRODROMAL AD VIA β-AMYLOID IMAGING: PLAQUE IMAGING

As mentioned, current approaches to β-amyloid imaging focus on β-amyloid fibrillar deposits. This is logical since the current gold standard for AD diagnosis is the postmortem visualization of amyloid plaques and neurofibrillar tangles. It has been suggested that levels of fibrillar β-amyloid in the form of plaque may correlate with neuronal function since fibrils have been shown to be neurotoxic both *in vitro* and *in vivo*[14–16] and it is established that plaque density correlates well with definitive AD diagnosis and this has been confirmed in PET imaging studies.[51,52] Nonetheless, it is still unclear if plaque density will correlate to the rate of progression or conversion to AD in a presymptomatic population.

Early studies that examined postmortem brains in clinically confirmed AD had difficulty making the correlation between total plaque burden and disease progression.[18–21] More recently, this phenomenon was tested in living subjects using PIB imaging and it was demonstrated that tracer uptake does not correlate to disease progression in patients already diagnosed with AD confirming earlier findings.[61] These data suggest that plaque may not be a causative factor in disease. Additionally, these data suggest that there is a steady-state level of plaque load that is achieved relatively late in disease progression, although cognitive function may continue to deteriorate. It is temping to speculate that imaging plaque prior to AD diagnosis, and presumably prior to steady-state plaque burden, will predict conversation to AD in patients who do not yet have overt clinical symptoms. Mild cognitive impairment (MCI) is a condition used to describe patients who have early cognitive deficits, and who are at risk of developing AD.[62] In a recent abstract, FDDNP has been used to follow the progression of a group of normals, MCI and AD cases. Five controls and four MCI cases were reimaged after a 2-year period. Two of the four MCI cases had converted to AD and one of the controls had progressed to MCI. In these three cases there was increased binding of FDDNP compared to the deposition of radioactivity seen at baseline. In the six other cases the scan remained unchanged.[63] MCI patients have also been followed by the Pittsburgh group, with images seeming to be grouped into either normal or AD like.[59] These data support the notion that tracer uptake, and presumably plaque burden, may indicate a predisposition to developing disease. Further longitudinal studies are being performed.

It is logical to speculate that plaque development requires long periods of time to manifest and at least some plaque burden will exist prior to the onset of any clinical cognitive symptoms. It should be noted that early studies that examined postmortem β-amyloid load identified the phenomenon of "high pathology controls" (patients with pathological levels of senile plaques who are cognitively normal).[21] Importantly, this observation was recently validated in a large-scale examination of cognitively normal subjects in which a remarkable 36% had levels of plaque that would be consistent with a neuropathologic criteria for the diagnosis of AD.[64] This further confirms that plaques do not correlate with disease. However, since it is well known that patients who have clinical AD typically have high plaque load, it is possible that high pathology controls may have a predisposition to converting to AD. Thus, plaque load may be used as a general risk factor for AD. Today, it is difficult to know whether this hypothesis will be viable. Obviously, postmortem studies are incapable of follow-up and thus conversion rates cannot be correlated. This only highlights the need for longitudinal studies using noninvasive plaque measures.

It is interesting to contemplate why some patients with high plaque loads similar to those who have AD can be completely cognitively normal. Although there are many potential theories including variation in neuronal plasticity, one hypothesis is that soluble β-amyloid is not present in high concentrations in these patients. It would be interesting to examine the levels of soluble β-amyloid in high pathology controls compared to patients with clinically confirmed AD.

## IDENTIFYING PRODROMAL AD VIA β-AMYLOID IMAGING: SOLUBLE OLIGOMERS

It has been suggested that a major reason for failure of a biomarker to act as true disease surrogate endpoint is the lack of a direct association between the biomarker and the causal mechanism of disease.[65] As stated above, the role of insoluble fibrillar plaques as a causative mechanism in AD is controversial and continues to be disputed. The clear association of soluble oligomers of β-amyloid to neurotoxicity in animal studies, as well as its correlation to cognitive dysfunction and synaptic density in humans, indicates that measuring soluble oligomers may hold more promise as a true surrogate biomarker for the clinical symptoms of AD. Further, since it has been established that fibrillar species are formed from lower ordered oligomers,[6] it is logical to speculate that neurotoxic forms of oligomers will precede the formation of plaques and therefore hold promise as early indicatorsss of prodromal disease. In line with the concept that plaques are ultimately derived from soluble β-amyloid, it is possible that plaque measures may be used as a surrogate marker for the levels of soluble β-amyloid. However, since β-amyloid accumulation is governed by a complex process that includes production, clearance, and aggregation, all of which may be independently controlled, the association of plaque and levels of soluble β-amyloid may not exist. Further, other studies suggest that oligomers and fibrils are formed from distinct pathways, which may disconnect the levels of each species.[66]

The lack of specific agents that can differentiate soluble oligomers from fibrillar forms of β-amyloid both *in vitro* and *in vivo* has hindered studies aimed at testing the correlation between oligomers and plaques and/or the relative clinical value of measuring different forms of β-amyloid species. The discovery and development of specific probes for soluble oligomers is greatly needed. Such probes will not only serve as potential PET tracers, but may be used in *ex vivo* postmortem studies to study the regional distribution of oligomers versus plaques. Such information would enable the correlation of neuronal loss with the spatial location of soluble oligomers and thus may accelerate the establishment of a true surrogate for the diagnosis of prodromal AD.

## THERAPEUTIC EFFICACY MONITORING VIA β-AMYLOID IMAGING: PLAQUE IMAGING

Several targeted therapeutic approaches that aim to reduce β-amyloid pathology are currently under evaluation in preclinical and clinical studies.[67–71] The ability to monitor the effectiveness of β-amyloid targeted therapy in a timely manner will be an important aspect for testing such approaches in the clinic. Unfortunately, tracking therapeutic efficacy using standard clinical cognitive tests will require long follow-up periods that translate into costly trials. For example, a recent clinical trial of active immunotherapy (vaccination) directed against β-amyloid required a minimum 1-year follow-up to observe clinically significant changes in treated versus control subjects.[72] This study confirms earlier animal studies that required long follow-up periods to observe changes in total plaque burden in PDAPP transgenic mice treated with passive immunotherapy.[13,31,73] The ability to monitor therapeutic efficacy early (prior to measurable symptomatic changes) will be necessary for clinical dose adjustments to delay or prevent onset of symptoms. Further, the prevention of adverse side effects and costly long-term treatment may be prevented with early therapeutic monitoring. Thus, there is a significant need to monitor amyloid therapies prior to measurable cognitive benefit.

In the context of tracking β-amyloid targeted therapy, it is important to realize that there are two major therapeutic approaches aimed at reducing β-amyloid load: (1) plaque clearance by active or passive immunotherapy (i.e., vaccination), or (2) inhibition of β-amyloid peptide production by beta or gamma secretase inhibition or clearance of monomeric β-amyloid by antibodies directed at this target (passive immunotherapy).[31,67,70,74] It is logical to speculate that therapies aimed at promoting plaque clearance, such as vaccination (active immunotherapy), may be expected to have a significantly rapid effect on β-amyloid plaque levels. A postmortem brain analysis from a patient immunized against β-amyloid found a striking absence of amyloid deposits compared to unimmunized AD controls.[68] Although such results are suggestive that plaque imaging may measure response to therapy, it is important to realize that significant differences must be observable prior to cognitive measures for plaque measures to be useful. Since other patients immunized in this study had a significantly improved rate of cognitive decline (compared to un-immunized controls) at 8–12 months post immunization, plaque changes would need to be observed less than 8 months post immunization.[72]

In contrast to vaccination, plaque sensitivity to secretase or antibody therapies will depend on the kinetics of the dissociation of monomers from fibrils and thus may not be an immediately sensitive measure of this therapeutic approach. Further, since the majority of amyloid in AD patients is in the form of insoluble fibrillar deposits,[21,23] immediate changes in production or clearance of monomer will be difficult to observe by monitoring total plaque load. This concept is supported by animal studies in which no change in total amyloid is seen (examined 6 weeks following therapy) in passively immunized mice that have high plaque burdens.[31] Interestingly, convincing support for the insensitivity of plaque measures to gauge inhibition of production was demonstrated by Jankowsky et al.,[95] which showed persistent plaque structures for up to 6 months following suppression of the APP transgene. These data confirm our early theoretical data generated from a computational simulation model of β-amyloid production and clearance in which higher ordered fibrillar concentrations required several months to drop appreciably following simulated gamma secretase inhibition (FIG. 3).[75] Conversely, these data show a dramatic fall in low molecular weight β-amyloid following identical therapeutic regimens.

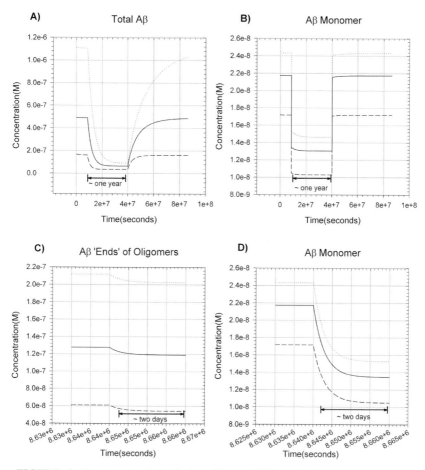

**FIGURE 3.** Computational simulation of β-amyloid-lowering therapy. Change in total β-amyloid oligomers (**A**) and monomer only (**B**) over 1 year of simulated therapy that reduces β-amyloid production by 40%. Change in total β-amyloid oligomers (**C**) and monomer only (**D**) over 2 days following initiation of the simulated therapy that reduces β-amyloid production by 40%. (*dotted line* = hippocampus; *solid line* = cortex; *dashed line* = cerebellum).[75] Reprinted with kind permission of Springer Science and Business Media.

It is important to note that kinetics of fibril formation *in vitro* and *in vivo* models may not accurately reflect that of human brains. Thus, it is still possible that the dynamics of plaque dissolution following secretase treatment may be rapid enough to measure using plaque-imaging techniques. Such studies must be performed to gain insights into the dynamics of plaque clearance following therapy.

## THERAPEUTIC EFFICACY MONITORING VIA β-AMYLOID
## IMAGING: SOLUBLE OLIGOMERS

β-amyloid plaque formation is a kinetically dynamic process that begins with self-aggregation of the β-amyloid peptide into large aggregates (FIG. 1).[6,8,9,76] Since soluble β-amyloid oligomers are near the initiation of this cascade it is likely that measures of soluble β-amyloid oligomers will be inherently more sensitive to inhibitors of amyloid production. A study that measured local brain levels of soluble β-amyloid in mice following gamma secretase-mediated β-amyloid inhibition showed dramatic changes in soluble β-amyloid levels within 3 h of treatment.[77] Interestingly, mice with greater amyloid loads (i.e., plaque) showed a delayed response, likely due to the large reservoir of β-amyloid that remains despite the inhibition of β-amyloid production, further confirming the inadequacy of plaque measures compared to soluble β-amyloid measures. As indicated above, our β-amyloid computational simulations are consistent with these observations (FIG. 3).

Others have found in animal models of passive immunotherapy (systemic injection of monoclonal antibody) that cognitive improvements precede measurable changes in *overall total* amyloid burden.[31] Interestingly, the authors provide evidence in other studies that this antibody binds soluble β-amyloid and may sink β-amyloid into systemic circulation, suggesting that removing small species of β-amyloid from the brain can improve cognitive function.[13,30,31] Since it is possible that soluble oligomers of β-amyloid are directly responsible for cognitive dysfunction, the levels of soluble β-amyloid may be validated as a surrogate for cognitive function. As mentioned above, several lines of evidence support this notion. Thus, if the level of soluble β-amyloid is a surrogate for cognitive function, then measuring soluble β-amyloid may have greater promise for monitoring therapeutic outcome regardless of the therapeutic approach. Studies aimed at correlating the levels of soluble β-amyloid oligomers to disease progression are needed to validate this concept.

## TECHNICAL FEASIBILITY OF DISCOVERING PROBES THAT
## ARE SELECTIVE FOR SOLUBLE β-AMYLOID OLIGOMERS

Unlike oligomers, our understanding of β-amyloid fibrils *in situ* is well established due, in part, to the widespread use of environmentally sensitive dyes, such as Thioflavin T or S, and Congo Red.[78-80] These dyes have been used to detect the spatial location, temporal kinetics, and the molecular environment of β-amyloid fibrils. Importantly, these dyes have been used on *ex vivo* postmortem brains to correlate the amount and location of plaques to disease progression. Further, current imaging tracers for β-amyloid plaques were developed through modification of these dyes such that they were suitable for noninvasive imaging. Thus, a hindrance to the more detailed study of β-amyloid oligomers, both *in vitro* and *in vivo*, is the lack of selective dyes or probes that can differentiate these forms of β-amyloid *in situ*.

Risks that are common to tracer discovery, such as sensitivity, specificity, target concentration, affinity, Bmax, and pharmacokinetics also apply to the discovery and development of a tracer for oligomeric β-amyloid. However, an additional technical risk that is unique to developing an oligomer-targeted tracer is the apparent lack of specific features in oligomers compared to fibrillar species. Since the primary amino acid sequence of β-amyloid is the same in both species, one must rely on the assumption that there are sufficient structural differences between the two species that will allow differential binding of small molecules. There are reasons to believe that such structural differences exist. For example, it is known that Thioflavin and Congo Red dyes, which bind to cross-beta sheets in fibrillar β-amyloid, do not bind as well to lower molecular weight β-amyloid, supporting the concept that oligomers exist in a distinct three-dimensional conformation that likely contains little β-sheet content.[8,81,82] Further, and more importantly, antibodies raised against soluble oligomers of β-amyloid have favored selectivity toward oligomers and indicate that distinct structural features may exist.[25,27,35] Lastly, molecular modeling data suggest that little similarities exist between fibrils and oligomers.[7,83,84] Combined, these data justify a screening program to identify compounds that may selectively bind oligomers and not fibrils. It is important to note that antibodies that have been reported in the literature to favor oligomers have been shown to bind fibrils under certain conditions and thus are not likely to accurately measure the different characteristics of fibrils from oligomers. Further, antibodies are more costly compared to small molecule probes and are unable to cross the blood–brain barrier thus limiting their use in brain imaging. Thus, a small molecular probe would have clear advantages over antibody-based approaches.

One way to find high affinity ligands that selectively bind soluble β-amyloid is by performing a competition screening assay. However, there are no ligands known to specifically bind soluble oligomers for use in competition assays. Another way is an antiaggregation assay (i.e., the displacement of β-amyloid peptide from preformed fibrils). However, it is unclear if antiaggregates work by binding to monomers, dimers, oligomers or in some cases bind β-sheets and cause disaggregation. Thus, we cannot rely on antiaggregation to yield information on specificity.

It has recently been shown that compounds with inherent fluorescent properties, can be screened against β-amyloid fibrils using a fluorescence method that eliminates the need to radiolabel compounds and mechanically separate free from bound ligand.[58,82] Preliminary screening performed in our laboratory indicates that some compounds may have specificity for soluble oligomers over fibrils. A novel *ex vivo* binding assay illustrates the selective nature of these probes (FIG. 4).

Oligomers                                    Fibrils

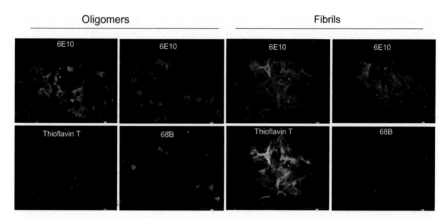

**FIGURE 4.** Selective binding of an oligomer-specific small molecule probe. β-amyloid oligomers or fibrils are incubated with either oligomers selective probe (68B) or Thioflavin T and imaged by fluorescence microscopy. 68B does not show any interactions with fibrils, but binds to oligomers. Staining of same sections with β-amyloid antibody 6E10 shows β-amyloid is present in each section. Note low binding of Thioflavin T to oligomers (Montalto *et al.*, manuscript in preparation).

## HUMAN BRAIN CONCENTRATIONS OF ENDOGENOUS SOLUBLE β-AMYLOID

Another key risk unique to developing oligomer-specific tracers is the apparent low levels of soluble amyloid present in the AD brain. For example, several reports indicate that soluble β-amyloid is present at 10 times lower concentration than fibrils.[20,23,24,32] This presents two challenges: (1) the tracer must have little or no binding affinity for fibrils while maintaining extremely high affinity for oligomers, and (2) even in the absence of background binding, the absolute concentration of soluble β-amyloid may not be sufficient to generate detectable signal for imaging. To address the first issue it would be important to include fibrils as a target in a screening assay and design subsequent libraries "away" from the chemical space that may mediate fibril binding. The second issue can only be addressed by gathering and analyzing published data available on levels of soluble β-amyloid in the brain. The best available studies indicate that soluble β-amyloid is present in the AD brain in the range 8 to 60 pmol/g, which is significantly elevated above normal by 3 to 10 times.[20,23,24,32] In all of these reports soluble β-amyloid levels were determined using an aqueous extraction procedure that includes a high-speed centrifugal step to remove insoluble debris and fibrillar β-amyloid. It is important to realize that high-speed centrifugation will also remove cellular bound proteins. It has recently been shown that soluble oligomers of β-amyloid can tightly associate with neuronal cell membranes,[27] indicating that the published concentrations of oligomers in the brain are likely underestimations.

Nonetheless, we have performed a computational PET imaging simulation to determine if pmol/g levels are detectable using targeted PET imaging. Our data show that rat hippocampal soluble β-amyloid is detectable at 30 pmol/g.[75] Thus, data available from the literature combined with our simulation models indicate that the levels of soluble β-amyloid oligomers do not preclude the possibility of measuring these levels via conventional PET imaging. Of course, many other factors, such as biodistribution, number of true binding sites (Bmax), and subcellular localization, may affect the ability to generate measurable PET signal above background. Such variables must be tested empirically.

In summary, the development of imaging techniques targeting β-amyloid plaques is rapidly evolving. Although neuroimaging studies using amyloid-binding ligands, such as PIB, are just beginning, there is evidence to justify studies aimed at diagnosing prodromal AD based on plaque imaging. Similarly, soluble β-amyloid oligomers are an attractive biomarker for presymptomatic AD and may provide an earlier measure of disease modification aimed to reduce levels of β-amyloid. Two key aspects that need to be addressed for development of an imaging agent against soluble oligomers are selectivity of the ligand and imageability of this biomarker. Data available indicate that some compounds can sufficiently differentiate soluble oligomers over fibrillar β-amyloid and that the levels of soluble β-amyloid oligomers do not preclude the possibility of measuring these levels by conventional PET imaging.

## ACKNOWLEDGMENTS

We thank Ken Fish and John Graf for contributing figures and data for this manuscript and Christoph Hergerberg for his critical review.

## REFERENCES

1. GLENNER, G.G. & C.W. WONG. 1984. Alzheimer's disease and Down's syndrome: sharing of a unique cerebrovascular amyloid fibril protein. Biochem. Biophys. Res. Commun **122:** 1131–1135.
2. MASTERS, C.L. *et al.* 1985. Amyloid plaque core protein in Alzheimer disease and Down syndrome. Proc. Natl. Acad. Sci. USA **82:** 4245–4249.
3. VASSAR, R. *et al.* 1999. Beta-secretase cleavage of Alzheimer's amyloid precursor protein by the transmembrane aspartic protease BACE. Science **286:** 735–741.
4. SINHA, S. *et al.* 1999. Purification and cloning of amyloid precursor protein beta-secretase from human brain. Nature **402:** 537–540.
5. KHACHATURIAN, Z.S. & M.M. MESULUM, Eds. 2000. Alzheimer's disease: a compendium of current theories. Ann. N. Y. Acad. Sci. **924:** 1–195.
6. BITAN, G., A. LOMAKIN & D.B. TEPLOW. 2001. Amyloid beta-protein oligomerization: prenucleation interactions revealed by photo-induced cross-linking of unmodified proteins. J. Biol. Chem. **276:** 35176–35184.

7. URBANC, B. *et al.* 2004. In silico study of amyloid {beta}-protein folding and oligomerization. PNAS **101**: 17345–17350.
8. INOUYE, H. & D.A. KIRSCHNER. 2000. A beta fibrillogenesis: kinetic parameters for fibril formation from Congo red binding. J. Struc. Biol. **130**: 123–129.
9. GORMAN, P.M. *et al.* 2003. Alternate aggregation pathways of the Alzheimer β-amyloid peptide: Aβ association kinetics at endosomal pH. J. Mol. Biol. **325**: 743–757.
10. IWATSUBO, T. *et al.* 1994. Visualization of A beta 42(43) and A beta 40 in senile plaques with end-specific A beta monoclonals: evidence that an initially deposited species is A beta 42(43). Neuron **13**: 45–53.
11. SHIBATA, M. *et al.* 2000. Clearance of Alzheimer's amyloid-ss(1-40) peptide from brain by LDL receptor-related protein-1 at the blood-brain barrier. J. Clin. Invest. **106**: 1489–1499.
12. GHERSI-EGEA, J.F. *et al.* 1996. Fate of cerebrospinal fluid-borne amyloid beta-peptide: rapid clearance into blood and appreciable accumulation by cerebral arteries. J. Neurochem. **67**: 880–883.
13. DEMATTOS, R.B. *et al.* 2002. Brain to plasma amyloid-beta efflux: a measure of brain amyloid burden in a mouse model of Alzheimer's disease. Science **295**: 2264–2267.
14. PIKE, C.J. *et al.* 1991. *In vitro* aging of beta-amyloid protein causes peptide aggregation and neurotoxicity. Brain Res. **563**: 311–314.
15. LORENZO, A. & B.A. YANKNER. 1994. Beta-amyloid neurotoxicity requires fibril formation and is inhibited by Congo red. Proc. Natl. Acad. Sci. USA **91**: 12243–12247.
16. DAHLGREN, K.N. *et al.* 2002. Oligomeric and fibrillar species of amyloid-beta peptides differentially affect neuronal viability. J. Biol. Chem. **277**: 32046–32053.
17. LI, Y.T., D.S. WOODRUFF-PAK & J.Q. TROJANOWSKI. 1994. Amyloid plaques in cerebellar cortex and the integrity of Purkinje cell dendrites. Neurobiol. Aging **15**: 1–9.
18. KIRKITADZE, M.D., G. BITAN & D.B. TEPLOW. 2002. Paradigm shifts in Alzheimer's disease and other neurodegenerative disorders: the emerging role of oligomeric assemblies. J. Neurosci. Res. **69**: 567–577.
19. NASLUND, J. *et al.* 2000. Correlation between elevated levels of amyloid beta-peptide in the brain and cognitive decline. JAMA **283**: 1571–1577.
20. MCLEAN, C.A. *et al.* 1999. Soluble pool of Abeta amyloid as a determinant of severity of neurodegeneration in Alzheimer's disease. Ann. Neurol. **46**: 860–866.
21. LUE, L.F. *et al.* 1999. Soluble amyloid beta peptide concentration as a predictor of synaptic change in Alzheimer's disease. Am. J. Pathol. **155**: 853–862.
22. KLEIN, W.L. 2002. Abeta toxicity in Alzheimer's disease: globular oligomers (AD-DLs) as new vaccine and drug targets. Neurochem. Int. **41**: 345–352.
23. KUO, Y.M. *et al.* 1996. Water-soluble Abeta (N-40, N-42) oligomers in normal and Alzheimer disease brains. J. Biol. Chem. **271**: 4077–4081.
24. WELLER, R.O. *et al.* 1998. Cerebral amyloid angiopathy: amyloid beta accumulates in putative interstitial fluid drainage pathways in Alzheimer's disease. Am. J. Pathol. **153**: 725–733.
25. BARGHORN, S. *et al.* 2005. Globular amyloid beta-peptide oligomer—a homogenous and stable neuropathological protein in Alzheimer's disease. J. Neurochem. **95**: 834–847.

26. KAYED, R. *et al.* 2004. Permeabilization of lipid bilayers is a common conformation-dependent activity of soluble amyloid oligomers in protein misfolding diseases. J. Biol. Chem. **279:** 46363–46366.

27. GONG, Y. *et al.* 2003. Alzheimer's disease-affected brain: presence of oligomeric A beta ligands (ADDLs) suggests a molecular basis for reversible memory loss. Proc. Natl. Acad. Sci. USA **100:** 10417–10422.

28. LAMBERT, M.P. *et al.* 1998. Diffusible, nonfibrillar ligands derived from Abeta1-42 are potent central nervous system neurotoxins. Proc. Natl. Acad. Sci. USA **95:** 6448–6453.

29. WALSH, D.M. *et al.* 2002. Naturally secreted oligomers of amyloid beta protein potently inhibit hippocampal long-term potentiation *in vivo*. Nature **416:** 535–539.

30. DEMATTOS, R.B. *et al.* 2001. Peripheral anti-A beta antibody alters CNS and plasma A beta clearance and decreases brain A beta burden in a mouse model of Alzheimer's disease. Proc. Natl. Acad. Sci. USA **98:** 8850–8855.

31. DODART, J.C. *et al.* 2002. Immunization reverses memory deficits without reducing brain Abeta burden in Alzheimer's disease model. Nat. Neurosci. **5:** 452–457.

32. WANG, J. *et al.* 1999. The levels of soluble versus insoluble brain Abeta distinguish Alzheimer's disease from normal and pathologic aging. Exp. Neurol. **158:** 328–337.

33. LESNE, S. *et al.* 2006. A specific amyloid-beta protein assembly in the brain impairs memory. Nature **440:** 352–357.

34. KIM, H.J. *et al.* 2003. Selective neuronal degeneration induced by soluble oligomeric amyloid beta protein. FASEB J. **17:** 118–120.

35. KAYED, R. *et al.* 2003. Common structure of soluble amyloid oligomers implies common mechanism of pathogenesis. Science **300:** 486–489.

36. KLYUBIN, I. *et al.* 2005. Amyloid beta protein immunotherapy neutralizes Abeta oligomers that disrupt synaptic plasticity *in vivo*. Nat. Med. **11:** 556–561.

37. MOHS, R.C., W.G. ROSEN & K.L. DAVIS. 1983. The Alzheimer's disease assessment scale: an instrument for assessing treatment efficacy. Psychopharmacol. Bull. **19:** 448–450.

38. FOLSTEIN, M.F., S.E. FOLSTEIN & P.R. McHUGH. 1975. "Mini-mental state." A practical method for grading the cognitive state of patients for the clinician. J. Psychiatr. Res. **12:** 189–198.

39. McKHANN, G. *et al.* 1984. Clinical diagnosis of Alzheimer's disease: report of the NINCDS-ADRDA Work Group under the auspices of Department of Health and Human Services Task Force on Alzheimer's Disease. Neurology **34:** 939–944.

40. PETRELLA, J.R., R.E. COLEMAN & P.M. DORAISWAMY. 2003. Neuroimaging and early diagnosis of Alzheimer disease: a look to the future. Radiology **226:** 315–336.

41. SILVERMAN, D.H. *et al.* 2001. Positron emission tomography in evaluation of dementia: Regional brain metabolism and long-term outcome. JAMA **286:** 2120–2127.

42. MOSCONI, L. *et al.* 2006. Visual rating of medial temporal lobe metabolism in mild cognitive impairment and Alzheimer's disease using FDG-PET. Eur. J. Nucl. Med. Mol. Imag. **33:** 210–221.

43. MOTTER, R. *et al.* 1995. Reduction of beta-amyloid peptide42 in the cerebrospinal fluid of patients with Alzheimer's disease. Ann. Neurol. **38:** 643–648.

44. HULSTAERT, F. *et al.* 1999. Improved discrimination of AD patients using beta-amyloid(1-42) and tau levels in CSF. Neurology **52**: 1555–1562.
45. CSERNANSKY, J.G. *et al.* 2002. Relationships among cerebrospinal fluid biomarkers in dementia of the Alzheimer type. Alzheimer. Dis. Assoc. Disord. **16**: 144–149.
46. MARUYAMA, M. *et al.* 2001. Cerebrospinal fluid amyloid beta(1-42) levels in the mild cognitive impairment stage of Alzheimer's disease. Exp. Neurol. **172**: 433–436.
47. KUNG, M.P. *et al.* 2002. Radioiodinated styrylbenzene derivatives as potential SPECT imaging agents for amyloid plaque detection in Alzheimer's disease. J. Mol. Neurosci. **19**: 7–10.
48. PODUSLO, J.F. *et al.* 1999. Receptor-mediated transport of human amyloid beta-protein 1-40 and 1-42 at the blood-brain barrier. Neurobiol. Dis. **6**: 190–199.
49. PODUSLO, J.F. *et al.* 2002. Molecular targeting of Alzheimer's amyloid plaques for contrast-enhanced magnetic resonance imaging. Neurobiol. Dis. **11**: 315–329.
50. KUNG, H.F. *et al.* 2003. Iodinated tracers for imaging amyloid plaques in the brain. Mol. Imag. Biol. **5**: 418–426.
51. SHOGHI-JADID, K. *et al.* 2002. Localization of neurofibrillary tangles and beta-amyloid plaques in the brains of living patients with Alzheimer's disease. Am. J. Geriatr. Psychiatry **10**: 24–35.
52. KLUNK, W.E. *et al.* 2004. Imaging brain amyloid in Alzheimer's disease with Pittsburgh Compound-B. Ann. Neurol. **55**: 306–319.
53. VERHOEFF, N.P. *et al.* 2004. In-vivo imaging of Alzheimer disease beta-amyloid with [11C]SB-13 PET. Am. J. Geriatr. Psychiatry **12**: 584–595.
54. NEWBERG, A.B. *et al.* 2006. Safety, biodistribution, and dosimetry of 123I-IMPY: a novel amyloid plaque-imaging agent for the diagnosis of Alzheimer's disease. J. Nucl. Med. **47**: 748–754.
55. KLUNK, W.E., R.F. JACOB & R.P. MASON. 1999. Quantifying amyloid $\beta$-peptide (A$\beta$) aggregation using the Congo red-A$\beta$ (CR-A$\beta$) spectrophotometric assay. Anal. Biochem. **266**: 66–76.
56. MATHIS, C.A. *et al.* 2003. Synthesis and evaluation of 11C-labeled 6-substituted 2-arylbenzothiazoles as amyloid imaging agents. J. Med. Chem. **46**: 2740–2754.
57. FARRAR, G. 2005. Challenges in the development of novel PET agents. Turku PET Symposium. Abstract 49.
58. AGDEPPA, E.D. *et al.* 2001. Binding characteristics of radiofluorinated 6-dialkylamino-2-naphthylethylidene derivatives as positron emission tomography imaging probes for beta-amyloid plaques in Alzheimer's disease. J. Neurosci. **21**: RC189.
59. VILLEMANGE, V. *et al.* 2006. 11C-PIB PET imaging in the different diagnosis of dementia. Society of Nuclear Medicine Annual Meeting. Abstact 209.
60. NEWBERG, A.B. *et al.* 2006. Use of 123I IMPY SPECT to differentiate Alzheimer's disease from controls. Society of Nuclear Medicine Annual Meeting. Abstact 220.
61. BLOMQVIST, G. *et al.* 2006. Imaging amyloid depositions and glucose uptake changes in Alzheimer's disease: a follow-up study. Presented at the Annual Conference of the Academy of Molecular Imaging. Mol. Imag. Biol. **8**: Abs no 88.
62. PETERSEN, R.C. 2003. Mild cognitive impairment clinical trials. Nat. Rev. Drug Discov. **2**: 646–653.
63. KEPE, V. *et al.* 2006. Detection of MCI-AD and control -MCI conversions in Alzheimer's disease patients with (F-18) FDDNP PET. Society of Nuclear Medicine Annual Meeting. Abstact 208.

64. BENNETT, D.A. *et al.* 2006. Neuropathology of older persons without cognitive impairment from two community-based studies. Neurology **66:** 1837–1844.

65. MANI, R.B. 2004. The evaluation of disease modifying therapies in Alzheimer's disease: a regulatory viewpoint. Stat. Med. **23:** 305–314.

66. BITAN, G. *et al.* 2003. Amyloid beta-protein (Abeta) assembly: Abeta 40 and Abeta 42 oligomerize through distinct pathways. Proc. Natl. Acad. Sci. USA **100:** 330–335.

67. WALSH, D.M. *et al.* 2002. Amyloid-beta oligomers: their production, toxicity and therapeutic inhibition. Biochem. Soc. Trans. **30:** 552–557.

68. NICOLL, J.A. *et al.* 2003. Neuropathology of human Alzheimer disease after immunization with amyloid-beta peptide: a case report. Nat. Med. **9:** 448–452.

69. PERMANNE, B. *et al.* 2002. Reduction of amyloid load and cerebral damage in a transgenic mouse model of Alzheimer's disease by treatment with a beta-sheet breaker peptide. FASEB J. **16:** 860–862.

70. DE FELICE, F.G. & S.T. FERREIRA. 2002. Beta-amyloid production, aggregation, and clearance as targets for therapy in Alzheimer's disease. Cell. Mol. Neurobiol. **22:** 545–563.

71. MAIORINI, A.F. *et al.* 2002. Potential novel targets for Alzheimer pharmacotherapy: I. Secretases. J. Clin. Pharm. Ther. **27:** 169–183.

72. HOCK, C. *et al.* 2003. Antibodies against beta-amyloid slow cognitive decline in Alzheimer's disease. Neuron **38:** 547–554.

73. WILCOCK, D.M. *et al.* 2004. Passive amyloid immunotherapy clears amyloid and transiently activates microglia in a transgenic mouse model of amyloid deposition. J. Neurosci. **24:** 6144–6151.

74. CONWAY, K.A. *et al.* 2003. Emerging beta-amyloid therapies for the treatment of Alzheimer's disease. Curr. Pharm. Des. **9:** 427–447.

75. SIMMONS, M.K. *et al.* 2005. A computational PET simulation model for imaging b-amyloid in mice. Mol. Imag. Biol. **7:** 69–77.

76. URBANC, B. *et al.* 1999. Dynamics of plaque formation in Alzheimer's disease. Biophys. J. **76:** 1330–1334.

77. CIRRITO, J.R. *et al.* 2003. *In vivo* assessment of brain interstitial fluid with microdialysis reveals plaque-associated changes in amyloid-beta metabolism and half-life. J. Neurosci. **23:** 8844–8853.

78. WESTERMARK, G.T., K.H. JOHNSON & P. WESTERMARK. 1999. Staining methods for identification of amyloid in tissue. *In* Amyloid, Prions, and other Protein Aggregates, Methods in Enzymology, vol. 309. R., Wetzsl, Ed.: 3–25. Academic Press, San Diego, CA.

79. STILLER, D. & D. KATENKAMP. 1975. Histochemistry of amyloid. General considerations, light microscopical and ultrastructural examinations. Exp. Pathol. Suppl. **1:** 1–116.

80. GLENNER, G.G. 1981. The bases of the staining of amyloid fibers: their physicochemical nature and the mechanism of their dye-substrate interaction. Prog. Histochem. Cytochem. **13:** 1–37.

81. LEVINE, H., III. 1993. Thioflavine T interaction with synthetic Alzheimer's disease beta-amyloid peptides: detection of amyloid aggregation in solution. Protein Sci. **2:** 404–410.

82. KUNER, P. *et al.* 2000. Controlling polymerization of beta-amyloid and prion-derived peptides with synthetic small molecule ligands. J. Biol. Chem. **275:** 1673–1678.

83. GEORGE, A.R. & D.R. HOWLETT. 1999. Computationally derived structural models of the beta-amyloid found in Alzheimer's disease plaques and the interaction with possible aggregation inhibitors. Biopolymers **50:** 733–741.

84. MA, B. & R. NUSSINOV. 2002. Stabilities and conformations of Alzheimer's beta -amyloid peptide oligomers (Abeta 16–22, Abeta 16–35, and Abeta 10–35): Sequence effects. Proc. Natl. Acad. Sci. USA **99:** 14126–14131.

85. AGDEPPA, E.D. *et al.* 2003. *In vitro* detection of (S)-naproxen and ibuprofen binding to plaques in the Alzheimer's brain using the positron emission tomography molecular imaging probe 2-(1-[6-[(2-[(18)F]fluoroethyl)(methyl)amino]-2-naphthyl]ethylidene)malono nitrile. Neuroscience **117:** 723–730.

86. ENGLER, H. *et al.* 2002. First human study with a benzothiazole amyloid-imaging agent in Alzheimer's disease and control subjects. Neurobiol. Aging **23:** S429.

87. BACSKAI, B.J. *et al.* 2003. Four-dimensional multiphoton imaging of brain entry, amyloid binding, and clearance of an amyloid-{beta} ligand in transgenic mice. Proc. Natl. Acad. Sci. USA **100:** 12462–12467.

88. OKAMURA, N. *et al.* 2004. Styrylbenzoxazole derivatives for *in vivo* imaging of amyloid plaques in the brain. J. Neurosci. **24:** 2535–2541.

89. SUEMOTO, T. *et al.* 2004. *In vivo* labeling of amyloid with BF-108. Neurosci. Res. **48:** 65–74.

90. ZHUANG, Z.P. *et al.* 2003. Structure-activity relationship of imidazo[1,2-a]pyridines as ligands for detecting beta-amyloid plaques in the brain. J. Med. Chem. **46:** 237–243.

91. ZHEN, W. *et al.* 1999. Synthesis and amyloid binding properties of rhenium complexes: preliminary progress toward a reagent for SPECT imaging of Alzheimer's disease brain. J. Med. Chem. **42:** 2805–2815.

92. SKOVRONSKY, D.M. *et al.* 2000. *In vivo* detection of amyloid plaques in a mouse model of Alzheimer's disease. Proc. Natl. Acad. Sci. USA **97:** 7609–7614.

93. HINTERSTEINER, M. *et al.* 2005. *In vivo* detection of amyloid-beta deposits by near-infrared imaging using an oxazine-derivative probe. Nat. Biotechnol. **23:** 577–583.

94. WENGENACK, T.M., G.L. CURRAN & J.F. PODUSLO. 2000. Targeting Alzheimer amyloid plaques *in vivo*. Nat. Biotechnol. **18:** 868–872.

95. JANKOWSKY, J.L. *et al.* 2005. Persistent amyloidosis following suppression of AB producyion in a transgenic model of Alzheimer's disease. PLoS Medicine 2: e355.

# Diffusion Tensor Imaging of Normal Appearing White Matter and Its Correlation with Cognitive Functioning in Mild Cognitive Impairment and Alzheimer's Disease

JUEBIN HUANG AND ALEXANDER P. AUCHUS

*University of Tennessee Health Science Center, Memphis, Tennessee, USA*

ABSTRACT: Diffusion tensor imaging (DTI) was used to examine the microstructural integrity of normal appearing white matter (NAWM) in subjects with mild cognitive impairment (MCI) and Alzheimer's disease (AD). Significant frontal, temporal, and parietal white matter diffusion tensor changes were demonstrated in MCI and AD compared with normal controls. These changes were correlated with cognitive functioning, and are consistent with a hypothesized loss of axonal processes in affected regions.

KEYWORDS: mild cognitive impairment; Alzheimer's disease; diffusion tensor imaging; Wallerian degeneration

## INTRODUCTION

Structural magnetic resonance imaging (MRI) studies on mild cognitive impairment (MCI) and Alzheimer's disease (AD) have largely focused on the brain's cortical gray matter. Although pathoanatomical and imaging studies have confirmed both microscopic and macroscopic white matter changes (WMC) in patients with AD and MCI, controversy exists regarding the relevance of WMC, the pathogenic mechanisms producing WMC, and the association of WMC with cognitive dysfunction.[1] The diffusion tensor imaging (DTI) technique provides increased sensitivity for detecting ultrastructural abnormalities of white matter *in vivo*.[2] Previous studies suggest that the pattern of white matter diffusion changes, as measured by fractional anisotropy (FA), water diffusivity parallel to axonal fibers (axial diffusivity: DA), and water diffusivity perpendicular to axonal fibers (radial diffusivity: DR), can be used

Address for correspondence: Juebin Huang, M.D., Ph.D., Department of Neurology, University of Tennessee Health Science Center, 855 Monroe Ave., Suite 415, Memphis, TN 38163. Voice: 901-523-8990; ext.: 7606; fax: 901-577-7273.

jhuang8@utmem.edu

Ann. N.Y. Acad. Sci. 1097: 259–264 (2007). © 2007 New York Academy of Sciences.
doi: 10.1196/annals.1379.021

to examine the underlying mechanisms of WMC secondary to myelin damage or axonal loss (e.g., as in Wallerian degeneration).[3,4]

In this study, we hypothesized that DTI would detect microstructural changes in areas of "normal appearing" white matter on traditional MR images, in MCI and early AD. We further hypothesized that these changes would correlate with measures of cognitive dysfunction.

# METHODS

## Subjects

Elderly subjects with normal cognition ($n = 6$), MCI ($n = 8$), and mild AD ($n = 4$) were recruited from the Alzheimer's Disease Research Center (ADRC) at Case Western Reserve University (CWRU). All MCI subjects met Petersen et al.'s criteria for amnestic MCI.[5] All AD subjects met the National Institute of Neurological and Communicative Diseases and Stroke–Alzheimer's Disease and Related Disorders Association (NINCDS–ADRDA)'s criteria for possible or probable AD.[6] Results of the Consortium to Establish a Registry for Alzheimer's Disease (CERAD) Neuropsychological Battery with Trail-making Test[7] examined within 1 year from enrollment were obtained from the ADRC database (TABLE 1). The study was approved by the Institutional Review Board of CWRU. Informed consent was obtained from all subjects.

TABLE 1. Descriptive demographics and cognitive test results*

|  | AD ($n = 4$) | MCI ($n = 8$) | NC ($n = 6$) |
|---|---|---|---|
| Age (years) | $73.75 \pm 6.08$ | $74.75 \pm 8.55$ | $71.17 \pm 5.74$ |
| Gender (Female/Male) | 2/2 | 4/4 | 4/2 |
| Education (years) | $14.25 \pm 1.71$ | $15.00 \pm 2.45$ | $14.0 \pm 2.10$ |
| Mini-mental state exam (MMSE) | $24.75 \pm 1.50^a$ | $26.63 \pm 2.56^a$ | $29.50 \pm 0.84$ |
| Verbal fluency (VF) | $10.50 \pm 1.92^{ac}$ | $16.50 \pm 3.62^a$ | $21.83 \pm 5.64$ |
| Boston naming (BN) | $13.25 \pm 0.50$ | $13.33 \pm 2.89$ | $14.33 \pm 0.82$ |
| Constructional praxis (CP) | $9.50 \pm 2.38$ | $9.33 \pm 2.88$ | $10.83 \pm 0.41$ |
| Word list memory total (WLM) | $14.75 \pm 5.56^a$ | $17.00 \pm 3.52$ | $22.67 \pm 4.37$ |
| Word list delayed recall (WLDR) | $2.25 \pm 1.50^a$ | $4.00 \pm 2.61^b$ | $8.40 \pm 1.20$ |
| Word list recognition (WLR) | $17.75 \pm 1.50^a$ | $18.67 \pm 1.37$ | $19.83 \pm 0.41$ |
| Constructional praxis recall (CPR) | $3.50 \pm 3.70^a$ | $7.17 \pm 3.43$ | $11.17 \pm 1.60$ |
| Trial making test, Part A (TMA) | $107.25 \pm 99.36^a$ | $44.17 \pm 17.53$ | $28.83 \pm 14.23$ |
| Trial making test, Part B (TMB) | $178.33 \pm 87.64^a$ | $118.39 \pm 62.55$ | $63.00 \pm 22.20$ |

$^aP < 0.05$ vs. Control; $^bP < 0.01$ vs. Control. $^cP < 0.05$ vs. MCI.
*M $\pm$ SD except Gender; AD = Alzheimer's disease; MCI = mild cognitive impairment; NC = normal control.

## MRI Acquisition Protocol

Conventional axial $T_1$, $T_2$, FLAIR, and DTI sequences were acquired along the AC-PC line with a 1.5 Tesla Siemens Symphony MR System. DTI images were acquired with a single shot, pulsed gradient, echo planar imaging protocol (TR = 8,000 ms, TE = 109 ms, Field of view = 240 × 240 mm, Matrix = 128 × 128, in-plane resolution 1.875 × 1.875, slice thickness 3 mm). Diffusion gradients were applied in 12 noncollinear directions with 2 b values (0 and 1,000 s/mm$^2$), Time per DTI acquisition = 7:06 min.

## DTI Processing

DTI dataset processing was performed using DTI Studio (Johns Hopkins University, Baltimore, MD http://cmrm.med.jhmi.edu). From 12 apparent diffusion coefficient maps, the maps of fractional anisotropy (FA) and three eigenvalues ($\lambda_1$, $\lambda_2$, $\lambda_3$) were determined. Normal appearing white matter (NAWM) was defined by normal signal intensity on standard $T_1$-weighted, $T_2$-weighted, and FLAIR images. Regions of interest (ROI) were placed bilaterally on images acquired without diffusion gradients (b = 0 s/mm$^2$). Small oval ROIs of 9~16 pixels (31.64~56.25 mm$^2$) were placed in the frontal, temporal, and parietal NAWM with 5 contiguous slices, and in the normal appearing occipital white matter with 3 contiguous slices. ROIs were then superimposed in identical slices on different tensor maps. FA, radial diffusivity ($[\lambda_2 + \lambda_3]/2$), and axial diffusivity ($\lambda_1$) for each ROI were recorded. For each subject, the measures of FA, DA, and DR were averaged across all the slices of each white matter area bilaterally.

## Statistic Analysis

Groups were compared using analysis of variance (ANOVA) or Kruskal–Wallis test as appropriate, with *post hoc* Scheffe or Mann–Whitney U test as appropriate. Correlations were evaluated by Spearman's ranks correlation.

## RESULTS

There were no significant differences in age, gender, and educational level between the three groups. Compared with normal controls, AD subjects scored significantly poorer on most cognitive tests, while MCI subjects demonstrated less degrees of cognitive impairment. (See TABLE 1).

Compared to normal controls, MCI subjects demonstrated decreased FA ($P = 0.008$) and decreased DA ($P = 0.01$) in temporal NAWM, while

AD subjects demonstrated decreased FA ($P = 0.01$), decreased DA ($P = 0.01$), and increased DR ($P = 0.01$) (See TABLE 2). In parietal NAWM, MCI showed decreased FA ($P = 0.001$), increased DR ($P = 0.003$), and AD showed increased DR ($P = 0.01$), compared to normal controls. AD also showed significantly increased DR ($P = 0.04$) in frontal NAWM compared to normal controls. Neither MCI nor AD showed any significant differences in diffusion tensor changes in occipital NAWM versus normal controls.

Since the MCI and AD groups did not differ from each other on any diffusion tensor measurement, we combined the two groups for correlation analyses with cognitive test results. Temporal NAWM diffusion measurements were significantly correlated with episodic memory (WLM with DR: $r_s = -0.68$, $P = 0.03$; WLDR with FA: $r_s = 0.66$, $P = 0.04$; WLDR with DR: $r_s = -0.77$, $P = 0.009$). Frontal WM diffusion measurements were significantly correlated with both episodic memory and executive function (WLM with DR: $r_s = -0.70$, $P = 0.03$; WLM with DA: $r_s = -0.75$, $P = 0.01$; WLDR with FA: $r_s = 0.65$, $P = 0.04$; WLDR with DR: $r_s = -0.77$, $P = 0.01$; TMA with DA: $r_s = 0.75$, $P = 0.01$; TMA with DR: $r_s = 0.69$, $P = 0.03$). Parietal WM DR was significantly correlated with general cognition as measured by MMSE total scores ($r_s = -0.66$, $P = 0.04$).

TABLE 2. Diffusion tensor measurements (Mean $\pm$ SD) of selected normal appearing white matter regions among AD, MCI, and normal control subjects

|  | AD ($n = 4$) | MCI ($n = 8$) | NC ($n = 6$) |
|---|---|---|---|
| Frontal NAWM |  |  |  |
| FA | $0.28 \pm 0.02$ | $0.30 \pm 0.04$ | $0.34 \pm 0.05$ |
| DA | $1.12 \pm 0.10$ | $1.04 \pm 0.06$ | $1.07 \pm 0.04$ |
| DR | $0.74 \pm 0.05^a$ | $0.68 \pm 0.05$ | $0.65 \pm 0.06$ |
| Temporal NAWM |  |  |  |
| FA | $0.41 \pm 0.02^a$ | $0.44 \pm 0.02^b$ | $0.51 \pm 0.05$ |
| DA | $1.21 \pm 0.04^a$ | $1.21 \pm 0.07^a$ | $1.30 \pm 0.03$ |
| DR | $0.64 \pm 0.04^a$ | $0.60 \pm 0.05$ | $0.55 \pm 0.05$ |
| Parietal NAWM |  |  |  |
| FA | $0.40 \pm 0.05$ | $0.40 \pm 0.03^b$ | $0.45 \pm 0.02$ |
| DA | $1.15 \pm 0.10$ | $1.11 \pm 0.04$ | $1.16 \pm 0.04$ |
| DR | $0.62 \pm 0.01^a$ | $0.61 \pm 0.02^b$ | $0.57 \pm 0.02$ |
| Occipital NAWM |  |  |  |
| FA | $0.45 \pm 0.03$ | $0.45 \pm 0.05$ | $0.44 \pm 0.07$ |
| DA | $1.22 \pm 0.03$ | $1.24 \pm 0.11$ | $1.23 \pm 0.12$ |
| DR | $0.60 \pm 0.03$ | $0.60 \pm 0.05$ | $0.60 \pm 0.07$ |

[a]$P < 0.05$ vs. Control; [b]$P < 0.01$ vs. Control. All DA and DR are in units of $10^{-9}$ mm$^2$/s.

NAWM = normal appearing white matter; FA = fractional anisotropy; DA = axial diffusivity; DR = radial diffusivity; AD = Alzheimer's disease; MCI = mild cognitive impairment; NC = normal control.

# DISCUSSION

In this study, we found evidence suggesting microstructural white matter changes in early AD and MCI in NAWM. These changes were present in brain regions serving higher cortical functions (temporal, parietal, and frontal lobes), but not in regions serving primary functions (occipital lobe). These findings are consistent with several previous DTI investigations that reported changes of anisotropy or diffusivities in the white matter of temporal, frontal, and parietal lobes.[8–10] The correlation between DTI parameters and cognitive functioning has not been analyzed comprehensively, although a few reports have demonstrated that performances in general cognition (MMSE) as well as delayed verbal recall test correlated significantly with changes of anisotropy and diffusivity of selected white matter regions.[8,11] This study confirmed previous observations and provided further specific information that the diffusion tensor abnormalities demonstrated in different brain white matter regions were associated with different cognitive dysfunction, for example, temporal diffusion tensor changes were correlated with episodic memory, frontal diffusion tensor changes were correlated with executive function and episodic memory, while parietal diffusion tensor changes were correlated with general cognition. These correlations suggested that the damage of white matter integrity might contribute to the loss of connectivity between different cortical functional regions in AD patients.

The pathogenic mechanisms of microscopic white matter damage in AD and MCI are unclear. Our results show that, in NAWM of the temporal lobe, the diffusivity parallel to the white matter fibers (DA) is significantly decreased, while diffusivity perpendicular to the white matter fibers (DR) is significantly increased in AD subjects. This pattern of diffusion change is characteristically observed with axon-related pathologies (e.g., as in Wallerian degeneration).[3] In contrast, myelin-related pathologies produce increased DR without changing DA.[4] However, we did not reveal similar patterns of diffusion changes in other brain regions, even though the parietal NAWM DA was also decreased compared with normal controls with borderline significance in the MCI group ($P = 0.07$). We may argue that because the pathology burden (especially neuronal loss) in other brain regions is not as severe as in the temporal lobe of MCI or early AD subjects, the typical diffusion features of Wallerian degeneration may not be detectable with our small sample size. And also, the pattern of diffusion change secondary to myelin-related or axon-related mechanisms also depends strongly on the preexisting regional architecture of white matter as well as other factors (e.g., vascular ischemic mechanism) that may change the amount and directional diffusivities of tissue water.[3]

This preliminary study suggested that DTI is a promising technique to identify microstructural white matter damage of AD and to test the hypothesis that Wallerian degeneration may be an important mechanism underlying these pathological changes.

## ACKNOWLEDGMENTS

This work was supported by grant from NIA (P50AG08012). The authors thank Sherye Sirrel for an outstanding job in recruiting participants in this study.

## REFERENCES

1. ENGLUND, E. 1998. Neuropathology of white matter changes in Alzheimer's disease and vascular dementia. Dement. Geriatr. Cogn. Disord. 9(Suppl 1): 6–12.
2. PIERPAOLI, C., P. JEZZARD, P.J. BASSER, et al. 1996. Diffusion tensor MR imaging of the human brain. Radiology 201: 637–648.
3. PIERPAOLI, C., A. BARNETT, S. PAJEVIC, et al. 2001. Water diffusion changes in Wallerian degeneration and their dependence on white matter architecture. Neuroimage 13: 1174–1185.
4. SONG, S.K., S.W. SUN, M.J. RAMSBOTTOM, et al. 2002. Dysmyelination revealed through MRI as increased radial (but unchanged axial) diffusion of water. Neuroimage 17: 1429–1436.
5. PETERSEN, R.C., R. DOODY, A. KURZ, et al. 2001. Current concepts in mild cognitive impairment. Arch. Neurol. 58: 1985–1992.
6. MCKHANN, G., D. DRACHMAN, M. FOLSTEIN, et al. 1984. Clinical diagnosis of Alzheimer's disease: report of the NINCDS-ADRDA work group under the auspices of the Department of Health & Human Services Task Forces on Alzheimer's Disease. Neurology 34: 939–944.
7. WELSH, K.A., N. BUTTERS, R.C. MOHS, et al. 1994. The Consortium to Establish a Registry for Alzheimer's Disease (CERAD). Part V. A normative study of the neuropsychological battery. Neurology 44: 609–614.
8. BOZZALI, M., A. FALINI, M. FRANCESCHI, et al. 2002. White matter damage in Alzheimer's disease assessed *in vivo* using diffusion tensor magnetic resonance imaging. J. Neurol. Neurosurg. Psychiatry 72: 742–746.
9. FELLGIEBEL, A., P. WILLE, M.J. MULLER, et al. 2004. Ultrastructural hippocampal and white matter alterations in mild cognitive impairment: a diffusion tensor imaging study. Dement. Geriatr. Cogn. Disord. 18: 101–108.
10. NAGGARA, O., C. OPPENHEIM, D. RIEU, et al. 2006. Diffusion tensor imaging in early Alzheimer's disease. Psychiatry Res. 146: 243–249.
11. FELLGIEBEL, A., M.J. MULLER, P. WILLE, et al. 2005. Color-coded diffusion-tensor-imaging of posterior cingulate fiber tracts in mild cognitive impairment. Neurobiol. Aging 26: 1193–1198.

# Enhanced Ryanodine-Mediated Calcium Release in Mutant PS1-Expressing Alzheimer's Mouse Models

GRACE E. STUTZMANN,[a] IAN SMITH,[b] ANTONELLA CACCAMO,[b] SALVATORE ODDO,[b] IAN PARKER,[b] AND FRANK LAFERLA[b]

[a]Department of Neuroscience, Rosalind Franklin University of Medicine and Science, The Chicago Medical School, Chicago, Illinois, USA

[b]Department of Neurobiology and Behavior, University of California, Irvine, California, USA

ABSTRACT: Intracellular $Ca^{2+}$ signaling involves $Ca^{2+}$ liberation through both inositol triphosphate and ryanodine receptors ($IP_3R$ and RyR). However, little is known of the functional interactions between these $Ca^{2+}$ sources in either neuronal physiology, or during $Ca^{2+}$ disruptions associated with Alzheimer's disease (AD). By the use of whole-cell recordings and 2-photon $Ca^{2+}$ imaging in cortical slices we distinguished between $IP_3R$- and RyR-mediated $Ca^{2+}$ components in nontransgenic (non-Tg) and AD mouse models and demonstrate powerful signaling interactions between these channels. $Ca^{2+}$-induced $Ca^{2+}$ release (CICR) through RyR contributed modestly to $Ca^{2+}$ signals evoked by photoreleased $IP_3$ in cortical neurons from non-Tg mice. In contrast, the exaggerated signals in $3 \times Tg$-AD and $PS1_{KI}$ mice resulted primarily from enhanced CICR through RyR, rather than through $IP_3R$, and were associated with increased RyR expression levels. Moreover, membrane hyperpolarizations evoked by $IP_3$ in neurons from AD mouse models were even greater than expected simply from the exaggerated $Ca^{2+}$ signals, pointing to an increased coupling efficiency between cytosolic $[Ca^{2+}]$ and $K^+$ channel regulation. Our results highlight the critical roles of RyR-mediated $Ca^{2+}$ signaling in both neuronal physiology and pathophysiology, and point to *presenilin*-linked disruptions in RyR signaling as an important genetic factor in AD.

KEYWORDS: IP3; endoplasmic reticulum; 2-photon; electrophysiology; calcium; Alzheimer; PS1; $3 \times Tg$-AD; transgenic; ryanodine; cortex; neuron

Address for correspondence: Grace E. Stutzmann, Ph.D., Department of Neuroscience, Rosalind Franklin University of Medicine and Science, The Chicago Medical School, 3333 Green Bay Road, North Chicago, IL 60064. Voice: 847-578-8540; fax: 847- 578-8515.
grace.stutzmann@rosalindfranklin.edu

Ann. N.Y. Acad. Sci. 1097: 265–277 (2007). © 2007 New York Academy of Sciences.
doi: 10.1196/annals.1379.025

## INTRODUCTION

Neuronal $Ca^{2+}$ signaling is tightly controlled to ensure proper operation of a myriad of $Ca^{2+}$-dependent processes.[1,2] Two major sources contribute to cytosolic $Ca^{2+}$ signals; an extracellular pool entering through plasma membrane channels, and an internal reservoir in the endoplasmic reticulum (ER) that is liberated by opening of inositol triphosphate- and ryanodine-receptor/channels ($IP_3R$ and RyR). The activation of both $IP_3R$ and RyR channels is promoted by cytosolic $Ca^{2+}$, resulting in a regenerative process of $Ca^{2+}$-induced $Ca^{2+}$ release (CICR).[3-5] The feed-forward action of $Ca^{2+}$ to enhance its own release through $IP_3R$ and RyR introduces considerable complexity in $Ca^{2+}$ signaling, and enables interactions between these different pathways.

Growing evidence implicates disruptions of $Ca^{2+}$ signaling in the etiology of neurological diseases.[6-8] In particular, mutations in *presenilin* (*PS*) genes associated with Alzheimer's disease (AD) increase $IP_3R$-evoked $Ca^{2+}$ release in a variety of cells.[9-11] Previous studies focused on responses evoked by elevating intracellular $IP_3$ either directly *via* flash photolysis of caged $IP_3$[10,11] or indirectly by agonist application,[9,12] and did not explicitly address the role of RyR in AD. Nevertheless, there is evidence pointing to RyR involvement. RyR expression levels are increased in cultured neurons expressing the $PS1_{M146V}$ mutation,[13,14] the RyR blocker dantrolene has been shown to reverse the elevated carbachol-induced $Ca^{2+}$ release seen in SH-SY5Y cells expressing a mutant *PS1*,[15] and the RyR agonist caffeine evokes larger $Ca^{2+}$ liberation in cultured neurons from transgenic AD mouse models.[14]

Here, we explore RyR involvement in neuronal functioning in both normal physiology, and during $Ca^{2+}$ signaling disruptions associated with AD. For the latter purpose we employed two mouse models of AD: the $PS1_{M146V}$ mutant knockin, and a triple-transgenic mouse model ($3 \times$Tg-AD).[16] Both transgenic mice display similarly exaggerated neuronal $Ca^{2+}$ signals to $IP_3$ at all ages, but whereas the $PS1_{KI}$ mice fail to show AD histopathology, the $3 \times$Tg-AD mice develop $\beta$A plaques and neurofibrillary tangles in an age- and a region-specific manner. We show that RyR activation contributes modestly to $Ca^{2+}$ signals in nontransgenic (non-Tg) control mice, but accounts for almost all of the exaggerated ER $Ca^{2+}$ signals in the $PS1_{KI}$ and $3 \times$Tg-AD transgenic mice models. Moreover, in all groups, $IP_3$-dependent membrane hyperpolarizations are regulated primarily through RyR, and the transgenic mice show hyperpolarizing responses even greater than expected from the enhanced $Ca^{2+}$ signals. Thus, RyR contribute largely to the exaggerated $Ca^{2+}$ signals associated with AD-linked mutations in *presenilin,* and may thereby present a target for therapeutic intervention.

# RESULTS

## *Exaggeration of IP₃-Evoked Ca²⁺ Signals in PS1_{KI} and 3×Tg-AD Neurons*

Individual neurons were loaded with caged $IP_3$ and fura-2 by dialysis through the patch pipette, and flashes of UV light of varying durations were applied to photorelease $IP_3$. The resulting ER $Ca^{2+}$ liberation was monitored by imaging fura-2 fluorescence from the soma (excluding the nucleus) and the proximal dendrites using a custom-built 2-photon imaging system, and by measuring changes in membrane potential resulting from activation of $Ca^{2+}$-dependent $K^+$ channels. In addition, depolarizing current pulses were applied to evoke action potentials and accompanying entry of $Ca^{2+}$ through VGCC.

FIGURE 1 A presents a scatter plot of individual $IP_3$-evoked responses evoked by selected flash durations, and FIGURE 1 B plots the mean amplitude of these responses as a function of flash duration (proportional to the amount of photoreleased $IP_3$) in the soma. The mean $Ca^{2+}$ responses in $PS1_{KI}$ and $3×Tg$-AD neurons were appreciably ($P < 0.05$) larger than in non-Tg control cells for all flash durations, with the greatest enhancement seen with 30 ms flashes (316% for $PS1_{KI}$ and 342% for $3×Tg$-AD neurons); but were not significantly different from one another. In marked contrast, no significant differences in spike-evoked $Ca^{2+}$ signals were apparent between non-Tg, $PS1_{KI}$, and $3×$ Tg-AD groups ($P = 0.24$).

## *Enhanced RyR-Mediated Ca²⁺ Release Predominates in ER-Ca²⁺ Dysregulation*

To ascertain the extent of the RyR-mediated component in the $IP_3$-evoked $Ca^{2+}$ signals, we first determined the relative RyR contribution by comparing somatic signals evoked by photoreleased $IP_3$ (FIG. 2 A, B) before and after bath-applying 10 μM dantrolene to block RyR. In non-Tg neurons dantrolene caused a modest ($20 ± 7\%$, $n = 6$) reduction in signals evoked by 50 ms flashes, and action potential-evoked $Ca^{2+}$ signals were reduced by $15 ± 5\%$. In marked contrast, dantrolene substantially reduced the $IP_3$-evoked $Ca^{2+}$ responses in $PS1_{KI}$ neurons (by $59 ± 11\%$, $n = 6$; $P < 0.01$) and in $3×Tg$-AD neurons (by $71 ± 9\%$, $n = 7$; $P < 0.01$). However, similar to non-Tg neurons, dantrolene produced only modest (15–20%) reductions of the spike-evoked $Ca^{2+}$ signals.

The effects of dantrolene on the dose-response relationship for $IP_3$-evoked $Ca^{2+}$ signals are shown in Figure 2 C. Responses in $PS1_{KI}$ and $3×Tg$-AD neurons were not significantly different from one another ($P > 0.05$), and we therefore combined these data (Tg) for analysis. Dantrolene strongly suppressed $Ca^{2+}$ signals in the pooled Tg neurons ($n = 19$) across the full range

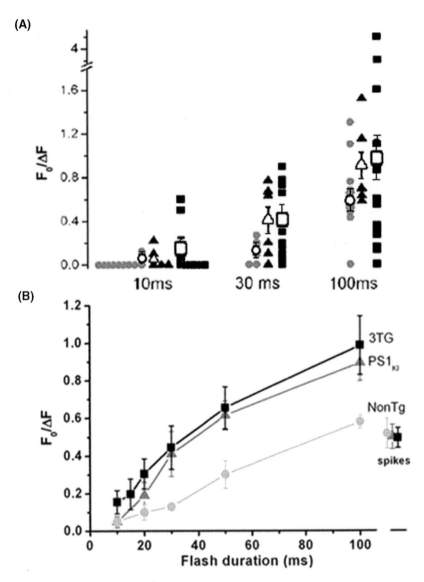

**FIGURE 1.** $IP_3$-evoked $Ca^{2+}$ signals are exaggerated in both $PS1_{KI}$ and $3\times Tg$-AD mice. (**A**) Peak amplitudes of $IP_3$-evoked somatic $Ca^{2+}$ signals evoked by photolysis flash durations of 10, 30, and 100 ms in individual non-Tg (*circles*), $PS1_{KI}$ (*triangles*), and $3\times Tg$-AD neurons (*squares*). Open symbols with error bars indicate corresponding means and standard errors. Average $PS1_{KI}$ and $3\times Tg$-AD $Ca^{2+}$ amplitudes were significantly ($P < 0.05$) larger for the 30 and 100 ms flash durations relative to the non-Tg values. (**B**) Mean peak amplitudes of somatic $Ca^{2+}$ signals as a function of photolysis flash duration; data are from 12–14 neurons for each group. Points at the right indicate mean $Ca^{2+}$ signals evoked by action potential trains. Data from non-Tg mice are indicated by *light-gray circles* (●), $PS1_{KI}$ mice by *dark-gray triangles* (▲), and $3\times Tg$-AD mice by *black squares* (■).

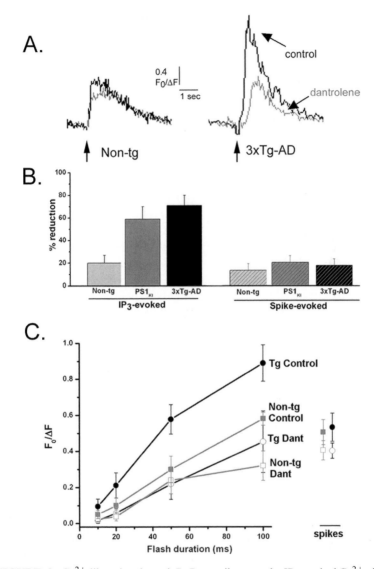

**FIGURE 2.** $Ca^{2+}$ liberation through RyR contributes to the $IP_3$-evoked $Ca^{2+}$ signals. (**A**) $IP_3$-evoked $Ca^{2+}$ signals are reduced by the RyR blocker dantrolene. Traces show $Ca^{2+}$ responses evoked by a 50 ms flash in control conditions (*black*) and in the presence of bath-applied dantrolene (*gray*), in representative non-Tg (*left*) and $3\times$Tg-AD (*right*) neurons. (**B**) Mean percentage reductions in amplitudes of $IP_3$-evoked $Ca^{2+}$ responses (50 ms flash duration) and spike-evoked $Ca^{2+}$ signals resulting from application of dantrolene (10 μM) in non-Tg ($n = 6$), $PS1_{KI}$ ($n = 6$), and $3\times$Tg-AD ($n = 7$) neurons. (**C**) Effect of dantrolene on the dose-response relationship of $IP_3$-evoked $Ca^{2+}$ signals. Points show measurements from non-Tg neurons ($n = 12$; *squares*) and pooled measurements from $3\times$Tg-AD and $PS1_{KI}$ neurons (Tg, $n = 25$, *circles*) before (*filled symbols*) and after (*open symbols*) applying dantrolene. Data at the right show respective spike-evoked $Ca^{2+}$ signals.

of flash durations tested (FIG. 2 C; circles), whereas the reduction in non-Tg neurons ($n = 6$) was less pronounced (FIG. 2 C; squares). Importantly, there were no significant differences ($P > 0.05$) between Tg and non-Tg groups in the $Ca^{2+}$ signals remaining in the presence of dantrolene, suggesting that $Ca^{2+}$ flux through the $IP_3R$ channels themselves is not appreciably enhanced by the AD-linked mutations, but rather that larger responses in the Tg neurons arises principally from greater CICR through RyR. In contrast to the $IP_3$-evoked $Ca^{2+}$ signals, spike-evoked $Ca^{2+}$ signals were reduced to a similar extent in both the non-Tg and Tg neurons.

### RyR Expression Levels Are Increased in Both PS1$_{KI}$ and 3 × Tg-AD Mice

We performed Western blot analyses of several $Ca^{2+}$ signaling-related proteins in the brains of non-Tg, PS1$_{KI,}$ and 3×Tg-AD mice at ages (4–6 weeks) equivalent to those used in the imaging studies. There were no significant differences ($P = 0.46$) in cortical expression levels of $IP_3R$, SERCA-2B, calsenilin, calbindin-D, or calreticulin (data not shown). However, RyR levels were significantly enhanced (FIG. 3; ~2-fold; ANOVA $F_{(2,8)} = 9.41$, $P \leq 0.01$) in the PS1$_{KI}$ and 3×Tg-AD mice relative to non-Tg controls (Fischer *post hoc* analysis, $P = 0.04$ and $0.005$, respectively). RyR levels in PS1$_{KI}$ and 3×Tg-AD mice were not different from each other ($P = 0.14$).

### IP$_3$-Evoked Membrane Hyperpolarization Is Driven by $Ca^{2+}$ Liberation through RyR

$IP_3$ evokes a membrane hyperpolarization in cortical neurons *via* activation of $Ca^{2+}$-dependent $K^+$ channels[17,18] and this hyperpolarization is enhanced in

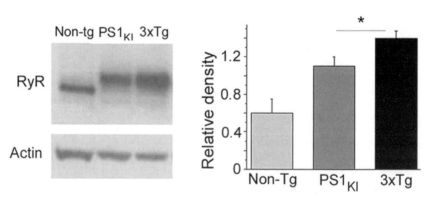

**FIGURE 3.** Tg neurons show enhanced expression of RyR and expression of mutant transgenes. *Left*: representative Western blots from homogenized non-Tg, PS1$_{KI,}$ and 3×Tg-AD cortices demonstrating differences in RyR levels relative to β-actin. *Right*: RyR levels in the PS1$_{KI}$ and 3×Tg-AD mice were significantly greater (~2-fold) than non-Tg levels ($P < 0.05$), but were not different from each other.

PS1$_{KI}$ mice.[18,19] Here, we sought to determine whether the K$^+$ channel regulation primarily involves Ca$^{2+}$ liberated through the IP$_3$R channels themselves, or is consequent to CICR through RyR channels.

Representative membrane potential responses to photorelease of IP$_3$ in non-Tg and 3×Tg-AD neurons are shown in FIGURE 4 A, and were appreciably smaller and of lower sensitivity in the non-Tg cells. These differences did not arise through differences in initial resting membrane potential (set to −60 mV by current injection) or input resistance. Strikingly, all responses

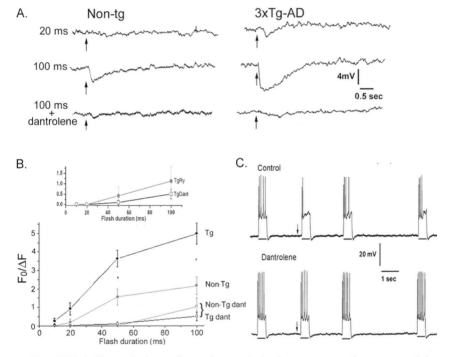

**FIGURE 4.** IP$_3$-evoked membrane hyperpolarizations are strongly suppressed by dantrolene. (**A**) Traces show (*from top to bottom*) changes in membrane potential in representative neurons from non-Tg (*left*) and 3×Tg-AD mice (*right*) following photolysis flashes of 20 and 100 ms duration, and the almost complete block of the response to a 100 ms flash in the presence of dantrolene (10 μM). (**B**) Relationships between photolysis flash duration and magnitude of the IP$_3$-evoked hyperpolarization. Main graph shows data from non-Tg (*n* = 17, *black squares*) and Tg neurons (*n* = 31, *gray circles*), before (*filled symbols*) and during (*open symbols*) dantrolene application. Inset: Mean data comparing effects of ryanodine in Tg neurons (*n* = 16; *closed circles*) with dantrolene in Tg neurons (*open squares*, same data as in the main graph). (**C**) IP$_3$-mediated reduction in spiking frequency is suppressed by dantrolene. The upper trace shows spikes evoked by periodic injections of depolarizing current. A photolysis flash (100 ms) was delivered at the arrow to photorelease IP$_3$, resulting in a reduced spiking frequency for several seconds. The lower trace was obtained using the same protocol in the same neuron while continually superfusing dantrolene (10 μM).

were substantially abolished by dantrolene (FIG. 4 A, lower traces), even in the $3 \times$ Tg-AD neuron following a strong (100 ms) flash. Mean data for non-Tg and Tg neurons in control and dantrolene conditions are plotted in FIGURE 4 B. Hyperpolarizing responses in both non-Tg and Tg neurons increased with increasing photorelease of $IP_3$ but, for a given flash duration, the responses in Tg neurons were nearly three times as large (3.04-fold with 50 ms flashes, $P <$ 0.01: and 2.7-fold with 100 ms flashes, $P \leq 0.01$). After adding dantrolene, only small $IP_3$-evoked hyperpolarizations remained with the strongest flashes, and were not significantly different between non-Tg and Tg neurons ($P >$ 0.05).

$IP_3$-evoked changes in membrane conductance strongly regulate spiking patterns, and photorelease of $IP_3$ caused a long-lasting reduction in numbers of action potentials evoked by depolarizing current pulses (FIG. 4 C, upper trace). This modulation was abolished by dantrolene (FIG. 4 C, lower trace).

### AD-Linked Mutations Affect the Coupling between RyR and Membrane $K^+$ Channels

The greater $IP_3$-evoked membrane hyperpolarization seen in neurons expressing AD-linked mutations might arise directly as a consequence of the enhanced ER $Ca^{2+}$ release. However, this appears not to be the sole mechanism, because scatter graphs plotting the relationship between $IP_3$-evoked hyperpolarization amplitude ($-\Delta mV$) and the accompanying $IP_3$-evoked $Ca^{2+}$ signals ($F_0/\Delta F$) revealed markedly different slopes between non-Tg and Tg neurons for both soma (FIG. 5 A) and dendrite (FIG. 5 B). That is to say, a given cytosolic $Ca^{2+}$ signal was associated with a larger membrane hyperpolarization in Tg neurons, suggesting that the AD-linked mutations modulate the "coupling efficiency" between cytosolic $Ca^{2+}$ signals and activation of membrane $K^+$ conductance, as well as enhancing the $Ca^{2+}$ signals.

To explore the mechanism underlying this effect, we constructed a similar scatter plot of hyperpolarization *versus* $Ca^{2+}$ signal amplitude after adding dantrolene to block RyR (FIG. 5 C). As noted before, both $Ca^{2+}$ and membrane potential signals were strongly reduced, requiring pooled measurements from the soma and dendrite to obtain sufficient data points. Regression lines showed a slope for non-Tg neurons that was not appreciably different from that in control conditions without dantrolene, whereas in Tg neurons the slope was dramatically reduced as a result of blocking RyR. Our findings are further summarized in FIGURE 5 D. Key points are: (1) The slope of the relationship between membrane hyperpolarization ($-\Delta V$) and $Ca^{2+}$ ($F_0/\Delta F$) was steeper (5.9) in Tg than in non-Tg neurons (3.15). (2) The slope in Tg neurons was greatly reduced by dantrolene, but was almost unchanged in non-Tg neurons. (3) The amplitudes of $IP_3$-evoked $Ca^{2+}$ signals (measured from the soma, averaged across all flash durations) in Tg neurons were approximately double that in

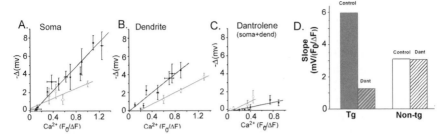

**FIGURE 5.** The relationship between the $IP_3$-evoked $Ca^{2+}$ signal and membrane hyperpolarization is steeper in Tg than in non-Tg neurons. (**A**) Scatter plot showing the relationship between $IP_3$-evoked $Ca^{2+}$ signal in the soma and the magnitude of the accompanying membrane hyperpolarization in neurons from non-Tg mice ($n = 14$; *open symbols, gray line*) and Tg mice ($n = 23$; *closed symbols, black line*). Points show means $\pm$ 1 SEM obtained after binning over selected ranges of fluorescence amplitudes. (**B**) Corresponding data for measurements in the proximal dendrites. (**C**) Corresponding data in dantrolene (10 $\mu$M), obtained after pooling data from soma and dendrites. (**D**) Dantrolene strongly reduces the slope of the relationship between $IP_3$-evoked membrane hyperpolarization and $Ca^{2+}$-fluorescence signal in Tg neurons, but has negligible effect in non-Tg neurons. Slope data were derived from the plots in (**A**, **B**, **C**).

non-Tg neurons, whereas membrane hyperpolarizations were more than three times larger. (4) Thus, RyR are critically involved in mediating the hyperpolarizing response evoked by $IP_3$. Moreover, AD-linked mutations appear to result in greater hyperpolarizing responses not only because they enhance the $Ca^{2+}$ signals, but also as a result of enhanced coupling efficiency between RyR and $Ca^{2+}$-activated $K^+$ conductance.

## DISCUSSION

### *Involvement of RyR in $IP_3$-Mediated Signaling in Neuronal Physiology and Pathophysiology*

The functional roles of intracellular $Ca^{2+}$ stores in neuronal signaling are becoming increasingly recognized, and include modulation of membrane excitability,[18,20] synaptic activity and plasticity,[21] and gene transcription.[22] To gain a more complete understanding of these intracellular $Ca^{2+}$ signaling mechanisms we attempted to parse their $IP_3R$ and RyR components so as to identify interactions between the two types of release channel and determine functions that may specifically be coupled to a particular channel.

Here, we show that $Ca^{2+}$ release evoked by $IP_3$ in cortical neurons from non-Tg mice arises primarily from $Ca^{2+}$ flux through $IP_3$ receptors themselves, with a modest additional component being added by $Ca^{2+}$ flux through RyR.

This balance, however, changes dramatically in transgenic mice expressing AD-linked mutations. *Presenilin* mutations are known to exaggerate ER-mediated $Ca^{2+}$ signaling in a variety of cell types, but this has implicitly been assumed to arise as a direct consequence of increased flux specifically through $IP_3R$ channels.[9-11] Instead, our results demonstrate that $Ca^{2+}$ flux through RyR accounts for the great majority of the exaggerated $IP_3$-evoked $Ca^{2+}$ response in AD transgenic mice. Consistent with this, neurons from AD transgenic mice showed larger $Ca^{2+}$ signals in response to the RyR agonist caffeine, and enhanced expression of cortical RyR levels. Interestingly, in the AD transgenic mice, the RyR component associated with VGCC activation was not different from the non-Tg. Thus, the enhancement of $Ca^{2+}$ signals by AD-linked mutations appears to arise primarily as a result of exaggerated $Ca^{2+}$ flux through RyR rather than through $IP_3R$, and specifically affects ER $Ca^{2+}$ signaling.

The RyR-mediated component of the intracellular $Ca^{2+}$ signals almost certainly arises because CICR through RyR is triggered by, and amplifies, the $Ca^{2+}$ liberated through $IP_3R$. Increased expression of RyR, as observed previously in cultured neurons[13,14] and in the brains of mice expressing the $PS1_{M146V}$ mutation,[19] provides a likely explanation for the exaggerated $IP_3$-evoked $Ca^{2+}$ signals. Moreover, CICR may be further enhanced by the actions of *PS1* mutations to enhance $Ca^{2+}$ filling of ER stores because elevated lumenal $[Ca^{2+}]$ is known to increase the sensitivity of RyR to both cytosolic $Ca^{2+}$ and caffeine.[23,24] Although increased store filling might also be expected to result in greater $Ca^{2+}$ flux through $IP_3R$—as has been observed in *Xenopus* oocytes, which lack RyR[10]—our present results may be reconciled if $Ca^{2+}$ stores in cortical neurons are enhanced sufficiently to sensitize RyR, while causing only a modest increase in $Ca^{2+}$ flux through $IP_3R$. Questions remain, however, as to why the $Ca^{2+}$ signals evoked by action potentials show relatively little RyR-mediated contribution; and why there is no appreciable enhancement of these signals in the transgenic mouse models of AD. An explanation may be that the voltage-gated $Ca^{2+}$ channels in the plasma membrane are located more distantly from RyR than are the $IP_3R$-channels, and are thus relatively ineffective in inducing CICR.

The mechanisms by which mutations in *PS* expression result in RyR up-regulation and exaggerated ER $Ca^{2+}$ release are presently unclear. One explanation draws on evidence showing that the *PS* mutations result in altered $\gamma$-secretase activity, which is responsible for the proteolysis of amyloid precursor protein (APP).[7] APP proteolysis generates several fragments, including the APP-intracellular domain fragment (AICD), which has been shown to regulate $IP_3$-mediated $Ca^{2+}$ signaling by possible transcriptional mechanisms.[25,26] Although the target proteins ultimately affected are not known in this case, the AICD transcriptional activity may serve to influence expression or function of the RyR.

## *Electrical Excitability Is Modulated by RyR*

Intracellular $Ca^{2+}$ plays an important role in modulating the electrical excitability of neurons, and AD-linked disruptions in $Ca^{2+}$ might thus be expected to have acute consequences for neuronal signaling, as well as for chronic disease pathology. Accordingly, we had found that hyperpolarizing responses to $IP_3$ are enhanced in $PS1_{KI}$ neurons,[11,19] probably because the enhanced cytosolic $Ca^{2+}$ signals evoke greater activation of $Ca^{2+}$-dependent membrane $K^+$ channels. We now show a similar exaggeration of $IP_3$-evoked hyperpolarizing responses in $3\times Tg$-AD neurons, and further demonstrate that in $3\times Tg$-AD, $PS_{KI}$, and non-Tg mice these membrane responses are mediated primarily by $Ca^{2+}$ liberated through RyR, rather than by the $Ca^{2+}$ directly liberated through $IP_3R$. In particular, blocking of RyR greatly reduced $IP_3$-evoked hyperpolarizations in both non-Tg and Tg neurons, resulting in almost identical membrane responses to a given flash duration.

The larger hyperpolarizing responses in the Tg neurons could most simply be accounted for as a direct consequence of the greater overall $Ca^{2+}$ signal. However, this appears not to be the sole explanation, because the membrane responses accompanying $Ca^{2+}$ signals of a given size were roughly twice as large in Tg versus non-Tg neurons: in other words, the Tg neurons showed a greater "coupling efficiency" between cytosolic $Ca^{2+}$ and activation of $Ca^{2+}$-dependent $K^+$ current. This may result if sites of $Ca^{2+}$ liberation through RyR are closer to the $Ca^{2+}$-dependent $K^+$ channels than are the sites of $IP_3R$-mediated $Ca^{2+}$ liberation. On this basis, the disproportionate hyperpolarization in Tg neurons arises because most of their exaggerated $Ca^{2+}$ signal arises through RyR; whereas after blocking RyR both Tg and non-Tg neurons show comparably small hyperpolarizations that are driven by the remaining $IP_3R$-mediated $Ca^{2+}$ liberation.

## CONCLUSIONS

Our results reveal important new aspects of $Ca^{2+}$ signaling disruptions associated with AD. Specifically, exaggeration of $IP_3$-evoked neuronal $Ca^{2+}$ signals is principally linked to mutations in *presenilin* and is largely independent of expression of $A\beta$ plaques or neurofibrillar tangles; these exaggerated signals are manifest throughout life and do not represent an acceleration of a normal aging process; and they arise principally through enhanced $Ca^{2+}$ flux through RyR, not $IP_3R$. Several crucial questions remain unanswered, including the mechanism by which mutations in *presenilin* modulate RyR-mediated signaling, and whether and how dysregulated $Ca^{2+}$ signaling may play a causative role in AD pathology. Nonetheless, these findings further strengthen the growing consensus that a calciumopathy may be at least partly responsible for neuronal degeneration in AD.

## REFERENCES

1. BERRIDGE, M., M. BOOTMAN & P. LIPP. 1998. Calcium—a life and death signal. Nature **395:** 645–649.
2. BERRIDGE, M., P. LIPP & M. BOOTMAN. 2000. The versatility and universality of calcium signaling. Mol. Cell Biol. **1:** 11–21.
3. FINCH, E., T. TURNER & S. GOLDIN. 1991. Calcium as a coagonist of inositol 1,4,5-triphosphate-induced calcium release. Science **252:** 443–446.
4. YAO, Y. & I. PARKER. 1992. Potentiation of inositol trisphosphate-induced $Ca^{2+}$ mobilization in Xenopus oocytes by cytosolic $Ca^{2+}$. J. Physiol. **458:** 319–338.
5. FRIEL, D.D. & R.W. TSIEN. 1992. A caffeine- and ryanodine-sensitive $Ca^{2+}$ store in bullfrog sympathetic neurones modulates effects of $Ca^{2+}$ entry on $[Ca^{2+}]_i$. J. Physiol. **450:** 217–246.
6. MATTSON, M. *et al.* 2000. Calcium signaling in the ER: its role in neuronal plasticity and neurodegenerative disorders. TINS **23:** 222–229.
7. LAFERLA, F.M. 2002. Calcium dyshomeostasis and intracellular signaling in Alzheimer's disease. Nat. Rev. Neurosci. **3:** 862–872.
8. STUTZMANN, G.E. 2005. Calcium dysregulation, $IP_3$, signaling and Alzheimer's disease. Neuroscientist **11:** 110–115.
9. GUO, Q. *et al.* 1996. Alzheimer's PS-1 mutation perturbs calcium homeostasis and sensitizes PC12 cells to death induced by amyloid beta-peptide. Neuroreport **8:** 379–383.
10. LEISSRING, M.A. *et al.* 1999. Alzheimer's presenilin-1 mutation potentiates inositol 1,4,5-trisphosphate-mediated calcium signaling in Xenopus oocytes. J. Neurochem. **72:** 1061–1068.
11. STUTZMANN, G.E. *et al.* 2004. Dysregulated $IP_3$ signaling in cortical neurons of knock-in mice expressing an Alzheimer's-linked mutation in presenilin1 results in exaggerated $Ca^{2+}$ signals and altered membrane excitability. J. Neurosci. **24:** 508–513.
12. ETCHEBERRIGARAY, R. *et al.* 1998. Calcium responses in fibroblasts from asymptomatic members of Alzheimer's disease families. Neurobiol. Dis. **5:** 37–45.
13. CHAN, S. *et al.* 2000. Presenilin-1 mutations increase levels of ryanodine receptors and calcium release in PC12 cells and cortical neurons. J. Biol. Chem. **275:** 18195–18200.
14. SMITH, I. *et al.* 2005. Enhanced caffeine-induced $Ca^{2+}$ release in the 3xTg-AD mouse model of Alzheimer's disease. J. Neurochem. **94:** 1711–1718.
15. POPESCU, B. *et al.* 2004. Gamma-secretase activity of presenilin 1 regulates acetylcholine muscarinic receptor-mediated signal transduction. J. Biol. Chem. **279:** 6455–6464.
16. ODDO, S. *et al.* 2003. Triple-transgenic model of Alzheimer's disease with plaques and tangles: intracellular Abeta and synaptic dysfunction. Neuron **39:** 409–421.
17. SAH, P. 1996. $Ca^{2+}$-activated $K^+$ currents in neurones: types, physiological roles and modulation. TINS **19:** 150–154.

18. STUTZMANN, G., F. LAFERLA & I. PARKER. 2003. $Ca^{2+}$ signaling in mouse cortical neurons studied by two-photon imaging and photoreleased inositol triphosphate. J. Neurosci. **23:** 758–765.

19. STUTZMANN, G.E. *et al.* 2006. Enhanced ryanodine receptor recruitment contributes to Ca2+ disruptions in young, adult, and aged Alzheimer's disease mice. J. Neurosci. **26:** 5180–5189.

20. DAVIES, P., D. IRELAND & E. MCLACHLAN. 1996. Sources of $Ca^{2+}$ for different $Ca^{2+}$-activated $K^+$ conductances in neurones of the rat superior cervical ganglion. J. Physiol. **495:** 353–366.

21. NAKAMURA, T. *et al.* 2000. Inositol 1,4,5-triphosphate ($IP_3$)-mediated $Ca^{2+}$ release evoked by metabotropic agonists and backpropagating action potentials in hippocampal CA1 pyramidal neurons. J. Neurosci. **20:** 8365–8376.

22. MELLSTROM, B. & J. NARANJO. 2001. Mechanisms for $Ca^{2+}$-dependent transcription. Curr. Opin. Neurobiol. **11:** 312–319.

23. SHMIGOL, A. *et al.* 1996. Gradual caffeine-induced $Ca^{2+}$ release in mouse dorsal root ganglion neurons is controlled by cytoplasmic and luminal $Ca^{2+}$. Neuroscience **73:** 1061–1067.

24. KOIZUMI, S. *et al.* 1999. Regulation of ryanodine receptor opening by lumenal $Ca^{2+}$ underlies quantal $Ca^{2+}$ release in PC12 cells. J. Biol. Chem. **274:** 33327–33333.

25. CAO, X., T.C. SUDHOF. 2001. A transcriptively active complex of APP with Fe65 and histone acetyltransferase Tip60. Science **293:** 115–120.

26. LEISSRING, M. *et al.* 2002. A physiologic signaling role for the gamma-secretase-derived intracellular fragment of APP. Proc. Natl. Acad. Sci. **99:** 4697–4702.

# Prospects for Prediction

## Ethics Analysis of Neuroimaging in Alzheimer's Disease

J. ILLES,[a] A. ROSEN,[b,c] M. GREICIUS,[d] AND E. RACINE[e]

[a]Stanford Center for Biomedical Ethics and Department of Radiology, Program in Neuroethics, Stanford, California, USA

[b]Department of Psychiatry and Behavioral Sciences, Stanford University, Stanford, California, USA

[c]Mental Illness Research Education and Clinical Center, Palo Alto VA Healthcare System, Palo Alto, California, USA

[d]Department of Neurology and Neurological Sciences, Stanford University, Stanford, California, USA

[e]Stanford Center for Biomedical Ethics, Program in Neuroethics, Stanford, California, USA

ABSTRACT: This article focuses on the prospects and ethics of using neuroimaging to predict Alzheimer's disease (AD). It is motivated by consideration of the historical roles of science in medicine and society, and considerations specifically contemporary of capabilities in imaging and aging, and the benefits and hope they bring. A general consensus is that combinations of imaging methods will ultimately be most fruitful in predicting disease. Their roll-out into translational practice will not be free of complexity, however, as culture and values differ in terms of what defines benefit and risk, who will benefit and who is at risk, what methods must be in place to assure the maximum safety, comfort, and protection of subjects and patients, and educational and policy needs. Proactive planning for the ethical and societal implications of predicting diseases of the aging brain is critical and will benefit all stakeholders— researchers, patients and families, health care providers, and policy makers.

KEYWORDS: neuroimaging; Alzheimer's disease; aging; prediction; neuroethics

Address for correspondence: J. Illes, Stanford Center for Biomedical Ethics, Program in Neuroethics, 701 Welch Rd., A1115, Stanford, CA 94304-5748. Voice: 650-724-6393; fax: 650-725-6131. illes@stanford.edu

Ann. N.Y. Acad. Sci. 1097: 278–295 (2007). © 2007 New York Academy of Sciences.
doi: 10.1196/annals.1379.030

# INTRODUCTION

The progressive deficits characterizing dementia in Alzheimer's disease (AD) ultimately destroy judgment and communication abilities. The deficits are particularly difficult to detect in early stages,[1] and true confirmation of this form of neurodegenerative disease is elusive without postmortem histological examination of the brain for neuronal loss, neurofibrillary tangles, and senile plaques. A consequence of the subtlety of these changes is that diagnostic criteria are conservative and diagnosis is delayed until there is significant functional disability (Diagnostic Statistical Manual IV, 1994). Given the late age of onset of AD and a growing elderly American population, the public health burden of this disease is significant. Estimates of the prevalence of Americans suffering from the condition today vary between 1.5 and 4 million, with projections increasing steadily through 2050.[2,3] Despite recent therapeutic advances, available treatments at present are aimed primarily at slowing progression of the disease rather than halting it completely or reversing its progression.

Imaging is one among a few tests, such as genetic markers, cerebrospinal fluid, and demographic risk factors that may predict AD. Original genetic studies in the early 1990s, for example, associated one gene that encodes apolipoprotein E with the disease. APOE is a plasma protein that binds and transports cholesterol.[4] The presence of the type 4 allele (estimated to occur in about 25% of the AD population)[5] is widely viewed as a risk factor. However, many individuals affected by AD do not have the allele, and others who do inherit it do not manifest AD. The development of imaging biomarkers and a discussion of accompanying ethical challenges are the focus of the present article.

## ROLES FOR CURRENT IMAGING CAPABILITIES AND IMAGING BIOMARKERS ON THE HORIZON

Neuroimaging techniques are poised to transform the process of diagnosis, prediction, and clinical management of AD and related dementias. The role of magnetic resonance imaging (MRI) and positron emission tomography (PET) in the diagnosis of dementia and investigation of cognitive impairment has been discussed at length by Knopman *et al.*[6] and Albert *et al.*[7] (www.alz.org/Research/Papers/Imaging_consensus_report.pdf). Currently, neuroimaging essentially serves the purpose of excluding alternate potential etiologies for cognitive dysfunction. For the future, there are three particularly important roles that neuroimaging may play: (1) increasing the sensitivity and specificity in diagnosing AD; (2) predicting who is likely to develop AD in the nondemented population; and (3) replacing clinical outcome measures in therapeutic trials (i.e., surrogate measures that have no direct relationship to a patient's clinical state but are presumed to substitute for a clinically important measure). With respect to diagnosis, current accuracy is already highly sensitive and specific as compared to the neuropathological standard. In contrast, there is much work needed to predict who will develop AD in the nondemented population. As a surrogate outcome measure in studies evaluating new treatments, neuroimaging has great potential to reduce the length and cost of clinical trials because it can be collected long before current clinical outcome measures are available. The 5-year public-private Alzheimer's disease neuroimaging initiative (ADNI) is an example of ongoing validation trial toward this goal[8] (http://www.loni.ucla.edu/ADNI).

Although brain imaging is not currently applied in a clinical context for diagnosing AD except as a means of ruling out other causes of dementia, such as strokes or tumors, it has been widely accepted that benefits would accrue to patients and individuals at risk with improved assessment of brain integrity; structural and functional imaging are likely candidates since they may provide more direct information than inferences based on behavior, genetics, or other systemic indicators, such as CSF metabolites.[9] As described in this volume and elsewhere, early detection of the disease has been a major focus of a variety of neuroimaging techniques, including fMRI, structural MRI, and PET. Recently, these techniques have also been found to be useful in monitoring cognitive and pathological progression of the disease, as well as monitoring response to clinical intervention and treatment.[10–14]

## MEETING ETHICAL CHALLENGES

With each new technique comes the burden of validation against current standards for diagnosis and disease state monitoring. The consensus report on the use of MRI and PET for Clinical Diagnosis of Dementia[7] provides guidelines based on the state-of-the-art and scientific research. This consensus report was developed to extend the current clinical standards as described by the American Academy of Neurology Guidelines[6] for the use of neuroimaging in clinical diagnosis. With each new application of a technique, there are ethical implications that must be addressed. To complement the other articles in this volume, the editorial board invited us to report on our examination of these implications. To do so, we explored them systematically according to five major themes:

1. overall medical and social consequences of predicting AD using functional neuroimaging,
2. differentiating different clinical subtypes of AD,
3. scanning protocols and modalities,
4. research and clinical ethics issues, and
5. key issues for education, counseling, and communication.

Our discovery and recommendations follow.

## Overall Medical and Social Implications of Predicting AD Using Functional Neuroimaging

As described previously[5] for genetic testing, the potential value of predicting AD must be considered in the context of the meaning of the disease for those affected and those around them. Unintended consequences and counseling further emerged as key areas under this theme.

### Meaning of Disease

- For predictive imaging, the meaning of disease will depend on the specificity of testing tools that are used.
- Changing technologies are going to have an impact on the nosology of the disease, for example, how the professional community classify it and assess significance.
- The value addition of imaging alone compared to other tools in the context of prediction is not clear-cut. A combination of different technologies—genetic testing, proteomics, and imaging interacting in different ways—is likely to achieve the best definition and predictions about AD and related diseases.
- AD may be increasingly viewed as a syndrome rather than a single disease. Advances in technology may lead to its further differentiation. As technologies become powerful and more predictive, the professional community can anticipate a proliferation of subclassifications of the syndrome.
- As presymptomatic testing becomes available, it is likely that people who are actually healthy now and will not manifest the disease for a long period of time will still be included within the classifications. This suggests the acute need for the development and introduction of early and effective interventions.
- It is imperative that research is conducted not only on the development of technology but on how it will be best used clinically and integrated with current health care practices.

### Unintended Social, Economic, and Ethical Consequences

A number of areas on which predictive imaging will have an impact may face unintended consequences. They are:

### Health Insurance

In the current health care system in the United States:

- Requirements by insurers for predictive testing must be articulated and vetted.

- Insurers could ask clients directly to take the test or, if there are laws that restrict that, they can ask people to voluntarily take tests or provide results of tests. If clients refuse to do so, insurers may act on that information. This is one strategy available to insurance companies for not violating certain legal restrictions.

*Stigma*

Because people live in a cognitively centered world, any information that raises questions about cognitive status of an individual may stigmatize that individual:

- Predictive imaging may expand the pool of disease to people who are much younger, and therefore expand the pool that is stigmatized.
- Both earlier prediction and stigma have the potential to reduce quality of life, including autonomy and the privilege to drive, and other daily functions.
- There may be medical discrimination against people at risk, for example, with respect to eligibility for organ transplantation.

We recognized that in spite of any stigma, some people will have psychological solace from the biologic information.

*Health care disparities*

Testing might exacerbate existing disparities, largely through access.

- If predictive imaging becomes commercialized, those who cannot afford tests may not be able to get them.
- If some interventions have a high impact on behavior—such as the demonstration that physical or cognitive exercise reduces risk—then knowing about that risk might affect behavior. Then those who cannot afford to pay out of pocket for these tests will not have those kinds of incentives.

*Counseling*

A great deal of expertise will be required of clinical providers who offer predictive imaging services. In this respect, a cohort of specialists may emerge especially since, recalling counseling in the history of genetic testing, guidelines fell away as primary care providers could not possibly keep up with demand.

- Before any test is offered clinically for which counseling will be needed, the validity of the test, including psychometric reliability and sensitivity, must be in place. Quality assurance analogous to CLIA laboratory guidelines may be one response to this recommendation. We note that the American Academy of Neurology currently vets tests and identifies those that are ready. Professional institutions have a responsibility to continue to meet and help clarify standard of care in this area.

• Since AD has a significant component of heritability and individuals with a first-degree relative and an ApoE4 allele are believed to have a 40% lifetime risk of developing AD, physicians should be aware of the implications for family members who may be present when testing results are disseminated. Physicians who convey test results to patients should be prepared to field questions from family members concerned about their own risk.

## Clinical Populations for Screening

Any discussion of the ethical issues at play for screening imaging for AD must take into account two important facts. The first is that treatments for AD currently have limited effectiveness and the disease is fatal. The second is that even the best imaging test will be prone to some degree of false positive and false negative results. The ethical issues pertaining to which clinical populations should be tested will depend largely on whether or not a definitive treatment becomes available. The screening of certain populations and the accompanying ethical issues will vary depending on whether such a treatment is effective at stemming the progression of AD or can actually reverse the pathologic changes and cure patients. Similarly, there will be a separate set of ethical questions if a treatment is developed that can prevent the disease from occurring when given to presymptomatic subjects. With these important caveats in mind we consider four specific scenarios for clinical screening as follows:

### Screen All Individuals for AD When They Reach 65 Years of Age

• Imaging tests could be added to the panoply of other screening tests (e.g., colonoscopy, mammogram) that are recommended as people grow older. The greatest concern for this scenario is that, even with prevalence rates approaching 10% in this age range,[15] there will be a significant number of false positives. In screening for AD, the benefit of a follow-up confirmatory biopsy or other gold standard procedure does not exist because brain biopsy is too risky. As such the imaging test may be the most definitive measure available and the one on which treatment decisions will be based.
• If relatively benign and effective treatments are developed, a relatively larger percentage of false positives in this scenario can be tolerated. However,

initial clinical trials of the β-amyloid vaccine, in which 6% of vaccinated patients developed a meningoencephalits,[16] serve to remind us that (potentially) potent therapies are rarely completely benign.

### Screen Patients Who Already Have Some Mild Cognitive Impairment

• The true prevalence of AD in the mild cognitive impairment population will be greater than in a sample of subjects without cognitive complaints. The positive predictive value of the test (the probability that a positive result is a true positive) will increase, giving clinicians greater confidence that a potentially potent but toxic treatment is being given to patients who actually have pathology.
• The rate at which cognitive and functional decline is likely to occur may be projected from this population.
• A downside to this scenario is that the AD pathology in this cohort of patients is already more advanced and may prove less amenable to treatment.

### Screen Asymptomatic Individuals with Risk Factors

The scenario to screen asymptomatic individuals with risk factors, such as family history, ApoE genotype, older age, or some combination of these variables, analyses represents the most typical of the cost-benefit analyses made by physicians considering testing a patient for a particular disease. Many patients and their families in this scenario may find it useful, in terms of planning for the future, to know with some certainty that the cognitive loss they are already suffering is due to AD. At the level of intervention, a physician might encourage or limit treatment, such as with a cholinesterase inhibitor, especially for an AD patient with limited means or multiple other medical conditions that can be treated more effectively. However:

• Given the lack of definitive treatment, the clinical value of making a diagnosis of AD is considerably reduced.
• Given the relatively slow course of the pathology and the persistent social stigma surrounding AD, there is more potential harm in making the diagnosis of AD in asymptomatic individuals who may not become ill for another 5 to 15 years.

### Screen Everyone Who Wants a Scan

A great deal of variability exists among consumers in the desire to be tested. This variability will exist as long as treatments are lacking, but will likely diminish as treatments become available. In light of this, and for this scenario as well as the others described above:

- Methods are needed for guaranteeing confidentiality of results.
- Guidelines are needed for defining who should have access to results of testing when they are purchased for reasons that are not medically indicated.
- Research is needed to assess the impact of results on personal liberty, self-image, job security, and patient-physician and family relationships.
- Currently unregulated methods for direct consumer advertising or direct physician advertising for imaging would benefit from professional self-regulation and guidelines for best practices.[17]

We further note that the greater predictive power combined with the growing number of people with AD might be the brick that breaks the back of the current health care system.

## *Scanning Modalities*

Efforts to improve the quality of imaging technologies are ongoing in a variety of domains, notably by increasing the availability of techniques and comfortable, well-validated clinical applications.

### *Patient Comfort*

- Making techniques maximally comfortable, fast, and efficient is essential to enable patients, who have difficulty tolerating medical procedures, to be evaluated. This includes rapid acquisition protocols that will make it easier for patients to remain still enough to undergo the procedures.

### *Standardization of Acquisition and Analysis Protocols*

- Standardization of acquisition and analysis protocols is vital to the replicability of data across sites, equipment, and software. Performing identical procedures does not ensure that acquisition routines result in comparable image quality with respect to parameters such as signal to noise.
- Quality assurance data should be collected on a regular basis.

### *Cost Reduction in Acquisition and Analysis*

The information contributed by neuroimaging techniques must improve in a manner that justifies its cost by increasing sensitivity and specificity of differential diagnosis for decision making.

- At the present time, only relatively few, elite centers are capable of performing reliable volumetric analyses on structural MRI images. PET imaging of radioligands is expensive. If neuroimaging begins to play a larger role in routine clinical standard of care in AD, cost-effectiveness must be demonstrated.[18] Early diagnosis that enables earlier treatment that in turn delays the placement of a patient in a nursing home is one measure of cost reduction.[19]
- Increased patient numbers and procedures will justify acquisition operations costs for more medical centers.

## Validation Studies for Diagnostic/Treatment Decision Making

### Individual Patients

- The majority of current studies of imaging techniques involve comparisons of groups of well-characterized subjects, but clinical decisions must be made for individuals. Standardized, reproducible protocols in which sensitivity and specificity of different measures are well established will be crucial in making decisions for individual patients.[20–22]
- Practices of disclosure of positive test information will need to take into account the nature of the experimentally or clinically validated test as well as the volunteer who may or may not wish to be informed of results.

### Diversity of Ethnicity and Age

Normative measures generated from one gender, ethnic, or age group may not generalize to all.

- Diverse populations should be included in all development efforts and this information should be routinely reported in normative samples.
- Clinical trials will be enriched by expanding study cohorts to include older adults in whom treatments that act on AD pathology are likely to show an effect.

### Populations with Comorbid Disease

- Patients in communities with inadequate preventive care often are at risk for comorbid illnesses, such as substance abuse, head injury, or vascular disease. Decision rules based on individually presenting diseases do not always easily apply. To enable generalization to these populations, studies are needed to assess the impact of comorbidities on decision-making rules.

## *Predictive Validity and Priorities for Imaging*

Unless an imaging biomarker has been tested to assess whether it is associated with later change through prospective longitudinal studies, it should be used with extreme caution.

- Errors in prediction could result in situations in which patients who need medication are denied it and patients who cannot benefit from medication are exposed to its risks.
- Once positive predictive value is achieved clinical trials over clinical management are favored as a priority given the information trials bring to clinical treatment of many patients.

## *Surrogate Markers for Speed and Cost-Effectiveness of Clinical Trials*

### *Surrogate Markers Are Viewed to Have Significant Potential Benefit.*

- Effective surrogate measures from MRI or PET that predict early clinical benefit would accelerate the pace of clinical trials.
- Surrogate biomarkers that are more sensitive and specific to the clinical progression of AD than current clinical measures[23] will yield more power to detect treatment effects and the need for fewer participants in clinical trials.

## *Incidental Findings in Predictive Neuroimaging*

Findings of possible clinical significance are detected in the brain both in clinical workup and in research. Previous studies of incidence suggest that the rate of occurrence of such findings is about 1–2% in the general population[24] and the data suggest that it may be substantially higher in older cohorts.[25]

- As reported elsewhere,[26] embedded in research imaging studies should be the anticipation of such findings and a protocol in place for managing them.
- In clinical medicine, findings are followed up routinely, although the rising cost-benefit ratio as in genomic testing has become a source of concern.[21]
- In the case of predictive imaging, however, much remains to be learned about functional anomalies. Current recommendations pertain only to anatomical images obtained for research and as yet, not to single subject metabolic measures.
- The greatest risk lies in misclassifying a finding as a positive indicator of disease.

*Therapeutic Benefits*

Although predictive neuroimaging has not yet reached its potential utility, we recognize future therapeutic benefits and procedures.

- To the extent that patients with various dementias will benefit differentially or experience different side effects from different medications, imaging in the future may enable selection of the optimal treatment or monitor progression more sensitively than is presently possible.
- It may become necessary to have secondary trials or repeated imaging of patients on medication after medications are released to the public.

## Research and Clinical Ethics

Neuroimaging research in AD raises a number of important well-known challenges in the domain of research ethics. These include issues such as informed consent, confidentiality, and privacy. The potential translation of neuroimaging research to clinical care intersects with a broader and significant number of potential ethical, legal, and social issues. In particular, it will yield sensitive personal information that will have to be handled with utmost ethical care. National and international laws and guidelines for research need to be carefully considered in the research design and recruitment phases of research given the current negative risk-benefit trade-off for individual AD volunteers often recruited from the pool of vulnerable volunteers (e.g., mentally disabled persons as alluded to in the Common Rule; Federal Policy for the Protection of Human Subjects; 45 CFR 46). Autonomy, cognitive privacy, and cultural sensitivity are of paramount importance. As stated in the *Belmont Report*, any participation of vulnerable volunteers, including patients with AD, should be based on the needs of science and for improving clinical care.

*Subjects with Decisional Capacity*

Many people suffering from AD remain capable of understanding and deciding whether they want to participate in a specific research project.

- It is the responsibility of PIs to ensure that the best conditions are met for the volunteer to be fully informed of the risks and benefits (if any) of a study.
- The setting must be free of coercion either from members of the research team or others (e.g., family member, health care provider) who can exert undue influence on a volunteer.
- Whenever feasible, AD volunteers who can consent to research should be recruited before those who cannot.

*Subjects with Limited Decisional Capacity*

Additional ethical complexity is created when volunteers cannot directly give informed consent either because they are declared legally incompetent in matters of research participation or lack the capacity to consent.

*Availability of Advanced Directives for Research*

When a volunteer has written specific advanced directives[27-29] for research participation, such as a research living will, guidance is available about prior autonomous wishes. These may be wishes, such as the willingness to participate in minimal risk research only or not to participate in research involving scanners. The pure autonomy standard, that is, precedence of previously expressed autonomous judgments, should apply.

*Absence of Advanced Directives for Research*

The absence of advanced directives for research is the likely case for most prospective research subjects. In the absence of specific directives:

- The volunteer may have designated, through a durable power of attorney, a proxy decision maker (sometimes called a research proxy) empowered to make research participation decisions. The decision lies in the hands of this formally designated research proxy based on the wishes of the volunteer and applicable legal provisions of the jurisdiction.
- In the absence of a research proxy, practices can vary depending on the circumstances and the applicable legal and regulatory context. An existing health care power of attorney may serve as a research decision maker. A legal guardian, i.e., a court-appointed legally authorized representative, or an informal decision maker (typically from the volunteer's family), may give consent for research participation. Following any of these options, the proxy decision maker should respect the previous wishes of the volunteer if known. Otherwise, when clear wishes are unknown, the proxy should use the best interest standard; that is, based on the values and prior wishes of the volunteer, judge what is in his or her best interests.
- When possible, the assent of the volunteer should be obtained even though assent is not a substitute for consent mechanisms. Signs of objection (dissent) from the volunteer should be considered a significant indication of refusal.

*Shared Databases*

Large neuroimaging consortia studying AD have created data banks that require specific security and deidentification measures.

- Deidentification measures have become especially important given that some cranial features acquired during imaging could possibly be used to reidentify volunteers.[30] Risks related to the crossing of information and the limits of deidentification and anonymization are considerable, even if the most effective methods are used.
- Further complicating the issue of brain databases is the discovery of incidental findings on secondary analysis of the data. Some of these issues are familiar to other areas of research, such as genetics. Cross-fertilization of approaches and standards are highly relevant but the practices of obtaining consent in AD and addressing some of the newer issues in the context of neuroimaging are still evolving and call for empirically evaluated practices.

*Hype versus Clinical Hope*

To date, FDG-PET has been approved by the Centers for Medicare and Medicaid Services to help distinguish AD from frontotemporal dementia. However, no neuroimaging procedure is currently used to rule-in, that is, definitively diagnose AD. The predictive power of neuroimaging remains to be proven despite positive impressions fueled hopes for technology transfer and commercialization and marketing practices.

- Once sufficiently validated for clinical use, however, conflicts of interest and tensions between academia and the private sector, and possibly within large academic consortia can be expected to rise.
- In spite of the current limited application of neuroimaging to health care in AD, discussion of the ethics of predictive neuroimaging should be encouraged given the prospects for clinical translation and the potential pitfalls of unattended risks for all parties involved.

**Education and Policy**

History predicts that the process of rolling out new technology, such as imaging, for an application such as detecting neurodegenerative disease, happens on a continuum. With off-label uses already in existence and active information dissemination throughout the media, Internet, and other sources, the full introduction of the technology can be anticipated. Working to maximize the generalizability of results is imperative. In the context of education and policy, therefore, four major considerations are key: the content of education, education about research, driving forces in utilization, and professional responsibility.

*Content of Education*

Key factors for education about the predicting AD with imaging are:

- Clarity about technical readiness and meaningfulness of data given a dynamic state of the art, breadth of uses including the use of imaging as an adjunct to clinical diagnosis and its predictive potential;
- Characteristics of imaging that differentiate this technology from others, including, for example, the potential to uncover latent disease;
- Relative degrees of specificity (e.g., genetic markers vs. individual brain regions), regulatory and access controlled at level of device;
- Individuality in methods and interpretation;
- Cost, time, invasiveness, and tempered promise.

*Education about Research*

The group recognized the importance of K-12 science education as first priority for education about science in our society. Beyond this:

- Informed consent, incidental findings, privacy, access to data and sharing are key priorities.
- Elucidating natural caveats of neuroimaging research defined by the process of discovery, and different types of altruism that might underlie participation by volunteers for diagnostic and predictive imaging research are also key ethical and educational challenges.
- All relevant groups will benefit from education about neuroimaging research, including physician, specialty societies, advocacy, national and local level, the media, patients, families, caregivers, conservators, insurers, trainees, funders, and government officials, such as Congress and the CDC.

*Utilization of Technology*

Many of the groups that represent cores for education also represent major driving forces in technology transfer and utilization.

- Constraints on utilization are access and cost, age of populations, time limitations of physicians, reimbursement for screening versus diagnosis, and ethnic differences.

- Advocacy groups can play a role in optimizing the transfer of technology into clinical use through objective education, dissemination of validated and vetted information, legislation, priority setting based on scientific and political pressure, and issue identification through short- and long-term planning.

*Professional Responsibility*

*Professional Responsibility Spans Both Funders and Investigators*

- Even as regulations are developed, the burden still rests on individual physicians to adopt guidelines responsibly and to engage in professional self-regulation modeled, for example, by the American Academy of Neurology.[6]
- Sponsors of research should continue to invest and create mechanisms for knowledge transfer. Communications liaisons for large-scale programs can serve the knowledge transfer role effectively.
- Taking into consideration all the factors discussed in this report, investigators themselves bear a significant burden to operationalize plans for information dissemination and transfer results from research on predictive imaging.
- A policy equivalent to the Genetic Nondiscrimination Act for insurance, eligibility for services, and employment is viable and may be needed for brain imaging.

## CONCLUSION

The goal of predictive neuroimaging is to improve upon the human condition in neurodegenerative disease by providing reliable information about treatment outcome, rate of decline, and possibly therapeutic benefit to slow or even halt its relentless progression. These worthy goals are challenged by the still relatively immature state of the technology. Past events in the history of neuroscience and clinical medicine have taught us that such challenges must further take into consideration how culture and values differ in terms of what defines benefit and risk, and who will benefit and who is at risk. Methods must be set in place to assure not only maximum safety, comfort, and protection of subjects and patients, but also the educational and policy needs of all stakeholders.

We explored many issues here, resolved some, and left others open. Clearly, we also left many completely untouched. Overall, we conclude that as ethical paths are followed right alongside the development of powerful imaging tools, the future will hold ever-greater promise for AD patients and their families.

## ACKNOWLEDGMENTS

This article is based on the results of a workshop held at Stanford University on May 16, 2006, that was independent of, but coincident with, the meeting at the New York Academy of Sciences on which this issue of the *Annals* is based. The specific themes described here were addressed in plenary sessions and in working groups comprising individuals from a diverse range of disciplines including bioethics, neuroscience, law, health policy, and education. This written product was prepared by the authors and refined based on feedback of participants by way of web-based open commentary and follow-up conference calls as needed. It does not reflect consensus or majority and minority opinions; rather it represents the issues, possible solutions or recommendations, and remaining ethical questions that participants felt were at the current heart of the state of the art in predictive imaging. The authors acknowledge the participation both of presenters and attendees. Presenters were: Susan Bookheimer (Department of Psychiatry and Biobehavioral Sciences, University of California, Los Angeles), Neil Buckholtz (National Institute of Aging, NIH), Henry T. (Hank) Greely (School of Law and Center for Biomedical Ethics, Stanford University), William Jagust (School of Public Health, University of California, San Francisco), Claudia Kawas (Department of Neurology and Neurobiology and Behavior, University of California, Irvine), Howard Rosen (Department of Neurology University of California, Berkeley). Invited participants were: Bruce Arnow (Department of Psychiatry and Behavioral Sciences, Stanford University), Laurence Baker (Health Research and Policy, Stanford University), Mildred Cho (Center for Biomedical Ethics, Stanford University), LaVera Crawley (Center for Biomedical Ethics, Stanford University), Ann Davidson (Stakeholder), Elizabeth Edgerly (Alzheimer's Association, Northern California and Northern Nevada), William Fisher (Alzheimer's Association, Northern California and Northern Nevada), Gary Glover (Department of Radiology, Stanford University), Victor Henderson (Department of Health Research and Policy, Stanford University), Agnieszka Jaworska (Department of Philosophy, Stanford University), Frank Longo (Department of Neurology and Neurological Sciences, Stanford University) David Magnus (Center for Biomedical Ethics, Stanford University), Micki Miller (Stakeholder) Ruth O'Hara (Department of Psychiatry and Behavioral Sciences, Stanford University), Peter B. Reiner (Department of Psychiatry and Brain Research Centre, University of British Columbia), David Salmon, Department of Neurosciences, University of California, San Diego), Navah Statman (National Alliance for the Mentally Ill), Joy Taylor (Department of Psychiatry and Behavioral Sciences, Stanford University), Tony Wyss-Coray (Department of Neurology and Neurological Sciences, Stanford University), Jerome Yesavage (Department of Psychiatry and Behavioral Science, Stanford University). The work was supported by NIH/NINDS RO1 045831. Sponsorship of the workshop was also provided by the Mental Illness Research Education and Clinical Center (MIRREC)

Palo Alto VA Healthcare System. The authors gratefully acknowledge Karen Renschler and Vivian Chin for conference and editorial assistance.

## REFERENCES

1. McKHANN, G. *et al.* 1984. Clinical diagnosis of Alzheimer's disease: report of the NINCDS-ADRDA Work Group under the auspices of Department of Health and Human Services Task Force on Alzheimer's Disease. Neurology **34:** 939–944.
2. EVANS, D.A. *et al.* 1989. Prevalence of Alzheimer's disease in a community population of older persons. Higher than previously reported. JAMA **262:** 2551–2556.
3. HY, L.X. & D.M. KELLER. 2000. Prevalence of AD among whites: a summary by levels of severity. Neurology **55:** 198–204.
4. STRITTMATTER, W.J. *et al.* 1993. Apolipoprotein E: high-avidity binding to beta-amyloid and increased frequency of type 4 allele in late-onset familial Alzheimer disease. Proc. Natl. Acad. Sci. USA **90:** 1977–1981.
5. McCONNELL, L.M. *et al.* 1999. Genetic testing and Alzheimer disease: Recommendations of the Stanford Program in Genetics, Ethics and Society. Genet. Test. **3:** 3–13.
6. KNOPMAN, D.S. *et al.* 2001. Practice parameter: diagnosis of dementia (and evidence-based review)—Report of the Quality Standards Subcommittee of the American Academy of Neurology. Neurology 56.
7. ALBERT, M. 2005. The use of MRI and PET for clinical diagnosis of dementia and investigation of cognitive impairment. Working Report: Neuroimaging Workgroup of the Alzheimer's Association.
8. MUELLER, S.G. *et al.* 2005. The Alzheimer's disease neuroimaging initiative. Neuroimag. Clin. N. Am. **15:** 869–877.
9. ROSEN, A.C. *et al.* 2002. Ethical, and practical issues in applying functional imaging to the clinical management of Alzheimer's disease. Brain Cog. **50:** 498–519.
10. MENTIS, M.J. *et al.* 1998. Increasing required neural response to expose abnormal brain function in mild versus moderate or severe Alzheimer's disease: PET study using parametric visual stimulation. Am. J. Psychiatry **155:** 785–794.
11. MIELKE, R. *et al.* 1995. Dysfunction of visual cortex contributes to disturbed processing of visual information in Alzheimer's disease. Int. J. Neurosci. **82:** 1–9.
12. THULBORN, K.R., C. MARTIN & J.T. VOYVODIC. 2000. Functional MR imaging using a visually guided saccade paradigm for comparing activation patterns in patients with probable Alzheimer's disease and in cognitively able elderly volunteers. Am. J. Neuroradiol. **21:** 524–531.
13. SMITH, C. *et al.* 2002. Women at risk for AD show increased parietal activation during a fluency task. Neurology **58:** 1197–1202.
14. BURGGREN, A.C. & S.Y. BOOKHEIMER. 2002. Structural and functional neuroimaging in Alzheimer's disease: an update. Curr. Top Med. Chem. **2:** 385–393.
15. HENDRIE, H.C. 1998. Epidemiology of dementia and Alzheimer's disease. Am. J. Geriatr. Psychiatry **6:** S3–S18.
16. ORGOGOZO, J.M. *et al.* 2003. Subacute meningoencephalitis in a subset of patients with AD after Abeta42 immunization. Neurology **61:** 46–54.
17. ILLES, J. *et al.* 2004. Advertising, patient decision-making, and self-referral to CT and MR imaging. Arch. Int. Med. **164:** 2406–2408.

18. McMahon, P.M. *et al.* 2000. Cost-effectiveness of functional imaging tests in the diagnosis of Alzheimer disease. Radiology **217:** 58–68.
19. Small, G.W. & F. Leiter. 1998. Neuroimaging for diagnosis of dementia. J. Clin. Psychiatry **59**(Suppl 11): 4–7.
20. Swets, J.A. & R.M. Pickett. 1982. Evaluation of Diagnostic Systems: Methods from Signal Detection Theory. Academic Press. New York.
21. Kraemer, H.C. 1992. Evaluating Medical Tests: Objective and Quantitative Guidelines. Sage. Newbury Park, CA.
22. Machulda, M.M. *et al.* 2003. Comparison of memory fMRI response among normal, MCI, and Alzheimer's patients. Neurology **61:** 500–506.
23. Jack, C.R., Jr. *et al.* 2003. MRI as a biomarker of disease progression in a therapeutic trial of milameline for AD. Neurology **60:** 253–260.
24. Katzman, G.L., A.P. Dagher, N.J. Patronas *et al.* 1999. Incidental findings on brain magnetic resonance imaging from 1000 asymptomatic volunteers. JAMA **281:** 36–39.
25. Illes, J. *et al.* 2004. Ethical consideration of incidental findings on adult MRI in research. Neurology **62:** 888–890.
26. Illes, J. *et al.* 2006. Incidental findings in brain imaging research. Science **311:** 783–784.
27. Stocking, C.B. *et al.* 2006. Speaking of research advance directives: planning for future research participation. Neurology **66:** 1361–1366.
28. Backlar, P. 1998. Advance directives for subjects of research who have fluctuating cognitive impairments due to psychotic disorders (such as schizophrenia). Comm. Ment. Health J. **34:** 229–240.
29. Berghmans, R.L. 1998. Advance directives for non-therapeutic dementia research: some ethical and policy considerations. J. Med. Ethics **24:** 32–37.
30. Mazziotta, J.C. 2000. Window on the brain. Arch. Neurol. **57:** 1413–1421.

# Index of Contributors